Complementary and Alternative Medicine:
Challenge and Change

Editors

Merrijoy Kelner *and* Beverly Wellman
University of Toronto, Canada

Associate Editors

Bernice Pescosolido, *Indiana University, USA*
Mike Saks, *De Montfort University, UK*

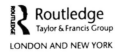

Routledge
Taylor & Francis Group

LONDON AND NEW YORK

First published 2000 by OPA (Overseas Publishers Association) N.V.
under the Harwood Academic Publishers imprint, part of the Gordon
and Breach Publishing Group.

Reprinted 2003 by Routledge
11 New Fetter Lane, London EC4P 4EE

Simultaneously published in the USA and Canada
by Routledge
29 West 35th Street, New York NY 10001

Routledge is an imprint of the Taylor & Francis Group

© 2003 Routledge, Taylor & Francis

British Library Cataloguing in Publication Data
A catalogue record for this book is available from the British Library

ISBN 90-5823-099-6 (pbk)

Complementary and Alternative Medicine

Canterbury College

110265

Table of Contents

Figures

Tables

The Social Dynamics of Medical Pluralism, Foreword

WAYNE JONAS
*Uniformed Services University of the Health Sciences,
Bethesda, USA*

We are all faced with illness at some time in our lives and most of us end up caring for a loved one who is ill. When illness comes, be it a minor or major problem, we all purport to want basically the same thing – a rapid, gentle treatment that cures us or at least can allay our fears and alleviate our suffering. Yet, despite this apparently common goal the social responses to disease and illness are remarkably varied and differences are often strongly held. Who we approach for help, what we decide is the best treatment for us, how we evaluate success, and when we look for alternatives – depend on many factors. These include how we conceive of health and illness, what we believe has gone wrong and why, and who we associate with and get advice from. In short, it depends on our models and perceptions of the world, the preferences and values we share, and the perceived benefit we get from associating with trusted others. Even in the age of modern science, decisions about the nature of humankind, health and illness, its meaning and how to prevent and treat it is primarily a social process. It is logical then that in order to understand the forces that shape any prominent change of behaviour toward health care – like the rising popularity of alternative medicine – we must carefully examine those social forces. This is the first book to do this in depth and is therefore essential reading for anyone who wants to understand this phenomenon, be they scientist or statesman.

During my tenure as the Director of the Office of Alternative Medicine at the National Institutes of Health, I recognized that 'unofficial' medicine has always been an important part of what the public uses in healthcare. Homeopaths and herbalists, folk practitioners and spiritualists provide a multiplicity of ways to address suffering. The public goes through periods of enchantment with unorthodox medicine. Homeopaths, herbalists, hypnotists, and various 'eclectics' were popular and public over a hundred years ago. At that time, orthodox physicians had little to no training and there was little regulation of practice. The popularity and use of the unorthodox would vary, depending on the perceived value of orthodox medicine, the needs of the public, and changing values in society. With the development of scientific medicine and its dramatic advances in the understanding and treatment of acute and infectious disease, these practices largely subsided (Gevitz, 1988).

The prominence of complementary and alternative medicine (CAM) is now rising rapidly. Two identical surveys of unconventional medical use in the United States done in 1990 and 1996, showed that CAM use by the public increased 45% over that six year period. Visits to CAM practitioners went from 400 million to over 600 million visits per year and the amount spent on these practices rose from $14 billion to $27 billion – most of it not reimbursed (Eisenberg *et al.*, 1998). The overwhelming effort now is toward an 'integration' of these practices into the mainstream. Seventy five medical schools in the United States have begun to teach about CAM practices (Wetzel *et al.*, 1998), hospitals have developed complementary and integrated medicine programs, health management organizations and health insurers are offering 'expanded' benefits packages that include CAM practitioners and services (Pelletier *et al.*, 1997). Biomedical research organizations are investing more into the investigation of these practices. For example, the budget of what was called the Office of Alternative Medicine at the U.S. National Institutes of Health rose from $3 million to $50 million in four years and changed from a co-ordination office to an independent center now called the National Center for Complimentary and Alternative Medicine (Marwick, 1998). It appears that complementary and alternative medicine has again 'come of age'.

This trend reflects not only changing behaviours but changing needs and values in modern society. It is the details of these changing values and behaviours that the scholars in this book examine. The book explores the psycho-social determinants of CAM use (Astin; Furnham and Vincent), the 'normalization' of users over time (Blais), how different concepts of the body influence health care practices (O'Connor), the relationship between the growing fitness movement and CAM (Goldstein), and the key role of the nature and quality of the therapeutic relationship in shaping health care preferences (Kelner). Chapters also address how CAM practices diffuse throughout society (Valente), and the role of health networks in influencing therapeutic choices (Wellman). Of note is that CAM practices, like most conventional practices, are adopted and 'normalized' long before scientific evidence has established safety and efficacy. Key differences in how this occurs, however, are that in conventional practice, procedures are usually introduced by professional bodies or industry rather than the public (McKinlay, 1981). This says something about the nature of public preferences and predicts that new unconventional practices will rise as current CAM groups become more professionalized and are adopted by the mainstream.

This is not the first time that the importance of unorthodox medical practices has risen in prominence. Orthodox medicine usually fights CAM practices by attacking them, limiting access to them, calling them quackery, and penalizing those who practice them. When they persist, mainstream medicine examines them, finding similarities with the orthodox and adopting them into normal medical practice (Worton, 1999). Medicine benefits from their selective integration by abandoning harmful therapies such as mercuralization, finding new drugs such as digitalis, and accepting more rigorous scientific methods with which to test them (Gevitz, 1988; Kaptchuk, 1998).

We now have sophisticated scientific methods for the application of basic science to clinical practice and for the management of acute and infectious disease. However, current methods for examining chronic disease or practices that have no explanatory model in western terms are not adequately informed by science (Linde and Jonas, 1999). CAM offers us the opportunity to debate and test new approaches for examining these areas as their importance increases in medicine (Pincus, 1997). Four authors in this book consider the role of science in informing us about CAM by examining use of the randomized control trial (Ernst), naturalistic inquiry (Glik), non-dichotomous models of conceptualizing and researching illness behaviour (Pescosolido), and the place of health services research in building a future of 'integrated' medicine (Best and Glik).

Other social factors are also influencing the growth in CAM use. These include: a rise in prevalence of chronic disease, increasing access to health information, increased democratization of medical care decision-making, a declining faith that scientific breakthroughs will have positive effects on personal health, and an increased interest in spiritualism (Fox, 1997; Starr, 1982). In addition, the public and professionals are increasingly concerned over the side-effects and escalating costs of conventional health care (Lazarou et al., 1998; Smith et al., 1998). As the publics' use of CAM accelerates, ignorance about these practices by physicians and scientists risks broadening the communication gap between the public and profession that serves them (Chez and Jonas, 1997; Eisenberg et al., 1998). This book addresses aspects of these broad influences by examining the re-emergence of pluralism in medicine (Sharma), the political consequences of CAM professionalization (Saks), and new strategies for a social and scientific research agenda for CAM (Best and Glik).

If we do not examine more closely the social and scientific forces that shape medicine we are destined to repeat many of the divisive tactics that have characterized the relationship between mainstream and non-mainstream practices of the past (Jonas, 1998). To adopt CAM without developing quality standards for its practices, products, and research is to return to a time in medicine when therapeutic confusion prevailed. Modern conventional medicine excels in the areas of quality healthcare and the use of science, and CAM must change to adopt similar standards. Conventional medicine is also the world's leader in the management of infectious traumatic and surgical diseases, in the study of pathology, and in biotechnology and drug development. All medical practices have the ethical obligations to retain these strengths for the benefit of patients (Chez and Jonas, 1997).

At the same time, there are important characteristics of CAM that risk being lost in its 'integration' with conventional care. The most important of these is an emphasis on self-healing as the lead approach for both improving wellness and the treatment of disease. All the major CAM systems approach illness first by trying to support and induce the self-healing processes of the person. If recovery can occur from this, the likelihood of adverse effects and the need for high-impact, high-cost interventions is reduced (Jonas, 1999). It is this orientation toward self-healing and health promotion (salutogenesis rather than pathogenesis) that makes CAM approaches to chronic disease especially attractive (Antonovsky, 1987).

The main "obstacles to discovery" writes Daniel Boorstin (1983), in his book *The Discoverers*, are "the illusions of knowledge". Humans fool themselves by making exaggerated claims of truth, clinging to unfounded explanations and denying observations they cannot explain. In addition, the complexity of disease and the powerful ability of the human body to recover often make it difficult to apply science to clinical medicine. K.B. Thomas (1994) demonstrated that nearly 80% of those who seek out medical care get better no matter what hand waving or pill popping we provide. I call this 'The 80% Rule', meaning that data collected on novel therapies delivered in an enthusiastic clinical environment will frequently yield positive outcomes in 70–80% of patients. Often our most accepted conventional treatments are shown to be non-specific in nature (Roberts *et al.*, 1993) or even harmful (Pratt, 1990) when finally studied rigorously. Their apparent effectiveness in practice is due to the powerful ability of the body to heal (with or without expectation), statistical regression to the mean (a measurement problem) and self-delusion (sometimes called bias; Jonas, 1994).

It is little wonder, then, that for the majority of physicians and patients there are many therapies both orthodox and unorthodox, that seem to work. Science has emerged as one of the few truly powerful approaches for mitigating this self-delusionary capacity. It will not continue to be a useful guide to medicine, however, unless we are willing to use it rigorously to examine both the social and the statistical forces that shape what we perceive and accept as reality. This book goes a long way in doing that for unorthodox medicine and also for orthodox medicine. Complementary and alternative medicine is here to stay. It is no longer an option to ignore it or treat it as something outside the normal processes of science and medicine. Our challenge is to move forward carefully, using both reason and wisdom, as we attempt to separate the pearls from the mud.

REFERENCES

Antonovsky, A. 1987. *Unraveling the Mystery of Health: How People Manage Stress and Stay Well.* San Francisco: Jossey-Bass.

Boorstin, D.J. 1983:xv. *The Discoverers.* New York: Random House.

Chez, R.A. and W.B. Jonas. 1997. 'The Challenge of Complementary and Alternative Medicine.' *American Journal of Obstetrics and Gynecology* 177:1156–1161.

Eisenberg, D.M., Davis, R.B., Ettner, S.A., Wilkey, S., Rompay, M. and R. Kessler. 1998. 'Trends in Alternative Medicine Use in the United States 1990–1997: Results of a Follow-up National Survey.' *Journal of the American Medical Association* 280:1569–1575.

Fox, E. 1997. 'Predominance of the Curative Model of Medical Care: A Residual Problem.' *Journal of the American Medical Association* 278:761–763.

Gevitz, N. 1998. *Other Healers: Unorthodox Medicine in America.* Baltimore: The Johns Hopkins University Press.

Jonas, W.B. 1999. 'Models of Medicine and Models of Healing.' In *Essentials of Complementary and Alternative Medicine* edited by W. Jonas and J. Levin. Philadelphia: Lippincott Williams & Wilkins.

Jonas, W.B. 1998. 'Alternative Medicine – Learning from the Past, Examining the Present, Advancing the Future.' *Journal of the American Medical Association* 280:1616–1618.

Jonas, W.B. 1994. 'Therapeutic labeling and the 80% Rule.' *Bridges* 5(1):4–6.

Kaptchuk, T.J. 1998. 'Intentional Ignorance: The History of Blind Assessment and Placebo Controls in Medicine.' *Bulletin of Historical Medicine* 72:389–433.

Lazarou, J. Pomeranz, B.H., and P.N. Corey. 1998. 'Incidence of Adverse Drug Reactions in Hospitalized Patients: A Meta-Analysis of Prospective Studies.' *Journal of the American Medical Association* 279:1200–1205.

Linde, K., and W.B. Jonas. 1999. 'Evaluating Complementary and Alternative Medicine: The Balance of Rigor and Relevance. In *Essentials of Complementary and Alternative Medicine* edited by W. Jonas and J. Levin. Philadelphia: Lippincott Williams & Wilkins.

Marwick, C. 1998. 'Alterations Are Ahead at the OAM.' *Journal of the American Medical Association* 280:1553–1554.

McKinlay, J.B. 1981. 'From "Promising Report" to "Standard Procedure": Seven Stages in the Career of a Medical Innovation.' *Millbank Memorial Fund Quarterly/Health and Society* 59:374–411.

Pelletier, K.R., Marie, A., Krasner, M. and W.L. Haskell. 1997. 'Current Trends in the Integration and Reimbursement of Complementary and Alternative Medicine by Managed Care, Insurance Carriers, and Hospital Providers.' *American Journal of Health Promotion* 12:112–123.

Pincus, T. 1997. 'Analyzing Long-Term Outcomes of Clinical Care Without Randomized Controlled Clinical Trials: The Consecutive Patient Questionnaire Database.' *Advances* 13:3–31.

Pratt, C.M. 1990. 'The Cardiac Arrhythmia Suppression Trial. Introduction; The Aftermath of the CAST – A Reconsideration of Traditional Concepts.' *American Journal of Cardiology* 65:1b–2b.

Roberts, A.H., Kewman, D.G., Mercier, L. and M. Hovell. 1993. 'The Power of Non-specific Effects in Healing: Implications for Psychological and Biological Treatments.' *Clinical Psychology Review* 13:375–391.

Smith, S., Freeland, M., Heffler, S., McKusick, D., *et al.* 1998. 'The Next Ten Years of Health Spending: What Does the Future Hold?' *Health Affairs* 17:128–140.

Starr, P. 1982. *The Social Transformation of American Medicine.* San Francisco: Basic Books.

Thomas, K.B. 1994. 'The Placebo in General Practice.' *The Lancet* 344:1066–1067.

Wetzel, M.S., Eisenberg, D.M. and T.J. Kaptchuk. 1998. 'A Survey of Courses Involving Complementary and Alternative Medicine at United States Medical Schools.' *Journal of the American Medical Association* 280:784–787.

Worton, J.C. 1999. 'The History of Complementary and Alternative Medicine.' In *Essentials of Complementary and Alternative Medicine* edited by W. Jonas and J. Levin. Philadelphia: Lippincott Williams & Wilkins.

List of Contributors

John A. Astin Department of Family Medicine, Complementary Medicine Programme, University of Maryland School of Medicine, Baltimore, USA

Allan Best Centre for Clinical Epidemiology and Evaluation, Vancouver Hospital, Vancouver, Canada

Régis Blais Department of Health Administration and Interdisciplinary Health Research Group, University of Montreal, Canada

Edzard Ernst Department of Complementary Medicine, University of Exeter, UK

Adrian Furnham Department of Psychology, University College London, UK

Deborah C. Glik UCLA School of Public Health, Los Angeles, USA

Michael S. Goldstein UCLA School of Public Health, Los Angeles, USA

Merrijoy Kelner Institute for Human Development, Life Course and Aging, University of Toronto, Canada

Bonnie B. O'Connor Department of Pediatrics, Brown University, Providence, USA

Bernice A. Pescosolido Department of Sociology, Indiana University, Bloomington, USA

Mike Saks Faculty of Health and Community Studies, De Montfort University, Leicester, UK

Ursula Sharma School of Education and Social Science, University of Derby, UK

Thomas W. Valente Department of Preventive Medicine, University of Southern California, Alhambra, USA

Charles A. Vincent Department of Psychology, University College London, UK

Beverly Wellman Institute for Human Development, Life Course and Aging, University of Toronto, Canada

Acknowledgments

Many people have helped us to create this book. Practitioners counseled us and provided opportunities to talk with their patients. Equally important was the contribution of patients who shared their health care stories with us so that we could understand the experience of people trying to cope with their health care problems. Without the financial support provided by the Social Science Humanities and Research Council of Canada, Health Canada, and the Office of Alternative Medicine at the National Institutes of Health, the book would never have come to fruition. We are also grateful to the Institute for Human Development, Life Course and Aging at the University of Toronto for providing us with the resources and space to do our work. We were assisted in that work by a number of people. Sivan Bomze performed a variety of tasks needed to prepare this manuscript. John Kroll and Barry Wellman gave us their support, advice, time and encouragement. Harwood Academic Publishers believed in this book from the beginning and gave us wise advice throughout.

Introduction
Complementary and Alternative Medicine: Challenge and Change

MERRIJOY KELNER AND BEVERLY WELLMAN

This book began years ago, long before complementary and alternative medicine (CAM) became so popular. In the 1970s, we began, separately and independently, academically and personally, to be involved in different forms of alternative care. One of us (Wellman) studied the Alexander Technique (postural re-education) while the other (Kelner) undertook a national study of chiropractors in Canada. These initiatives led us both to the offices of CAM practitioners. As we spent time sitting in these offices awaiting our turn for treatment, we both observed that the composition of the clientele was undergoing changes. At the outset, the patients consisted of a narrow slice of society. People attracted to the Alexander Technique were almost entirely artists. They were either dancers, musicians or actors; people who used their bodies strenuously. Those who were drawn to chiropractic, on the other hand, were largely people who did hard physical labour and had injured their backs in some way.

Over time, the range of people who sought both kinds of care began to expand and diversify. The artists were joined by truck drivers, academics and people who were resisting the recommendation for surgery they had received from their physicians. Similarly, chiropractic patients included more and more patients who wanted a treatment that was less invasive than surgery. Contrary to the stereotype of CAM patients as poor and uneducated, these more recent patients were obviously well dressed, well educated, affluent, and sophisticated in their approach. We asked ourselves: What is going on? Why are these people coming here when they must pay out of their own pockets instead of going to a doctor who is reimbursed by the government? And how are they learning about these options?

These types of questions led to our meeting and a decision to pursue social scientific research together that would help us find the answers. When we began the research, it was considered exotic by our colleagues and friends.

They were skeptical, dismissive and interested, all at the same time. They asked lots of questions but remained unconvinced about the utility of CAM and the academic merits of researching it. Later, people began coming up to us at social gatherings and confiding that they had decided to try some form of CAM. What did we know about it? And could we recommend somebody? The pace of inquiries kept accelerating as did the attention paid to CAM by television, newspapers, magazines and later on, by the Internet. We recognized that a personal and academic interest had become a public phenomenon. This book reflects the convergence of our personal, intellectual, and scholarly worlds and also draws on an international frame of reference, primarily covering the United States, Canada and Britain. This comparative perspective is also represented in the international editorial team which has been instrumental in putting together this volume. This includes Merrijoy Kelner and Beverly Wellman from Canada, Bernice Pescosolido from the United States and Mike Saks from Britain.

Complementary and alternative medicine is not new. Unorthodox therapies such as homoepathy, acupuncture and herbalism have been around before the advent of scientific medicine. Most societies have historically been medically pluralistic (Wallis and Morley, 1976). What we are seeing today, however, is a new kind of medical pluralism. People from various backgrounds and socio-economic groups are choosing to consult CAM practitioners for a range of conditions while at the same time continuing to use medical services. The popularity of CAM therapies has become increasingly widespread since the 1960's, as more and more people in Western societies have developed an interest in using them. In the United Kingdom (Ernst, 1996a; Thomas *et al.*, 1991), in the United States (Astin *et al.*, 1998; Eisenberg *et al.*, 1993, 1998), in Canada (Kelner and Wellman, 1997a; Blais *et al.*, 1997; Millar, 1997; Verhoef and Sutherland, 1995), and elsewhere in the industrialized world (Fisher and Ward, 1994; MacLennan *et al.*, 1996), the use of CAM is clearly on the rise.

This book uses social science research to examine the emergence of this dynamic change in the pattern of health care services. While the mass media have showered an avalanche of attention on non-orthodox therapies and healers, scholarly knowledge has lagged far behind. Some reliable information is being amassed. Epidemiologists such as Eisenberg and his colleagues (1998) and Paramore (1997) have been conducting research on the use of CAM in the U.S. which shows it now to be widespread and extensive. Similar surveys have been done in the U.K., Europe, Australia and Canada. These surveys show that in spite of the insurance for medical services available in many of these countries, people are still choosing to pay (out of pocket) for CAM services. Clinical scientists have also begun to turn their attention to examining why and how CAM influences the state of health. Under the aegis of the Office of

Alternative Medicine now the National Center for Research on CAM (U.S. National Institutes of Health) a series of studies have been initiated to test questions such as the usefulness of acupuncture for treating drug addiction, the efficacy of alternative approaches to pain control and the effectiveness of CAM treatments for cancer. Physicians in some leading North American hospitals are conducting experiments to test the impact of CAM therapies such as therapeutic touch and energy healing on the rate of recovery after surgery. Rigorous tests of efficacy are being conducted in the United Kingdom where researchers are investigating issues such as the utility of acupuncture in the treatment of asthma and the effect of homeopathy on chronic headaches.

The social sciences provide yet another way of understanding the phenomenon of CAM, using the large canvasses of sociology, anthropology and politics as well as the more detailed brush strokes of psychology. In the pages of this book, a multidisciplinary, cross-national group of social scientists apply their research experience and theoretical expertise to building a valid knowledge base. They employ social science concepts and research findings to clarify the social context in which CAM has created such popular interest. This includes explanations of who uses these therapies, why they choose to consult CAM practitioners and how they find their way to their offices. The book also encompasses the key issues of research and policy in response to user demands.

Less developed in the book is analysis of the characteristics, aspirations and motivations of CAM practitioners and physicians who elect to use CAM therapies in their practice. This is because less work has been done in this area to date. In the future social scientists will undoubtedly focus more attention on practitioners and their potential for winning professional recognition and a more central role in the overall health system.

In an environment where so much of the knowledge has been anecdotal and subject to the biases and claims of various camps, this book offers important information, new perspectives and creative models for thinking about a significant social development. The readers of this book can be confident that they will find here a compilation of knowledge and ideas that reflect the work of reputable scholars. Here we lay out some of the most complex questions currently troubling scholars. The first issue we grapple with is the basic question of how to define CAM.

DEFINING CAM

The definition of CAM is open to many interpretations, making it difficult to ensure a common understanding. This lack of consistency is not surprising in a field that has such diverse cultural and historical roots, and is evolving so rapidly. There is confusion about which therapies to include or exclude from the definition and how to classify the multitude of therapies in some coherent way. There is confusion even about what such therapies should be called – alternative, complementary, holistic, unorthodox, unconventional, non-scientific, and marginal are only some of the many descriptors in the literature. Indeed, the borders between orthodox medicine and CAM are themselves unclear as particular CAM therapies such as osteopathy and chiropractic continue to gain wide acceptance and it becomes increasingly difficult to decide where to place them. Moreover, practices which are considered 'alternative' by the majority of people in Western society, are thought of as conventional and mainstream by people in other societies. As Millet (1999) observes 'The problems of vocabulary and confusion turn out to be problems of history, sociology, and power.' As the field continues to develop, trying to achieve a clear definition of CAM is like struggling to hit a moving target.

The goal, however, must be to find a definition that expresses the essential nature of CAM. The definition must apply fully to all kinds of alternative therapies yet not delineate too broadly or too narrowly. Clarity and care are essential since how the description is framed will influence the choice of data for study. The challenge here is to find appropriate language for description in an area where there is still so much controversy around value conflict and political dominance.

A panel convened by the Office of Alternative Medicine in 1995 to define and describe CAM, struggled with the difficulties outlined here and came up with the following general definition:

> Complementary and alternative medicine (CAM) is a broad domain of healing resources that encompasses all health systems, modalities, and practices and their accompanying theories and beliefs, other than those intrinsic to the politically dominant health system of a particular society or culture in a given historical period. CAM includes all such practices and ideas self-defined by their users as preventing or treating illness or promoting well-being. Boundaries within CAM and between the CAM domain and the domain of the dominant system are not always sharp or fixed (1997, p. 50).

Such a definition treats both conventional medicine and CAM on an equal footing and avoids negative connotations. It also takes into account the existence of multiple healing systems which have various degrees of dominance and influence in the United States, Canada, Britain and other western societies.

Regardless of how they are defined, it is important to recognize that conventional medicine and CAM tend to operate under very different paradigms of theory and practice. In fact, Kuhn (1970) would probably describe them as 'incommensurate', since they are based on different assumptions. Conventional medicine typically treats disease as a breakdown in the human body that can be repaired by direct biochemical or surgical intervention. The theoretical underpinning is frequently claimed to be rational and scientific. The model on which it is based conceives illness as arising from specific pathogenic agents, and views health as the absence of disease. The concept of CAM, on the other hand, covers a diverse set of healing practices, which do not normally fit under the scientific medical umbrella. Instead, these practices emphasize the uniqueness of each individual, integration of body, mind and spirit, the flow of energy as a source of healing, and disease as having dimensions beyond the purely biological (Berliner and Salmon, 1979). The life force is very commonly seen as a crucial element of the healing process and strong emphasis is placed on the environment, the subjective experience of patients, the healing power of nature, and health as a positive state of being (Goldstein, 1999).

One way to think about the definition of CAM is to see it as a social creation that depends on the perspective of the individual who is doing the defining. For most medical scholars, CAM is defined by its location 'outside accepted medical thought, scientific knowledge, or university teaching.' (Ernst, 1996b; p. 244). In other words, the definition is derived from its differences to the dominant mode of health care which is conventional medicine. But this *residual* form of definition does not do justice to the healing capacities of CAM. Social scientists like O'Connor (1995) define CAM based on its alternative *belief system* with its distinctive views of the body, of health, and of the causes of illness. A third way of defining CAM is as a complementary adjunct to medical care. The term *complementary* implies the possibility of cooperation with conventional medicine and recognizes the widespread research finding that users of CAM also consult physicians on a regular basis (Kelner and Wellman, 1997b). The term *alternative* highlights the fact that CAM stands on the edges of the established health care system and receives almost no support from the medical establishment or the government (Saks, 1992). This definition points to the political dominance of medicine and its role in controlling research funding, and limiting inclusion of CAM in the basic medical curriculum.

Quoting from Menger (1928, p. 76), Popper (1959, p. 55), reminds us: 'Definitions are dogmas; only the conclusions drawn from them can afford us any new insight.' Each definition is arbitrary; each has its own consequences and requires its own methodological decisions. For the purposes of this book, a composite definition of CAM has been chosen to provide an extensive opportunity to analyze the various forms of health care described here. CAM is conceived as an approach to health care that while different from conventional medicine, is sometimes complementary to it and at other times is distinctly alternative. The book focuses mainly on patient contacts with CAM practitioners rather than the many informal alternative health care activities that people employ such as use of megavitamins, special diets, folk remedies, herbal supplements and meditation.

Up to now, we have referred to CAM as a homogenous phenomenon. This is misleading, however, since individual therapies vary according to philosophy, terminology, practice, the degree of public acceptance, and the extent of efficacy. There have been several attempts to classify and categorize the various CAM therapies. One of the best known has been developed by Fulder (1996) who proposes a typology of five categories: ethnic medical systems (acupuncture, Chinese medicine and Ayrurveda), manual therapies (chiropractic, reflexology and massage therapy), therapies for mind/body (hypnotherapy, psychic healing and radionics), nature- cure therapies (naturopathy and hygienic methods), and non-allopathic medicinal systems (homeopathy and herbalism).

Here we suggest a different form of classification that arranges CAM therapies according to the context in which they are delivered. The categories are: (1) clinical forms (chiropractic, homeopathy, acupuncture and naturopathy); (2) psychological/behavioural forms (yoga, dance therapy, and biofeedback); and (3) social/community forms (faith healing and folk medicine). Another useful way to classify CAM therapies is based on the extent of legitimacy and public acceptance: (1) top of the hierarchy (osteopathy, chiropractic and acupuncture); (2) middle range (naturopathy and homeopathy); (3) bottom of the hierarchy (rebirthing and Reiki). CAM therapies can be categorized in still other ways; for example, according to the extent of scientific evidence for their efficacy, or whether or not they involve touching patients. The important point here is that these classifications are not permanent; they will continue to shift according to clinical, cultural, political and economic developments. Scholars have to choose their typologies according to the particular questions they are addressing at a given point in time.

What is important is to recognize that CAM is a complex and constantly changing social phenomenon which defies any arbitrary definition or classification. As social scientists design CAM research, it is not necessary or even possible that there be one agreed upon definition.

DESIGNING RESEARCH ON CAM

When social scientists think about research methods, they need first to establish the research question being asked. It is the question rather than the paradigm which should drive the design, data collection and data analysis used in the study. It is worth remembering that we do not live in a single, objective reality; there are various ways of looking at the world. Research questions emanate from a variety of social contexts and cannot be separated from the environment in which they are situated. This means that in order for research paradigms to be appropriate, they need to reflect the social and cultural setting of the question being investigated.

To date, most social science research on CAM has been based on models of health care which were developed to study peoples' use of medical care. These models make the assumption that people act in rational ways when they make health care decisions. They are also focused exclusively on individuals, thus neglecting the larger social context in which people negotiate their health care options. This approach has yielded reliable data concerning the extent to which people use CAM, their motivations for doing so and something about the nature of their encounters with CAM practitioners. New and different models are needed to open up this research area to other kinds of questions and the use of innovative investigative strategies. This is one of the major purposes of this book.

One such strategy is based on social networks (Wellman, 1988). Network analysis is a technique for mapping the people in an individual's network. It measures the frequency of contact, the closeness of the bonds, and the relationships of the people in each person's network. Network analysis enables social scientists to answer questions such as: who people turn to when they have a health problem, who gives them recommendations to CAM therapies and therapists, and who gives them constructive assistance with their health care. Another perspective, communication research, allows us to explore the diffusion of an innovation such as CAM. This makes it possible for social scientists to chart the rate and extent to which new ideas and practices are adopted by the society at large.

Building on these research strategies, the Network Episode Model which Pescosolido describes in chapter 10, presents a dynamic approach which views all illness behaviours as embedded in day to day life. It includes diverse kinds of health care rather than studying any particular one in isolation. While previous models have been solely based on rational choice of health care, this model also includes a social component. It focuses on the illness episode as a dynamic process, rather than on decision-making about health care at any one point in time. This more inclusive approach views the individual as operating within a multidimensional context of shifting treatment options and service delivery systems. While the Network Episode Model adds depth to current research parameters, it also highlights the need to rethink the concepts and research strategies now being used to examine the use of CAM.

The field of anthropology provides an additional way of conceptualizing health care and in particular, researching the use of CAM as illustrated in chapter 2 by O'Connor. The ethnographic approach to studying CAM relies on evaluative field studies in naturalistic settings and stresses the importance of the patient's perspective and self-reports. These are the settings that best reveal the dynamics of social processes and their impact on health care decisions. For example, observational studies on folk or spiritual healing show that it is important to consider both the social location and the cultural relevance of healing practices. These considerations can not only help to explain why people are attracted to CAM therapies but also why they may be effective. Clinical studies certainly have an important place in evaluating health outcomes, but they tell only one part of the story. Adding real world conditions and focusing on structure, process and outcomes of care, makes it possible to gain a broader view of the healing process as a social intervention.

The crucial question is, where should we go from here? Longitudinal, prospective research is one obvious direction that would fill the present knowledge gap. The cross-sectional data that has been compiled to date, present a picture taken at only one point in time. Retrospective studies, while valuable, are also limited in their usefulness by the need for respondents to reconstruct their experiences over time. Health care is a process which needs to be captured at different points over a long period. Moreover, health status is a changing condition; only longitudinal, prospective studies can adequately capture these changes. With a longitudinal approach, for example, scholars can chart the beliefs and attitudes of patients who have left the practitioners they were using (leavers), and compare their views with those who have stayed (stayers) or moved back and forth among several practitioners (floaters).

Multi-dimensional research designs can also enrich future understandings of the use of CAM. While individual determinants of CAM use and the models that have been used to explain it have given us descriptive profiles of users, there is more to the total picture. In order to grasp the complexity of the larger health care context, researchers need to include different levels of analysis, from the individual to the cultural and societal. Future research should include a focus on dimensions such as personal experience, political and economic opportunities and constraints, availability of resources, and the *zeitgeist* of the times, in a model that integrates them all.

Another way to think about the future of CAM research is to take a global perspective. As the number of scholars taking an interest in CAM increases around the world, it becomes possible to carry out high quality international research and to make cross-country comparisons. Such comparisons could identify the effects of distinctive socio-political conditions and cultural influences on the use of CAM. [This book is an example of collaboration between scholars from different countries and different disciplines. It can help to develop and test new, more inclusive approaches.] Application of new models to various settings can help to refine the fit between theory and reality.

EVALUATING CAM

There is a widespread assumption among the general public that CAM is natural, and therefore safe. Many people are making use of CAM services and practitioners without evidence-based assurances of safety or efficacy. At the same time, growing numbers of health care providers and policy makers are calling for accountability and regulation. There is currently a lively and unresolved controversy about how best to assure the safety and test the effectiveness of CAM therapies (Ernst, 1996; Mitchell and Cormack, 1998). There is considerable debate whether alternative health practices can be studied in the same way that standard medical practices are assessed. Cant (1996) suggests that the philosophical foundations of some alternative health practices make it impossible to judge them by the same standards as conventional medicine. Others argue that existing methodological strategies are not useful for evaluating CAM therapies such as massage therapy. A Quantitative Methods Working Group convened in 1995 at the National Institutes of Health in the USA concluded that these problems could be overcome. They found that there were existing methodologies and data analysis procedures which were quite capable of addressing the majority of study questions related to evaluating CAM (Levin et al., 1997).

Some attempts at evaluation are already underway. In the United States, the Office of Alternative Medicine has been funding major tests of efficacy primarily through university departments around the country. In Europe, there have been evaluation studies on various forms of acupuncture, chiropractic, homeopathy and other CAM practices (for example, Meade et al., 1990). Worldwide, the Cochrane Collaboration has become important (Sackett, 1994). It is including CAM in its goal of assessing the evidence base in all fields of medicine. In Canada, evaluation research has also begun. An Office of Natural Health Products has recently been established to ensure that medicinal herbs and vitamins are safe for consumers to use (Globe and Mail, March, 1999). These efforts represent the initial steps in what will undoubtedly evolve into a systematic program in evaluative research.

At the moment, the randomized clinical trial (RCT) is considered to be the gold standard of research design, the one by which all other clinical studies are judged as Ernst argues in chapter 9. This is a procedure in which research subjects are matched for similar illnesses as well as demographic characteristics, and are then randomly assigned to two or more groups. One group receives the intervention, for example, a drug thought to be useful for their condition, while the other group is untreated and serves as the control. Usually, those who are not being treated are given a placebo so that they will believe they are also receiving treatment. If the treated group improves significantly (as determined by statistical procedures) as compared to the control or placebo group, the intervention is judged to have a positive therapeutic effect. Ideally, those who administer the treatment and/or placebo and those who evaluate the results of the study are blinded; that is they are not aware of who has received the treatment and who has not.

RCTs have proven to be the method of choice for assessing the effectiveness of new drugs. When used to evaluate other kinds of therapies, however, they have some definite limitations. The problem is that many therapies are incompatible with this approach and do not lend themselves to evaluation by RCTs. For example, surgery and psychotherapy are two instances of conventional medicine in which it is extremely difficult to blind the therapists or to simulate the therapy. CAM therapies that use hands-on-techniques like acupuncture and chiropractic present similar difficulties. Another difficulty lies in the nature of CAM treatments; they are customarily tailored to the individual patient rather than standardized for a specific condition. In addition, most CAM practitioners see the placebo effect as something to be used in a constructive fashion, rather than taking the medical view that the placebo should be eliminated from consideration to assure scientific rigour (Pietroni, 1991). These limitations on the use of RCTs to study alternative therapies have prompted Levin *et al.* (1997) in their Methodological Manifesto to proclaim that: 'Clinical trials are not the only game in town' (p. 1086).

The dominance of RCTs has meant that many alternative therapies have been ignored or dismissed by the medical establishment because their efficacy has not been demonstrated by this particular research strategy (for example, British Medical Association, 1986). RCTs work best for simple interventions with diseases that are easily definable and capable of being quantified. But this tactic is not always suited to CAM therapies which take a holistic approach to treatment. A holistic research strategy requires a broad view that can encompass elements of the healing process such as the role of patients, the impact of the therapeutic relationship and the non-technical aspects of treatment

In addition to these methodological problems, the RCT has important economic and political ramifications. It is an enormously expensive process that entails vast resources and is usually undertaken by drug companies willing to invest large sums in the expectation that they will reap big rewards when the successful drugs are marketed. The same kind of financial incentives do not apply to substances and practices that cannot be patented. Moreover, it is wise to remember that many conventional medical techniques, including a number of diagnostic and surgical techniques and treatments, have never been subjected to double-blind controlled clinical trials (Saks, 1994). Furthermore, numerous medical remedies including aspirin and penicillin became widely used long before experts knew how they worked (see, for instance, MacEoin, 1990). Critics of CAM often apply a double standard, showing more enthusiasm in their efforts to discredit unevaluated CAM therapies than they do in questioning the safety and efficacy of conventional medicine.

It seems clear that RCTs cannot and should not be applied to all procedures and substances. The power of the medical profession, however, may make it difficult to move away from the heavy reliance on RCTs that medicine has normally insisted on for testing the efficacy of CAM therapies. Medicine's ways of knowing are grounded in a strong background in the biomedical sciences. Medical research tends to be based on the premise that biomedicine is impartial and empirically verifiable and that there is only one objective picture of reality and one valid empirical method of verifying it. This claim leaves little room for more flexible definitions of health, more complex pictures of reality and hence more pluralistic views of how evaluation should be conducted.

Rather than distorting CAM to fit the preexisting conventions of RCTs, it makes sense to adapt current evaluation methods in ways that fit with the underlying premises of CAM. The following examples illustrate the range of other research methodologies that have been suggested by a number of scholars (Glik, 1993; Canter and Nanke, 1993; Black, 1996; Aldridge, 1993; Moss, 1992; Levin *et al.*, 1997; Cant and Sharma, 1996).

(1) Basic biological research – This applies biological research to CAM healing therapies by assessing the effect of these therapies on physiological changes in the body. For example, looking at the effect of acupuncture treatment on blood pressure, the level of certain chemical messengers between the brain and the body, or the effects of healing energies on adhesion of cultured cells and haemodialysis of blood cells.

(2) Long term assessment – Tracing the long term effects of different forms of treatment on specific groups, controlling for length of time in treatment. It is also important, where appropriate, to ensure that treatments are given by the same practitioner.

(3) Co-operative inquiry – The patient, the researcher and the therapist all form a team which works together to explore the ways in which the treatment affects both patient and practitioner. This method is useful for demonstrating the effects of factors such as patients' lifestyle and the therapeutic relationship on treatment.

(4) Single case study design – This method treats the patient as his/her own control. It allows a patient to be monitored over time using diverse treatments including a placebo. Such an approach can yield valuable detailed information about the outcome of specific treatments.

(5) Outcome studies – For evaluating CAM therapies, the conception of outcomes should be broad enough to include considerations such as

'feeling better', more energy, increased mobility, relief of pain, and greater capacity to cope with the demands of daily life.

(6) Cost benefit analysis – At the individual level, it is fairly easy to document what people are spending and what benefits they feel they are receiving. At the societal level, however, it is exceedingly difficult to assess with any degree of accuracy whether government expenditures on health care are reduced as a result of CAM therapies. Morbidity and mortality statistics usually form the basis for such an analysis. Quality-of-life measures are not customarily included in cost/benefit analyses even though CAM therapies may have their greatest impact on this aspect of health.

Other new methods for evaluating CAM therapies will undoubtedly be developed as more practitioners/researchers are attracted to this phenomenon and acknowledge the need to protect the health and safety of those who use CAM. The argument that new, imaginative evaluation methods are required, that take into account CAM's special characteristics, in no way negates the necessity for rigorous standards and peer review. One single standard of evaluation for both CAM and medicine is needed. Competent researchers should carry out well designed experiments to ensure that their results have both validity and reliability. All evaluation studies of CAM therapies should be able to withstand the skeptical scrutiny of CAM's harshest critics.

SOCIAL SCIENTISTS MEET CAM

This book is divided into four sections. Section One addresses the question of why people choose to consult CAM practitioners. The growing number of people turning to CAM has aroused the curiosity of researchers trying to make sense of this social change in health care patterns. Section Two examines social and health characteristics of CAM users and analyzes their pathways to care. Section Three opens up new avenues for doing research. Beginning with established, clinical methods, this section presents new research strategies rooted in the social sciences. Section Four uses social science knowledge and concepts to make projections about how CAM will develop in the future and how it might fit into the overall health care system.

Section One

This section explores the myriad explanations that have been offered for the widespread popularity of CAM at this particular point in time. Michael Goldstein, in chapter one, highlights the correspondence between fitness, health promotion and the use of CAM. He argues that people who are actively concerned with fitness and health promotion are more likely to be users of CAM, since they share many significant assumptions and beliefs about the body and about health. Goldstein emphasizes the importance of the market-place in promoting these assumptions. Health, he argues, has become a com-modity sold by corporations who see fitness and CAM as a money-making opportunity. He concludes by predicting that we can expect an increasing synergy between fitness and CAM in the future.

In chapter two, Bonnie Blair O'Connor recognizes that the use of CAM is not a new phenomenon. Historically, the way people conceive of the body has had a major influence on their decisions to incorporate CAM into their health care. She points out that at various points in the history of the United States, nonmedical conceptions of the body and CAM approaches to maintaining health were widely popular. Earlier in the 20th century, medicine became the dominant force in health care. Today, she explains the resurgence of CAM by the argument that alternative conceptions of health and of the body are more congruent with people's experiences of illness than are the assumptions of the biomedical model.

Adrian Furnham and Charles Vincent, in chapter three, address the question of why people choose CAM when there is so little evidence that it works. They examine a number of empirical studies that have been carried out in an effort to answer this complex question. Furnham and Vincent then identify nine pos-sible reasons why people seek out CAM practitioners, depending on the motives and the academic disciplines of those who ask the question. They con-clude by observing that it is too simple to think in terms of patients who are either 'pushed' or 'pulled' toward CAM by their particular health histories; larger considerations such as environmental concerns also shape peoples' health care decisions.

Merrijoy Kelner, in chapter four, explores the notion that it is the distinctive kind of therapeutic relationship that exists between CAM practitioners and their patients that accounts for the upsurge of interest in CAM. She looks at the three main models that have been used to explore the doctor- patient- rela-tionship and applies them to patient relationships with alternative practition-ers. By examining the relationships experienced across five kinds of treatment groups: family physicians, chiropractors, acupuncturists/traditional Chinese doctors, naturopaths and Reiki healers, she finds that all groups of patients place most value on the shared decision-making model of care, but that this approach is more commonly found among CAM practitioners and provides one explanation for their growing popularity. Kelner's research also shows that most people who use CAM have highly pragmatic motivations; they seek relief from long-term chronic problems and will continue to try new options in the hope of finding one that works.

Section Two

The second section of the book addresses two key questions: what kinds of people use CAM and how do they find their way there? In chapter five, John Astin describes the psycho-social characteristics of CAM users based on a national survey of adults in the United States. He goes beyond epidemiological identifiers such as social class and gender (Eisenberg *et al.*, 1993; 1998) to include specific cultural values, previous health care experiences and particular world-views. In the end, however, Astin concludes that it is people who have been unable to find relief from continuing pain or discomfort who are most likely to seek out CAM therapies.

The sixth chapter by Régis Blais is based on two health surveys carried out at different periods of time, thus providing a longitudinal analysis of people who use CAM. Blais finds that between the years of 1987 and 1993 the number of persons in Quebec, Canada using CAM has increased, the type of CAM practitioners consulted has diversified and the reasons for consultation have expanded. Overall, however, the demographic profile of CAM users did not change. His description of CAM users corresponds to the findings of other researchers in North America and Europe; they are mainly female, young, well educated and affluent.

Thomas Valente, in chapter seven, uses diffusion of innovation theory to explain how people decide to adopt CAM use. He distinguishes between the various types of CAM users, ranging from a few early adopters through to the mass of majority adopters to the few laggards at the end of the cycle. He associates progress through these stages of diffusion with changes in personal perceptions and also with the influence of the media. For early adopters, it is personal or situational factors that are the most persuasive. Whereas for majority and late adopters it is network influences that are most directly responsible for the decision to seek an alternative practitioner.

In chapter eight, Beverly Wellman uses network analysis to examine the health ties of patients who consult either family physicians or some form of CAM practitioner. She examines the nature of health information and support that these patients receive from kin, friends, physicians and alternative practitioners. In all the treatment groups in the study, people have close health confidants who are influential in determining where people go for their health care. The difference is that the health networks of the alternative patients are broader and more inclusive than those of the family physician patients, thus providing access to more kinds of health care options.

Section Three

Section three of the book delves into the controversial issues surrounding research on CAM. Different approaches are taken by scholars from a range of disciplines and their different backgrounds influence the shape of the models they propose. In chapter nine, Edzard Ernst urges that the safety and efficacy and effectiveness of CAM become paramount issues for researchers. He makes the point that although some forms of CAM may be considered 'natural', that does not mean that they are necessarily safe. With few exceptions, specific effectiveness for CAM therapies has not been firmly established. Ernst argues that double blind, clinical trials in defined situations are the best way to test the effectiveness of CAM therapies. Where sufficient numbers of good quality trials do not yet exist, systematic reviews or meta-analyses are needed. He concludes that what is required is high-quality and appropriate research and that without rigorously derived evidence, the public should be wary of embracing CAM therapies.

In chapter ten, Bernice Pescosolido, a sociologist, presents a network episode model for understanding illness behaviour and the use of CAM therapies. This model combines individual determinants of health care decision-making with social considerations. She emphasizes that the underlying mechanism of this model is interaction in social networks. Illness behaviour is seen as a dynamic process, rather than a choice of health care at any one point in time. She conceives of the health care system as a changing set of providers and services with which individuals may come into contact when they become ill.

Deborah Glik, a social anthropologist, argues in chapter eleven that there has been a bias toward studying professionalized forms of care, to the neglect of indigenous or folk healing. She makes a case for research models that include a broad range of societal factors such as the therapeutic context and the cultural values of patients. She contends that research conducted in naturalistic settings using evaluative field methods is just as valuable as more clinical approaches. Glik illustrates her argument by drawing on studies of spiritual healing groups and patients of homeopathic practitioners.

Section Four

This final section of the book focuses on the future of CAM. In chapter twelve, Ursula Sharma argues that the continuing re-emergence of CAM in the UK and other western countries should be understood in the context of a wider web of relationships, for example, the organization of other health care professions. She points out that medical pluralism of one kind or another is the norm in countries around the world and that biomedicine does not enjoy a natural priority. She envisions a more pluralistic health care system in the future. But this pluralism, Sharma points out, is not the same as the medical pluralism that was evident before the rise of biomedical hegemony. In the UK today, some CAM therapies are situated in the public sector and at the same time there is a flourishing market for private consumption of CAM. Sharma predicts that while some types of CAM therapies will remain on the margins and need to be purchased in the private market place, other types will be recognized as legitimate and be incorporated into the government supported health system.

In chapter thirteen, Mike Saks explores the political implications of the increasing efforts of alternative practitioners to win professional acceptance. He points out that over the last century in Britain, Canada and the United States, the profession of medicine has had a legally underwritten monopoly in the marketplace. Since the 1960s, however, many CAM practitioner groups have strengthened their position *vis-à-vis* medicine through political lobbying and professionalization. This trend has sharpened competition for those physicians who wish to incorporate CAM into their practices as well as posing a substantial challenge to the dominance of the medical establishment. Saks suggests that the potential for CAM therapists to gain professional standing may be limited in scope. This is due in part to the success of the medical establishment in incorporating CAM therapies, and thus reducing the threat of losing its dominance. Finally, Saks examines the question of whether professionalization of CAM is desirable and deserves support by the state.

In the last chapter of the book, Allan Best and Deborah Glik present a conceptual framework that positions CAM research as health services research. They argue that such an approach can help to meet the escalating public interest in using CAM therapies and also guide the process of reforming health care. The authors believe that in order to promote appropriate integration of CAM, research must examine issues of utilization, cost-effectiveness and the evidence base for practice. The chapter provides a working model for research on integrative health services which outlines three distinct strategies: healing, learning and research, to provide the data required for making decisions about health reform. The need for development of measures is also discussed and the authors sketch a provisional conceptual map for organizing key constructs and relevant variables. They make a case for establishing three areas of research priorities: conceptualization, design, and analysis, and application. The chapter concludes with recommendations for integrative research and emphasizes that partnerships between the producers of research and the consumers of this research are essential if the promise of better health services is to become a reality.

CHALLENGE AND CHANGE

We are seeing dramatic changes in the delivery of health care in industrialized society today. Consumer demand is increasingly driving the shape of health care which is becoming more and more pluralistic in nature. The health care system is experiencing widespread restructuring influenced in part by the growing dominance of corporate interests. The future place of CAM in all of this is not yet determined. It seems likely that insurance companies, managed care organizations, national health insurance schemes and hospitals will incorporate some aspects of CAM into their practices and policies. Medical schools are also adding courses on CAM to their curricula and more research funds are beginning to be directed by governments toward the study of CAM treatments.

We can expect that the demand for CAM will continue to expand. Indeed, CAM has already become a viable business for many of its practitioners and even more so for the companies that produce products associated with it. The big question for the future is whether the practices of CAM will be integrated into the mainstream of health care. Already, some doctors are adding elements of CAM therapies to their own practices while others are recommending it to some of their patients. If integration is to occur, issues of licensure, credibility, and education will need to be seriously pursued. One change that seems unlikely is that people will turn away from conventional medicine. The medical model still has a pervasive influence as does the infrastructure that supports it. The question is, whether CAM will be able to coalesce across therapies and develop its own organizational structure independent of medicine. Or will it eventually be incorporated into the conventional medical system?

Changes of this magnitude pose a series of challenges for the delivery of health care. One challenge is to thoroughly map the area called CAM. While some of the therapies and practices are well known, there are a myriad of others available for use but little known. In addition to ascertaining what is out there, it will be essential to understand what the different therapies offer and how their practices work. In an era of evidence-based medicine, rigorous research on issues of safety, efficacy and cost benefits is imperative. This kind of knowledge will help to facilitate the appropriate integration of CAM with conventional medicine, making it complementary rather than alternative. If both systems can learn to work together in a synergistic whole, the outcome can only be positive. The scientific expertise of medicine and CAM's emphasis on prevention, holism and personal responsibility can combine to truly make the definition of health mean more than the absence of illness.

Incorporation into the existing health care system will entail the challenge of educating doctors and CAM practitioners in each others' specialized knowledge. Furthermore, CAM practitioners need to put aside differences and unite to establish practice standards that will invite the trust of the public. They will need to be licensed and accountable so that the public perceives them as safe, reliable, and competent and physicians will be willing to work with them as partners. A challenge for CAM practitioners will be to co-exist in the new health care system without losing their distinctive ways of practicing. Finally, the challenge for society as a whole is to decide, if and when CAM therapies have been shown to be effective and safe, how they can be made available to everyone who needs them in the most responsible way.

APPENDIX

There are by now a plethora of books on aspects of CAM, but most are not based on systematic research. A few books have been based on research dealing with individual therapies such as homeopathy (Ernst and Hahn, 1998; Jonas and Jacobs, 1996), chiropractic (Kelner et al., 1980; Smith-Cunnien, 1998), and acupuncture (Saks, 1992). Books like these provide descriptive detail that is beyond the scope of this book. Here we take a broader perspective which encompasses the whole phenomena of CAM and address the reasons for its current popularity. Listed below and presented in chronological order is a representative sample of the work done thus far by social scientists interested in CAM.

One well-known, early effort to map the terrain was Warren Salmon's edited book on *Alternative Medicines: Popular and Policy Perspectives* (1984). He reports the popular resurgence of interest and activity in CAM in the United States and Europe. The book provides an understanding and an overview of selected CAM therapies and offers a range of viewpoints on their public acceptance and related policy issues. Stephen Fulder's The *Handbook of Complementary Medicine* (1988) was published later with classifications and explanations of a wide range of therapies including their philosophies and practices. He draws portraits of patients of CAM in the United Kingdom at that time and also describes the backgrounds of the therapists. Included in the book is an international overview of the social and legal position of the therapies in countries in Europe and elsewhere. Norman Gevitz (1988) in his edited book, *Other Healers: Unorthodox Medicine in America,* takes a scholarly perspective on CAM groups and practices in the United States. The book outlines a number of different types of therapies and uses historical perspectives and descriptive analyses to explain their growing public acceptance. Included in the book is an examination of spiritually oriented healing movements as well as contemporary folk medicine.

Meredith McGuire (1988) in her book *Ritual Healing in Suburban America,* reports an in-depth study of several different types of ritual healing groups frequented by suburban Americans in a small town in New Jersey. The people involved in the groups, either as leaders or followers, were interviewed in detail about their beliefs, attitudes and experiences with healing. She found that orthodox medicine was only one among many kinds of health care being used. People were becoming 'contractors of their own care' and making choices between mainstream medicine and CAM therapies on the basis of their beliefs about what would help them most. The people she studied viewed health, illness, and healing from a perspective which went far beyond the bio-medical model. Her research suggested that there was a strong link between health and healing and broader socio-cultural issues.

Rosalind Coward accounts for the surge of interest of CAM in the United Kingdom in *The Whole Truth: The Myth of Alternative Health* (1989). She describes the dramatic change in public attitudes which now regard good health as an ideal state which is one's personal responsibility to pursue. She contends that alternative therapies are based on a new philosophy of nature, health and the body and that this new philosophy has captured the popular consciousness. Coward is particularly interested in the implications of these views for the ways in which people think of themselves in both social and political terms. She regards CAM therapies both as a spearhead and as a symptom of wide-spread changes in attitudes and argues that individuals are attracted to the new mythology about nature and health which surrounds these practices. Coward concludes that while the new philosophy is critical of excesses of industrialization, modernity and impersonality, these criticisms rarely extend to a more complete challenge to the structures of a capitalist society. She describes CAM as essentially an individualistic approach in which each person assumes responsibility for their own health and well-being.

As the public interest in CAM has risen, the number and types of practition-ers have also increased. With this increase have come problems created by the diverse nature of the numerous alternative practitioners and therapies, which make it difficult for CAM to coalesce around a central organizing thrust. Despite these differences, many CAM practitioners are seeking professional recognition and legitimation. Mike Saks, in an edited book entitled *Alternative Medicine in Britain* (1992), was one of the first to write about the political and social context in which CAM practitioners are attempting to go from a mar-ginal to a central role in the British health care system. He identifies the obsta-cles in the path to full professional acceptance of CAM practitioners, and highlights the difficulties posed by the power and self protective interests of the medical profession. Saks argues that the success experienced by the medical profession in the mid-nineteenth century in attaining its dominant role in the health care division of labour has served to underwrite the current position of biomedicine as the basis of medical orthodoxy.

As the use of CAM has become more prevalent, the issue of 'efficacy' (that is, does it work?) has assumed critical importance. The disparate nature of CAM techniques creates serious problems for evaluation procedures. Furthermore, it has become clear that while conventional clinical trial methods are the 'gold standard' for evaluating efficacy, there are difficulties in assessing all CAM procedures using this one methodology. George Lewith and David Aldridge (1993) edited *Clinical Research Methodology for Complementary*

Therapies, a book which addressed this problem. They outline a range of possibilities for evaluating the efficacy of CAM including not only clinical trials but also longitudinal studies of health care practice, co-ordinated single case designs, and other social science research methods. They conclude that with health care demands accelerating, it is imperative to investigate new options which may serve to reduce costs and encourage prevention.

Bonnie Blair O'Connor (1995) in her book *Healing Traditions: Alternative Medicine and the Health Professions* focuses on 'vernacular' health belief systems in the United States. She looks at the ways in which people's experiences, beliefs, and values influence their choice of health care. Her book addresses the issues of how people define health and illness; how and why people believe they become sick; how they decide what to do about it; who they go to for which kinds of care; and the implications of these beliefs and decisions for health professionals in the 'conventional western' medical system. She cites as examples belief systems that have originated in a wide range of cultural contexts and geographical locations. She shows for example, that in the case of HIV/AIDS, conventional medical treatment is augmented by elaborate vernacular treatment strategies, particularly for middle and upper middle class white men. It is they who largely comprise the organized gay community, which in turn has served as a CAM information-sharing network. Finally, O'Connor points out that patients evaluate options for health care that go far beyond the conventional medical system. Today, in America, vernacular health belief systems are strongly influencing the kinds of health care resources that are being used and have significant implications for conventional medical education and health care delivery.

Ursula Sharma (1995) conducted research on users and practitioners of CAM in *Complementary Medicine Today: Practitioners and Patients*. She carried out her study in a community in the Midlands in England and identified a profile of typical CAM users. The people who were most likely to consult CAM practitioners were female, middle-aged and younger, well educated, well to do, with high occupational status. This profile corresponds to the findings of similar studies in Europe, Australia, United States, and Canada. Sharma analyzed how people decided to use CAM for the first time; their patterns of use; their complementary use of orthodox medicine; how they learned about CAM; and the motivations which led them to the offices of CAM practitioners. The second half of her book deals with the practice of CAM. She studied the practitioners, examined the national context, and analyzed the political arena in which CAM is being delivered.

In *Professions and the Public Interest: Medical Power, Altruism and Alternative Medicine* (1995), Saks uses the example of acupuncture in Britain to illustrate how CAM therapies were initially rejected by organized medicine which used its professional power to keep acupuncture in a marginal position. In the first half of the nineteenth century acupuncture had flourished and medicine had responded in a relatively positive manner to consumer demand for this popular lay practice. The state extended the monopoly rights of medicine so that the medical rejection of acupuncture was legally reinforced. At present, as more and more patients seek acupuncture therapy, the position of medicine has started to shift from outright rejection to limited incorporation. Medicine has responded by attempting to co-opt the practice of acupuncture, using it as a supplement to orthodox medical treatment and for a limited range of conditions.

In 1995, Carole Damiani published *La Medecine Douce: Une Analyse De Pratiques 'Holistes' En Sante* (Alternative Medicine: An Analysis of Holistic Health Practices). Her study describes and analyzes the emergence of alternative therapies in Canada in the province of Quebec by focusing on the practitioners. She traces their backgrounds including education and training, establishes a portrait of their practices and identifies the socio-cultural context in which they practice. She finds an eclectic group of practitioners who are orienting themselves toward professionalization and future integration into the larger health care system. She concludes that CAM practitioners and patients are found throughout Quebec society and patients are using CAM therapies for a wide range of health problems.

In their 1996 book, *Complementary and Alternative Medicines: Knowledge and Practice*, two anthropologists, Sara Cant and Ursula Sharma have compiled a series of articles which deal with the legitimation of CAM knowledge and practices. The book highlights the fact that the boundaries between orthodox and CAM medicines are far from fixed and that a growing number of doctors are actually offering CAM therapies in some form. The questions raised here focus on the public legitimation of certain forms of knowledge such as medical knowledge and the discreditation of others. The authors argue that expert knowledge has become a fundamental resource of social life and is closely associated with power. CAM therapists today are struggling to establish their credentials as 'experts' in order to gain legitimacy and authority. Cant and Sharma describe the current environment as one of 'intense contestation' between biomedicine and diverse healing modes, in which we can expect to see the emergence of strategic realignments.

Charles Vincent and Adrian Furnham in *Complementary Medicine: A Research Perspective* (1997) focus on the research that has been done on CAM. They examine the existing evidence for and against therapies such as acupuncture, spinal manipulation, herbalism, homeopathy, and naturopathy. They suggest research strategies which can evaluate specific types of CAM therapies and recommend research priorities including training in basic research methods for the CAM community. They underscore the need for a range of studies, from small scale analyses of practice procedures, to large scale surveys of the use of CAM, through to more tightly controlled clinical research.

The authors of *Alternative Health Care in Canada: Nineteenth-and Twentieth-century Perspectives*, view the current preoccupation with CAM as a social movement (Crellin *et al.*, 1997). They examine a selection of CAM practices both past and present with a view toward understanding their historical development. They also address aboriginal traditional medicine and what they refer to as 'ethnic' practices and examine the interface between these forms of care and CAM practices. The book emphasizes the challenges posed to CAM by orthodox medicine throughout history and in the current environment of shifting health care priorities. The book concludes that while CAM has gained a significant place in Canadian society, the future growth of CAM remains uncertain unless it establishes rigorous standards and regulations for its practices.

Most recently Michael Goldstein (1999) in *Alternative Health Care: Medicine, Miracle or Mirage?* makes the case that a fundamental change is taking place in society's orientation to health and healing. Alternative health care, he argues, represents a true paradigm shift. The author outlines six points that he believes represent the core of alternative medicine. These six points are: (1) a belief in holism, (2) an emphasis on the integration of body, mind and spirit, (3) a view of health as a positive state on a continuum with illness, (4) a belief that the body is suffused with the flow of energy, (5) a belief in vitalism, and (6) a distinctive view of the healing process. Goldstein acknowledges the difficulties in defining alternative medicine and prefers to regard it as an identity movement, driven by massive demand. All of this is occurring within a context of corporate dominance of health care in the United States. Large corporations are entering the health care market and influencing the nature and delivery of conventional medical care. At the same time, the rapid growth of alternative medicine has made it attractive to big corporations. In the future, Goldstein sees the forces of consumer demand, combined with the pressures from managed care, government and the media, combining to bring alternative health care into the mainstream.

These books have made important contributions to our understanding of the psycho-social context of CAM. There remain, however, significant unexplored issues and contentious unresolved areas in the knowledge that social scientists have yet been able to develop.

REFERENCES

Astin, John A. 1998. 'Why Patients Use Alternative Medicine: Results of a National Study.' *JAMA* 279:1548–53.

Aldridge, D. 1993. 'Single Case Research Designs.' in *Clinical Research Methodology for Complementary Therapies*, edited by G.T. Lewith and D. Aldridge. London: Hodder and Stoughton.

Berliner, Howard S., and J. Warren Salmon. 1979. 'The Holistic Movement and Scientific Medicine: The Naked and the Dead.' *Socialist Review* 43:31–52.

Black, N. 1996. 'Why We Need Observational Studies to Evaluate the Effectiveness of Health Care.' *British Medical Journal* 312:1215–1218.

Blais, Régis, Aboubacrine Maiga, and Alarou Aboubacar. 1997. 'How Different Are Users and Non-Users of Alternative Medicine?' *Canadian Journal of Public Health* 88:159–162.

Cant, Sarah, and Ursula Sharma (Eds.). 1996. *Complementary and Alternative Medicines: Knowledge in Practice*. London: Free Association Books.

Canter, D., and L. Nanke. 1993. 'Emerging Priorities in Complementary Medical Research.' in *Clinical Research Methodology for Complementary Therapies*, edited by D Aldridge and George T.Lewith, London: Hodder and Stoughton.

Coward, R. 1989. *The Whole Truth: The Myth of Alternative Health*. London: Faber and Faber.

Crellin, J.K., R.R. Andersen, and J.T.H. Connor (Eds.). 1997. *Alternative Health Care in Canada: Nineteenth and Twentieth Century Perspectives*. Toronto: Canadian Scholars Press.

Damiani, Carole. 1995. *La Medecine Douce: Une Analyse De Pratiques Holistes En Sante*. Montreal-Nord: Editions Saint-Martin.

Eisenberg, David M., Roger B. Davis, Susan L. Ettner, Scott Appel, Sonja Wilkey, Maria Van Rompay, and Ronald C. Kessler. 1998. 'Trends in Alternative Medicine Use in the United States, 1990–1997: Results of a Follow-up National Survey.' *The Journal of the American Medical Association* 280:1569–1575.

Eisenberg, David M., Ronald C. Kessler, Cindy Foster, Frances E. Norlock, David R. Calkins, and Thomas L. Delbanco. 1993. 'Unconventional Medicine in the United States: Prevalence, Costs and Patterns of Use.' *New England Journal of Medicine* 328:246–252.

Ernst, Edzard. 1996a. 'Complementary Medicine: From Quackery to Science?' *Journal of Laboratory Clinical Medicine* 127:244–245.

Ernst, Edzard (Ed.). 1996b. *Complementary Medicine: An Objective Appraisal*. Oxford: Butterworth Heinemann.

Ernst, Edzard, and Eckhart G. Hahn. 1998. *Homeopathy: A Critical Appraisal*. Oxford: Butterworth Heinemann.

Fisher, P., and A. Ward. 1994. 'Complementary Medicine in Europe.' *British Medical Journal* 309:107–111.

Fulder, Stephen. 1988. The Handbook of Complementary Medicine. 2nd ed. Oxford: Oxford University Press.

Fulder, Stephen. 1996. *The Handbook of Alternative and Complementary Medicine*, 3rd edition. Oxford: Oxford University Press.

Gevitz, Norman (Ed.). 1988. *Other Healers: Unorthodox Medicine in America*. Baltimore: Johns Hopkins.

Glik, Deborah. 1993. 'Methodological Pitfalls in the Design of Randomized Clinical Trials to Assess Alternative Medicine: The Case of Classical Homeopathy.' Paper presented at the *American Sociological Association*. Miami Beach, Florida.

Goldstein. Michael, S. 1999. *Alternative Health Care: Medicine, Miracle or Mirage?* Philadelphia: Temple University Press

Jonas, Wayne B., and Jennifer Jacobs. 1996. *Healing with Homeopathy: The Natural Way to Promote Recovery and Restore Health*. New York: Warner Books.

Kelner, Merrijoy, Oswald Hall, and Ian Coulter. 1980. *Chiropractors, Do They Help?* Toronto: Fitzhenry and Whiteside.

Kelner, Merrijoy, and Beverly Wellman. 1997a. 'Health Care and Consumer Choice: Medical and Alternative Therapies.' *Social Science and Medicine* 45:203–212.

Kelner, Merrijoy, and Beverly Wellman. 1997b. 'Who Seeks Alternative Health Care? A Profile of the Users of Five Modes of Treatment.' *Journal of Alternative and Complementary Medicine* 3:1–14.

Kuhn, T.S. 1970. *The Structure of Scientific Revolutions*. Chicago: University of Chicago Press.

Levin, J.S., T.A. Kushi Glass, J.R. Steele Schuck, and W.B. Jonas. 1997. 'Quantitative Methods in Research on Complementary and Alternative Care.' *Medical Care* 35:1079–1094.

Lewith, George T., and David Aldridge (Eds.). 1993. *Clinical Research Methodology for Complementary Therapies*. London: Hodder & Stoughton.

MacCoin, D. 1990. 'The Myth of Clinical Trials.' *Journal of Alternative and Complementary Medicine* 8(8):15–18.

MacLennan, A.H., D.H. Wilson, and A.W. Taylor. 1996. 'Prevalence and Cost of Alternative Medicine in Australia.' *Lancet* 347:569–573.

McGuire, Meredith. 1988. *Ritual Healing in Suburban America*. New Brunswick: Rutgers University Press.

Meade, T. Dyer, S. Browne, W., Townsend, J. and Frank, A. 1990. "Low Back Pain of Mechanical Origin: Randomised Comparison of Chiropractic & Hospital Outpatient Treatment", *British Medical Journal* 300: 1431–37.

Menger, Karl. 1928. *Dimensionstheorie*. Leipzig, Germany: B.G. Teubner.

Millar, W.J. 1997. 'Use of Alternative Health Care Practitioners by Canadians.' *Canadian Journal of Public Health* 88:154–158.

Millet, Stanley. 1999. 'Personal Commentary: Reflections on Traditional Medicine.' The Journal of Alternative and Complementary Medicine 5(2):203–05.

Mitchell, Annie, and Maggie Cormack. 1998. *The Therapeutic Relationship in Complementary Health Care*. London: Churchill Livingstone.

Moss, F. 1992. 'Quality in Health Care.' *Quality in Health Care* 1:1–3.

OAM (Office of Alternative Medicine, NIH) Committee on Definition and Description. 1997. 'Defining and Describing Complementary and Alternative Medicine.' *Alternative Therapies in Health and Medicine* 3(2):49–57.

O'Connor, Bonnie Blair. 1995. *Healing Traditions: Alternative Medicine and the Health Professions*. Philadelphia: University of Pennsylvania Press.

Paramore, L.C. 1997. 'Use of Alternative Therapies: Estimates from the 1994 Robert Wood Johnson Foundation National Access to Care Survey.' *Journal of Painful Symptom Management* 13:83–89.

Pescosolido, Bernice, and Jennie J. Kronenfeld. 1995. 'Health, Illness, and Healing in an Uncertain Era; Challenges from and for Medical Sociology.' *Journal of Health and Social Behaviour*: 5–33.

Pietroni, P. 1991. *The Greening of Medicine*. London: Victor Gollancz.

Popper, Karl Raimund. 1959. *The Logic of Scientific Discovery*. Toronto: University of Toronto Press.

Sackett, D. (Ed.). 1994. *The Cochrane Collaboration Handbook*, Oxford: The Cochrane Collaboration.

Saks, Mike (Ed.). 1992. *Alternative Medicine in Britain*. Oxford: Clarendon Press.

Saks, Mike. 1994. "The Alternative to Medicine". pp. 84–103 in *Challenging Medicine*, edited by Gabe, J. Kelleher, D. and Williams, G. Routledge.

Saks, Mike. 1995. *Professions and the Public Interest: Medical Power, Altruism and Alternative Medicine*. London: Routledge.

Salmon, J.W. (Ed.). 1984. *Alternative Medicines: Popular and Policy Perspectives*. New York: Tavistock.

Sharma, Ursula. 1995. *Complementary Medicine Today: Practitioners and Patients, 2nd edition*. London: Routledge.

Smith-Cunnien, Susan L. 1998. *A Profession of One's Own: Organized Medicine's Opposition to Chiropractic*. Maryland: University Press of America.

Thomas, Kate J., Jane Carr, Linda Westlake, and Brain T. Williams. 1991. 'Use of Non-orthodox and Conventional Health Care in Great Britain.' *British Medical Journal* 302:207–210.

Verhoef, Marja J. and Lloyd R. Sutherland. 1995. 'General Practitioners' Assessment of and Interest in Alternative Medicine in Canada.' *Social Science and Medicine* 41(4):511–515.

Vincent, Charles, and Adrian Furnham. 1997. *Complementary Medicine: A Research Perspective*. Chichester, England: John Wiley & Sons.

Wallis, Roy, and Peter Morley (Eds.). 1976. *Marginal Medicine*. London: Peter Owen.

Wellman, Barry. 1988. Chapters 1 and 2. In Social Structures: A Network Approach edited by Barry Wellman and Steve D. Berkowitz. Cambridge, UK: Cambridge University Press.

Section 1: Why CAM Now?

This is the question social scientists frequently ask about a social phenomenon. Why at this particular point in time does a trend become pervasive? In the case of CAM, there are many answers. The rise of the consumer movement and the accompanying distrust of experts has often been cited (Haug and Lavin, 1983; Goldstein, 1999; Kronenfeld and Schneller, 1997). The influence of the womens' health movement has also had an impact. Woman have expressed their dissatisfaction with aspects of conventional medical care which has lead to a search for alternative strategies (Boston Women's Health Collective 1984; Shorter, 1991). The holistic health movement along with a new and broader definition of health created a climate conducive to the use of CAM (Epp, 1986). The rise of the self-help movement in the 1970s was powerful in shifting. responsibility for health care from professionals to individuals and their support groups (Kelner, 1985). Today the Internet is empowering people by providing them with enormous amounts of information on health and illness, and also where to go for care (Clarke and Hoffman-Goetz, 1999). The chapters in this section reflect on the reasons for the popularity of CAM at the end of the 20th century.

Boston Women's Health Collective. 1984. *The New Our Bodies, Our Selves.*New York: Simon and Schuster.

Clarke, Juanne N., and Laurie Hoffman-Goetz. 1999. 'Information Technologies as a Source of Medical Information.' in *Trends Conference*. Ottawa.

Epp, Jake. 1986. *Achieving Health for All: A Framework for Health Promotion.* Ottawa: Ministry of National Health and Welfare.

Goldstein, Michael S. 1999. *Alternative Health Care: Medicine, Miracle, or Mirage?* Philadelphia: Temple University Press.

Haug, Marie R., and Bebe Lavin. 1983. *Consumerism in Medicine: Challenging Physician Authority.* Beverly Hills: Sage.

Kelner, Merrijoy. 1985. 'Community Support Networks: Current Issues.' *Canadian Journal of Public Health* 76:69–70.

Kronenfield, Jennie.J and Schneller. 1997. 'The Growth of a Buyer Beware and Consumer Practitioners Model in Health Care: The Impact of Managed Care on Changing Models of the Doctor-Patient Relationships.' presented at the Annual Meetings of the American Sociological Association, August, Toronto, Canada.

Shorter, Edward. 1991. *Women's Bodies: A Social History of Women's Encounter with Health, Ill Health, and Medicine.* New Brunswick: Transaction Publishers.

CHAPTER 1

The Culture of Fitness and the Growth of CAM

Michael S. Goldstein

Throughout North America and Western Europe the promotion of health and fitness is a widespread and growing phenomenon. In the United States almost one third of adults own stationary exercise cycles (Darnay, 1998:589). Almost two thirds of the smokers in the nations which comprise the European Community have tried to stop at least once (Commission on the State of Health, 1996:32). In Canada the rate of participation in physical activity among adults rose from 21% to 37% between 1981 and 1995 (Active Living Canada, 1999). Although many, if not most, advocates and participants in these efforts to promote health and fitness may not view their activities as part of complementary and alternative medicine (CAM), there is nonetheless, an increasing connection between fitness and CAM. Each shares a set of crucial underlying values and assumptions as well as a skepticism toward conventional medicine, and an affinity with the growing commodification of health.

This paper will set out six important values shared by both advocates of CAM and those who regularly participate in activities to remain fit. Next, the chapter examines the increasing level of skepticism toward, and commodification of conventional medicine. Each of these trends acts synergistically to reinforce the affinities between CAM and fitness. I conclude that the growing emphasis being placed on fitness throughout Western societies is likely to be a major entry point to the world of CAM.

SHARED VALUES

An emphasis on fitness and use of CAM are conceptually compatible, since they share six basic assumptions about the individual, health and healing:

1) Health as Wellness, Not the Absence of Symptoms
The notion that an individual's health is not synonymous with the mere absence of illness or symptoms is perhaps the most fundamental assumption

within the world views of those who advocate CAM as well as health and fitness. From this perspective, 'health' is about maximizing one's potential, and is applicable to everyone, regardless of their physical condition. The belief is that despite the limits on a person, arising from genetics, symptoms, or ways of thinking, it is always possible to be healthier. A quality of striving, typified by the phrase 'achieving high level wellness', permeates both attempts to become more fit, and CAM approaches to chronic illness (Dunn, 1973; Goldstein, 1992; Chopra, 1989:236–7; Johnston, 1991).

Efforts to reach wellness are unique to each individual, and are derived from one's particular goals, needs, and status in life. Thus, in efforts to keep fit, as in the use of CAM, the meaning of health is different for everyone. Achieving health or wellness does not mean reaching an arbitrary, preset goal, Rather, it is an ongoing process, which demands active participation and effort. An overriding concern with striving to transcend whatever one's current situation (losing a few more pounds, refraining from smoking for another day, keeping one's tumor, asthma, or genital herpes in check, etc.) is a key point of convergence for CAM and for efforts to be fit.

2) Personal Responsibility for Health

Although the idea of being responsible for one's health is not a new one in western, and particularly, American society, it has received new vigor and prominence (if not omnipresence) within the worlds of both fitness and CAM (Reiser, 1985). It is a theme drawn upon by every major exponent or spokesperson in the world of fitness, and a key component of most approaches within CAM. This emphasis on personal responsibility comes in many different versions. Moderate or mainstream approaches, such as the classic statements by John Knowles, past President of the Rockefeller Foundation, simply emphasize that '99% of us are born healthy' and that it is our own 'misbehavior' that renders us unfit or ill later in life (Knowles, 1977). More radical or far reaching versions go beyond the behavioural level, and stress the mental states, under one's own control, that are seen as essential to maintaining health, and even curing illness (Pelletier, 1979; Ferguson, 1987; Chopra, 1993). These mental states are said to operate in two ways: indirectly, by fostering the behavioral changes needed to get and stay healthy, and directly, by exerting an independent physiological impact throughout the body. While only a few of the better known exponents of CAM, such as Hay (1987) and Jampolsky (1989) go so far as to suggest that the individual is responsible for absolutely everything that happens to him or her, others like Deepak Chopra are not far behind.

For our purposes, the importance of this common emphasis on personal responsibility is that those who have been involved with fitness and health promotion are likely to be quite familiar with notions of personal responsibility that are strikingly similar to those within the world of CAM. Individuals who have succeeded in their efforts to become more fit are apt to be strongly committed to these beliefs. The fact that numerous research reports by mainstream scientists (especially in the field of psychoneuroimunology) have validated the view that the mind can produce chemical changes at the cellular level throughout the body, has given a strong boost to the importance of these beliefs for both CAM and health promotion.

3) The Interpenetration of Mind, Body and Spirit

A third major tenet common to both the worlds of CAM and fitness is the inextricable connection between these three dimensions of life; each of which can have a causal impact upon the others. Again, we find something that is not in any way a new belief, but rather a traditional belief given new vigour, as well as a broadened emphasis, by its importance in both CAM and fitness. What is of particular interest here is not only the idea that the mind and body have a potentially strong influence over each other. Rather, it is the inclusion of 'spirit' as a co-equal partner in the equation (Levin, 1996; Dossey, 1993). Most major approaches in CAM, such as Traditional Chinese Medicine (T.C.M.) and Ayurveda have religious origins, as well as an important spiritual dimension (Beinfeld and Korngold, 1991; Frawley, 1990). Many others, such as chiropractic, naturopathy, and homeopathy have strong religious roots which have become relatively neglected at the present time (Fuller, 1989; Kaptchuk, 1997). For these, and for many of the newer modes of CAM, the ill defined, non-denominational term 'spirituality' has replaced religion. Still, for most of the CAM healing practices there is a crucial dimension of life that goes beyond both the body and the mind.

The spiritual component of a heightened concern with health and fitness may not be immediately apparent. Yet, history demonstrates that an emphasis on physical fitness has often been an important part of religious movements and revivals in both the U.S. and Europe (Whorton, 1982; Dubos, 1959). Today, numerous advocates of fitness have stressed its spiritual aspects. Spiritual or 'peak' experiences are often cited as the outcome of intense physical exertion (running in a marathon, completing an AIDS Ride, climbing a mountain, etc), as well as the motivation for continuing efforts to become even more fit. Again, we find an important overlap in the basic beliefs of CAM and those promoting an interest in health and fitness.

4) Health as Harmony with Nature

In *Mirage of Health*, Rene Dubos (1959) described two competing Greek deities and their approaches to achieving health. Hygeia symbolized health through discovering and following the laws of nature, while Aescalapius represented health through the triumph of human intervention aimed at limiting the ravages of existing illnesses. While the image and ideology of Aescalapius have dominated conventional medicine in this century, it is Hygeia whose approach is the key to most approaches in CAM, as well as to the worlds of fitness and health promotion. Prevention of future illness and disability is the ultimate goal of both. In this quest each emphasizes the need, not to control 'nature', but to align ourselves more with 'nature's laws'.

The roots of this view are similar both for CAM and health promotion. The early advocates of fitness in America, (Jefferson, Thoreau, Benjamin Rush, Thomas Paine, etc.) and the masters of TCM, Ayurveda, and many other modes of CAM did not distinguish between what nature taught about something purely physical, such as what to eat, and something social or political, such as how to behave with one's friends or family. It is all a seamless web of choices which flow from knowledge of nature's (god's) laws (Rosen, 1974). To see this seamless web in today's CAM practices, simply examine the catalog of choices at one of the thriving centers of CAM training, such as the Omega Institute, north of New York City, or any other place where advocates of CAM gather. The courses, symposia, and workshops typically aim to bring health, healing, work life, family life, and fitness all into closer harmony with nature. Or, conversely, read any of the popular books on running, aerobics, or dieting, and see how the author grounds both the motivation for engaging in the activity, as well as the successful outcome, in terms of coming closer to living 'naturally'.

A central image offered in both CAM and the fitness movement is the (re)creation of 'naturalness' in ourselves and the larger world. Eating natural foods, allowing natural healing processes to take place, accepting our natural emotions, and keeping our bodies in their natural state by avoiding drugs, alcohol and tobacco, are all part of this worldview.

5)   Ambivalence Toward Science and Technology

For many fitness advocates the notion that people can maintain their unhealthy lifestyles, and then be 'saved' by some technological breakthrough is problematic (Dubos, 1959; Illich, 1976; Gusfield, 1981). Similarly, exponents of CAM typically feel that a reliance on high tech medicine runs counter to the lessons that their particular school of therapy has to offer. Both groups agree that relying on a 'technological fix', such as artificial sweeteners to replace sugar, will not only fail (the sweeteners themselves may cause ill health or disease), but that they epitomize a mind set opposed to all the other values central to the group. For example, an emphasis on scientific medicine frequently leads to a reliance on physicians, which runs counter to the idea of taking responsibility for one's health. The 'wisdom of the body', as opposed to the expertise of professionals is likely to be the guiding force of both CAM and the advocates of health promotion.

6) Transcendence, Restraint, and Vigilance

A final area where the underlying values of both CAM and advocates of fitness come together is their joint focus on the need for people to direct their energies toward transcending their current state of health and reaching for something higher; something beyond where they are now. This is not an easy thing to do. But, with sufficient commitment, effort, attention, and restraint from things that are unhealthy, it can be done. There are people in wheelchairs who race in marathons, and there are people with every known 'terminal' illness who far outlive the normal curve. It usually turns out that most of the things that must be done to transcend to a higher level of health or wellness involve rejecting things that the dominant consumer culture presents as good: an excess of materialism, hedonism, and impulsiveness. CAM practitioners often present moderation and balance as the ultimate health producing values. The goal of treatment is often simply to allow natural, 'vitalistic' forces to reign, both within the body and between people (Gordon, 1980; Jahnke, 1990). Thus, both serious efforts to remain fit, as well as much of the participation in CAM practices require a major, ongoing change in lifestyle.

At the conceptual level, it is clear that someone who has been involved in sustained efforts to become or remain fit will be familiar with many of the underlying premises of CAM. They will not seem remote or 'foreign'. Rather, they will appear to be a natural progression or outgrowth of those same values and attitudes which already inform the individual's sense of who they are, how their body works, and how the two interact.

SKEPTICISM TOWARD CONVENTIONAL MEDICINE

Continuing participation in health promotion and fitness activities is likely to result in skepticism and distancing toward conventional medicine. This is the case even if such activities were initially prompted by conventional physicians. There is an ironic aspect to this, as much of the research validating the importance of fitness has emerged from the mainstream medical research establishment. Physicians are increasingly likely to accept the findings from this research, and the overall biopsychosocial definition of health, with its very positive attitude toward fitness (Engel, 1997). Still, the day to day premises and practices of mainstream medicine are often not conducive to motivating people to actually make the effort to be more fit, nor to supporting those who do try. The ideology of biomedicine, and the dominant professional ethos of physicians, remains one of curing, not preventing (Calnan, Boulton, and Williams, 1986).

The decision to actively engage oneself in becoming fit is, from the point of view of the person, primarily a mind-body issue. Generating motivation, and sustaining it through all the tribulations involved (pain, boredom, denial of pleasure, etc.) are all matters of psychology. Yet, conventional medicine has been dominated by a Cartesian dualism that precludes it from seeing the human being as an organic whole. Many, if not most, mainstream practitioners have little in their training and experience to help those patients who wish to become more fit with the mental difficulties they face. If the patient wants or needs anything beyond verbal support for their efforts, they often find they must get it somewhere else. On the other hand, most CAM approaches and practitioners are highly responsive to these needs.

Today, mainstream medicine offers a rhetorical stance which recognizes and promotes the value of fitness more than at any time in the past. Yet, these changes are dwarfed by another set of changes taking place in western medicine. The health care systems in North America and much of Europe are in a state of rapid transformation; some would say crisis or even revolution. The immense absolute and relative costs of health care services, and the inability to demonstrate that the expenditures yield a commensurate gain in health status (Evans and Stoddard, 1990; Wolfe, 1986), along with a set of broader political changes, have led to the rise of 'managed care' and corporate medicine. In the U.S., government funding has been cut back, providers have consolidated, often under the ownership of huge profit-driven corporations, and employers have become much more aggressive in controlling the cost of health insurance (Drake, 1997). All this has created an environment in which health care has become more like other commodities. As medicine is rationalized by those paying the bills (insurers and employers), medical decision-making and clinical practices are more apt to be assessed just like any other business decision. Restrictions are being increasingly placed on the availability of doctors, the time spent per visit, referrals, and the opportunity to use the fullest range of drugs and ancillary services.

All these developments are reflected by a growing disenchantment with conventional medicine (Kilborn, 1997). There is a sense that doctors don't know as much (especially about chronic illness) as they 'should', and that the way care is organized limits the availability and utility of what they do know. The amount of coverage the mass media give health care topics has mushroomed. The effect of much of this attention is to make people more aware of medicine's ambiguities, if not failures. The 'magic bullets' and other medical wonders that are sometimes described in the press often feel remote from peoples' everyday experiences of medicine.

The feminist health movement is one of many social movements that have emphasized a combination of skepticism toward conventional medicine, combined with themes that are similar to the shared values of fitness and CAM. The preface to the popular and influential book, *The New Our Bodies, Ourselves* (Boston Women's Health Collective, 1984) begins by stressing the theme of personal responsibility for one's health. Most of the book, which by now has sold many millions of copies, presents the necessity of synthesizing mind, body, and spirit (termed 'feminism') when dealing with any of the full range of health problems and issues that affect women. The authors are clear that the development of a feminist identity and collective action is dependent upon the utilization of the same core values of holism and the integration of body, mind, and spirit which permeate CAM. Skepticism about the medical profession and, especially high technology diagnosis and treatment is omnipresent, along with a strong emphasis on dietary change and exercise as a means of remaining healthy and resisting illness.

A similar critical distancing and distrustful or skeptical consumerism toward conventional medicine is frequently found among fitness advocates (Emanuel and Emanuel, 1992). They are likely to know that conventional medicine has little concern for prevention, and little to offer those who want to know the practical 'nuts and bolts' of how to do it. These individuals, both those who have succeeded in their fitness goals and those who have repeatedly failed but who still want to succeed, are quite likely to be open to the sort of model or paradigm offered by CAM. While society's and medicine's de-emphasis or disregard for health, prevention, and fitness may once have been seen as simply inevitable, if unfortunate, it is now seen as a wrong to be righted; a grievance.

THE COMMODIFICATION OF HEALTH

A third major factor in bringing active participants in health promotion and fitness into the world of CAM is the fact that the mass media and other powerful economic interests increasingly present them in a commodified context where health promotion, fitness and alternative medicine appear as an integrated, synergistic entity.

Conventional medicine, CAM, and fitness have all increasingly become part of the economic mainstream in western industrialized nations, especially the United States (McKinlay and Stoekle, 1989). Traditionally, conventional and alternative medicine were both similar in that they operated as small businesses; individual practitioners received compensation for services they rendered to individual clients. Of course, mainstream providers made much more money in absolute terms, and were more likely to deal with intermediaries such as insurance companies. Still, the basic economics of practice were similar. In this system physical fitness advocates were almost nonexistent as economic actors (Gevitz, 1988; Young, 1961; Goldstein, 1999).

Today the situation has changed greatly, and remains in constant flux. Although the traditional entrepreneurial form of CAM practice is widespread and remains dominant, new patterns have emerged. There is growing consolidation of distributors such as health food stores (in the U.S. two rapidly growing chains now dominate the market), as well as suppliers (two producers of homeopathic remedies have driven scores of smaller local firms out of business). CAM is fast becoming part of big business. In the U.S., sales of medicinal herbs were almost 4 billion dollars in 1999, up from less than 1 billion in 1991, and are estimated to be growing at a rate of 18% per year (Brody, 1999). Between 1989 and 1994 the sales of organically grown fruits and vegetables almost doubled to nearly 8 billion dollars. Homeopathic remedies (over 100 million dollars per year) are now sold by most of the major chain pharmacies.

Some practitioners (Chopra, Weil, etc.) have become able to generate immense amounts of money through their publications, and have expanded into product lines, periodicals, videos, seminars, and other areas. The significance of all this goes far beyond the huge incomes these practitioners earn. Rather it lies in the fact that mainstream corporations have become aware of CAM's potential to generate revenue as mass marketed products and pathways to other products they sell. Media conglomerates like Time-Warner, Disney/CBS, the New York Times Company, and many others have been quick to see this potential, and they are reshaping the face of CAM in America.

The pattern with regard to health and fitness has been much the same. Like most things in an advanced capitalist society, health and fitness have come to be commodified. Their potential to generate profit has been another important factor in their recent promotion. Health foods, health clubs, exercise clothing and shoes, newsletters and magazines, websites, personal trainers and sporting goods are just some of the highly profitable businesses that have blossomed under the fitness banner. The mass media are a particularly important industry that has become enamored of health and fitness. Many large newspapers now have daily columns or weekly sections devoted to the topic, as well as extensive news and feature coverage. Information about how to become and stay fit is sold in the form of books, videotapes, and many other media. The publishing industry is so successful in selling books on health that they (along with others on self help and related topics) are now tallied on separate best seller lists so as not to completely overwhelm the traditional fiction and nonfiction categories.

Selling information about keeping healthy and fit has become a mainstay of the information industry. The corporate purveyors of all this information do not, for the most part, distinguish between fitness and CAM. The substance of what is offered in the books sold in the new megastores, or found on the search engines of the Internet, or in the health section of the daily newspaper is all a market driven mix of conventional and alternative approaches. Those seeking information and advice about fitness will almost inevitably be exposed to favorable information about CAM. When someone who seeks to remain fit purchases vitamin supplements at a large chain supermarket and sees homeopathic and herbal remedies stocked right alongside, the effect is to legitimize the latter while blurring the distinction between them. They are all just products.

The emphasis on economic efficiency and profit making which now dominates mainstream American medicine has proven quite amenable to many modalities within CAM (Landmark Healthcare, 1996). This is due to the fact that many types of CAM are relatively low cost, as well as because health care corporations often see the inclusion of CAM in the packages they provide as an effective marketing tool to gain members who are middle class and interested in taking care of themselves. In this environment it is hard to assess whether CAM is being integrated into the medical mainstream or co-opted by it (Carlson, 1979). Still, one clear outcome of these developments is that growing numbers of individuals who are oriented to being fit gain exposure to CAM. Chiropractic, naturopathy, yoga, massage therapy, and nutritional counseling have all achieved a degree of acceptance in the world of managed care that they never had in traditional fee-for-service American medicine.

The commodification of health and illness, be it through the rise of managed care, or the inclusion of CAM in the agenda of large corporations and media conglomerates, combined with the immense number of people concerned with being healthier, has resulted in an environment where CAM and information about fitness are frequently presented as part of an integrated whole.

THE GROWING CONSENSUS OVER FITNESS

It is clear that an emphasis on physical fitness and health promotion is highly congruent with exposure to, openness toward, and involvement with CAM. Changes occurring in the contexts in which many health care systems are currently operating make it is equally apparent that this compatibility will increase in the coming years.

Throughout the industrialized world, health care systems are becoming more concerned with promoting health and fitness. In large part this is due to the growing acceptance by physicians and health policy makers that the prevention and amelioration of chronic problems can partly be achieved through the adoption of healthier behaviors earlier in life. Changes in the way health care services are organized and financed have also led to the belief by some (largely unsubstantiated) that an emphasis on fitness will lead to a reduction in overall health care expenditures, as well as prove to be a marketing advantage for those who offer them (Turner, 1995; Ornish, 1995:88).

Perhaps the most important reason for the growing popularity and concern with fitness and health promotion is the growing recognition that a healthy lifestyle is, in fact, associated with lessened mortality and morbidity from scores of chronic illnesses, reduced symptoms, higher levels of functioning, and better mental health. Although some social science accounts may dismiss or minimize such claims, the evidence in their support is strong. Not smoking, a reduced intake of fats, regular vigorous exercise, a reduction in perceived stress, and moderation (if not elimination) of alcohol are all correctly under-stood as highly rational goals by many people in society (Department of Health and Human Services, 1991).

While it is clear that there is more societal concern devoted to health and fitness, the outcome of this heightened attention on peoples' health status is not as certain. In the United States the picture is decidedly mixed. Rates of cigarette smoking have generally declined, although there is geographic varia-tion, and recent indications are that smoking among young people may be rising. Obesity and overweight have increased, especially among young people, while the proportion of the population who engage in a sedentary lifestyle has remained constant over the past decade (Office of Technology Assessment, 1993:80) This pattern is also observed throughout western Europe (Commission on the State of Health, 1996). In eastern Europe the picture is considerably worse. These figures may mask some important differences between ethnic and income groups. It is fair to say that knowledge about, and attitudes toward health and fitness have been heightened on a society-wide basis, but corresponding behaviour changes have been largely restricted to those in the upper-middle classes and those who believe themselves to be at particularly high risk for a given condition.

Despite these caveats, it is reasonable to assert that concern with health and fitness is a significant element in contemporary American culture. To the extent that American culture is coming to permeate much of the world, it is likely that these values and attitudes toward physical fitness will assume a greater importance throughout the rest of North America and Europe as well.

CONCLUSION

Due to a variety of economic and social factors, discontent, distancing, and skepticism toward conventional medicine, the use of CAM is likely to grow. Managed care and evidence based medicine are likely to become even more decisive in how people receive their care, leading to patients spending even less time with physicians to talk about matters like keeping fit, and receiving less attention to 'mind-body' issues. At the same time, the aging of the population has brought higher rates of chronic illness, along with an increasing level of knowledge about the risk factors which predispose individuals to such conditions. More people will feel the need to become fitter, even as they suffer from chronic illness or disabilities. More will be known about what it means to be fit (specific dietary changes, exercise regimens, ways of relieving stress, etc.). But conventional medicine will be no more, and perhaps even less, able to assist people in becoming fit. CAM, on the other hand, will be able to help them with their fitness goals. Thus, it is likely that the future will be marked by an increasing synergy between fitness and alternative medicine. Participation in efforts to be fit, and to reduce the risk of chronic illness will continue to be a key entry point into the world of CAM.

REFERENCES

Active Living Canada. 1999. *Toward an Active, Healthy Canada*. URL http://activeliving.ca/activeliving/alctoward_summary.html (visited 2/8/99).

Beinfeld, Harriet, and Efram Korngold. 1991. *Between Heaven and Earth: A Guide to Chinese Medicine*. New York: Ballentine Books.

Boston Women's Health Collective. 1984. *The New Our Bodies, Ourselves*. New York: Simon and Schuster.

Brody, Jane. 1999. Americans Gamble on Herbs as Medicine. *New York Times*. 9 February: D1,7.

Calnan, Michael, Boulton, M., and Williams, A. 1986. Health Education and General Practitioners: A Critical Appraisal. pp. 183–203 in *The Politics of Health Education: Raising the Issues*, edited by S. Rodnell and A. Watt. London: Routledge and Kegan Paul.

Carlson, Rick. 1979. "Holism and Reductionism as Perspectives in Medicine and Patient Care." *Western Journal of Medicine*. 131: 466–470.

Chopra, Deepak. 1989. *Quantum Healing: Exploring the Frontiers of Mind-Body Medicine*. New York: Bantam Books.

_____. 1993. *Ageless Body, Timeless Mind: the Quantum Alternative to Growing Old*. New York: Harmony Books.

Commission on the State of Health in the European Community. 1996. *Report From the Commission*. Brussels, Luxembourg.

Darnay, Arsen, J. (ed.) 1998. *Statistical Record of Health and Medicine*. Detroit: Gale Publishing Co.

Department of Health and Human Services. 1991. *Healthy People: National Health Promotion and Disease Prevention Objectives*. Washington, D.C. U.S. Government Printing Office. Publ. No. 91–50212.

Dossey, Larry. 1993. *Healing Words: The Power of Prayer and the Practice of Medicine*. San Francisco: Harper Collins.

Drake, David, F. 1997. Managed Care: A Product of Market Dynamics. *Journal of the American Medical Association*. 277:560–563.

Dunn, Halbert, L. 1973. *High Level Wellness*. Arlington, VA.: R. W. Beatty Co.

Dubos, Rene. 1959. *The Mirage of Health*. London: Allen and Unwin.

Emanuel, E. and Emanuel, L. 1992. Four Models of the Patient-Practitioner Relationship. *Journal of the American Medical Association*. 267:2221–2226.

Engel, George, L. 1997. The Need for a New Medical Model: A Challenge for Biomedicine. *Science*. 196(4286):129–136.

Evans, Robert, W. and Stoddard, Gregory, L. 1990. Producing Health, Consuming Health Care. *Social Science and Medicine*. 31:1347–1363.

Ferguson, Marilyn. 1987. *The Aquarian Conspiracy*. Los Angeles: J.P. Tarcher.

Frawley, David. 1990. *Ayurvedic Healing*. Salt Lake City: Morson Publ.

Gevitz, Norman. 1988. *Other Healers: Unorthodox Healers in America*. Baltimore: The Johns Hopkins University Press.

Goldstein, Michael, S. 1992. *The Health Movement: Promoting Fitness in America*. New York: Twayne/Macmillan.

_____. 1999. *Alternative Health Care: Medicine, Miracle, or Mirage?* Philadelphia: Temple University Press.

Gordon, James, S. 1980. The Paradigm of Holistic Medicine, pgs. 3–38 in *Health for the Whole Person,* edited by Arthur C. Hastings, James Fadiman, and James S. Gordon. Boulder, CO: Westview Press.

Gusfield, Joseph. 1981. *The Culture of Public Problems: Drinking-Driving and the Symbolic Order.* Chicago: University of Chicago Press.

Hay, Louise. 1987. *You Can Heal Your Life.* Santa Monica, CA.: Hay House.

Illich, Ivan. 1976. *Medical Nemesis.* New York: Random House.

Jahnke, Roger. 1990. *The Most Profound Medicine.* Santa Barbara, CA: Health Action Books.

Jampolsky, Gerald, G. 1989. Pg. 156 in *Healers on Healing,* edited by Rick Carlson and B. Shield. Los Angeles: Tascher/Putnum.

Johnston, Linda. 1991. *Everyday Miracles: Homeopathy in Action.* Van Nuys, CA: Christine Kent.

Kilborn, Peter. 1997. Dissatisfaction is Growing with Managed Care Plans: quality of services is doubted, survey says. *The New York Times.* September 28:12.

Knowles, John. 1977. *Doing Better and Feeling Worse: Health in the United States.* New York: Norton.

Landmark Healthcare. 1996. The Landmark Report on Public Perceptions of Alternative Care. Report. Sacramento, CA.

Levin, Jeffrey, S. 1996. How Prayer Heals: A Theoretical Model. *Alternative Therapies.* 2(1):66–73.

McKinlay, John, and Stoeckle, John. 1989. Corporatization and the Social Transformation of Doctoring. *International Journal of Health Services.* 18:191–205.

Office of Technology Assessment. 1993. *International Health Statistics: What They Mean for the United States.* Washington, D.C. U.S. Government Printing Office. Publ. No. OTA-BP-H-116.

Ornish, Dean. 1995. Healing the Heart, Reversing the Disease. *Alternative Therapies.* 1(5):84–92.

Pelletier, Kenneth. 1979. *Holistic Medicine: From Stress to Optimum Health.* New York: Delacorte Press.

Reiser, Stanley. 1985. Responsibility for Personal Health: A Historical Perspective. *Journal of Medicine and Philosophy.* 10:7–17.

Rosen, George. 1974. *From Medical Police to Social Medicine: Essays on the History of Health Care.* New York: Science History Publications.

Turner, S. 1995. Taking Health to Heart. *Hospitals and Health Networks.* 69:79–80.

Weil, A. 1995. *Spontaneous Healing.* New York: Fawcett Columbine.

Whorton, James, C. 1982. *Crusaders for Fitness: The History of American Health Reformers.* Princeton, NJ: Princeton University Press.

Wolfe, B.L. 1986. "Health Status and Medical Expenditure: Is There a Link?" *Social Science and Medicine.* 22: 993–999.

Young, James, H. 1961. *The Toadstool Millionaires: A Social History of Patent Medicine in America Before Regulation.* Princeton, NJ: Princeton University Press.

Conceptions of the Body in Complementary and Alternative Medicine

BONNIE B. O'CONNOR

INTRODUCTION

The broad domain of health belief and practice now referred to as complementary and alternative medicine (CAM) represents an extraordinarily diverse collection of theories, actions, individual modalities, and complex systems directed at promoting or restoring health and maintaining wellness. In the Anglo-European context, the CAM domain (OAM Committee, 1997) is typically characterized – by scholars and participants alike – in terms of its distinctions from, and sometimes incongruities with, conventional Western biomedicine and the conventional medical model of normal human functioning, pathologic processes, and preventive and therapeutic approaches to disease. The basis of this differentiation is a core set of fundamental concepts about the nature of persons and of health, together with the practices that logically derive from them. These core concepts are shared in broad form among CAM constituents, but are absent from the conventional medical worldview.

Among the distinctions that set CAM approaches to health care apart from the domain of biomedicine are a range of conceptions of the body that differ significantly from the anatomical and physiologic constructions of the conventional medical model. Non-biomedical conceptions of the body have been a central feature of CAM systems throughout their histories, whatever their places and periods of origin.[1] This is an important feature of CAM systems, for at least two reasons. Firstly, conceptions of the body are inextricably interconnected with definitions of health and illness, with constructions of disease etiology, and with corollary notions of appropriate care. Secondly, the conceptualizations of the body found in CAM systems resonate strongly, both philosophically and experientially, for large numbers of people and this helps to account for the current and rising public popularity of CAM.

A close look at understandings of the body found in three historic-ally, culturally, and conceptually disparate examples of CAM systems will lay the groundwork for the discussion that follows. Each illustrates both system-specific conceptions of the body and measures for maintaining its health, as well as general principles found in common across several CAM systems.

THE BODY AND HEALTH: THREE EXAMPLES

Popular Health Reform in Victorian America

The decades of the 1830s through the 1850s were a time of great philosophical ferment in the United States, a period in which the nature and perfectability of humanity – both individual persons, and through them in sufficient numbers, human society – were topics of much sectarian discussion and theorizing. The human body and human nature were focal points of intense scrutiny, and were conceptualized as the instruments of both potential perfection and potential destruction. In a moralist Christian ideological framework of Protestant perfectionism, the health reform movement of this period framed the human body as the strong and perfect product of divine design (Morantz, 1977; Whorton, 1988; Fuller, 1989). Human nature, by contrast, was seen as imper-fect, dangerous, and readily subject to depravity. Good health was the natural and God-given condition of humankind. The path to its maintenance and pro-motion lay in the willful control of instincts and desires (aspects of imperfect human nature) that, when indulged, led through inevitable excess to physical, mental, and moral ruin.

A prominent figure in this movement was William A. Alcott, who coined the term and formulated the discipline of 'physical education.' Alcott held that each individual had a moral duty to 'understand the structure and function of the body he [had] been given and to adopt the diet, activities, dress, and other habits that [would] keep that body working at its maximum disease-thwarting, God-glorifying efficiency' (Whorton, 1988:60). Alcott considered it essential to well-being that people curb their appetites and their 'non-rational' (or instinctual) impulses. Such discipline constituted both a fundamental principle of moral behaviour and a critical step in the maintenance of health and avoidance of disease. Temperance and moderation were thus alloyed as both morally and physiologically desirable goals. Perhaps better known to the general American public in current times is Sylvester Graham, who together with Alcott, helped to build a popular hygiene movement of national scope and appeal, whose legacy is still apparent to this day.

The popular hygiene movement incorporated certain conventional medical health promotion recommendations of the day – avoidance of excesses in food, drink, and tobacco use, plus regular exposure to the salutary effects of fresh air and moderate physical exercise. These reformers had a distinctive physiological interpretive framework that set them apart from the medical establishment, however, and they carried the medical message of moderation to the point of severity and extreme abstinence. Important to the philosophical foundation of the popular hygiene movement was the theory of pathology expounded by François Broussais, a renowned French physician of the 1820s. Broussais contended that 'all disease results from excessive stimulation of some body tissue (especially the digestive tract), that repeated stimulation leads to irritation and inflammation, and that the local inflammation can be transmitted through the nervous system to any other part of the body,' causing systemic weakness and breakdown (Whorton, 1988:61). Interpreting Broussais, Graham conceived of the stomach as the physiological source for delivery of 'vital power,' necessary for health and healing, to the rest of the body. Pure and proper foods, he believed, kept the stomach supplied with nutrients essential for this work. It was equally important that the stomach not be overstimulated, for that would lead to inflammation and disturb its core vital function (Fuller, 1989).

Broussais' theory referred specifically to physical stimulants and irritants. The health reform movement ideology of the mid-nineteenth century, however, extended the concept of 'stimulation' to include activities and ideation that could arouse animalistic cravings or diminish civilized inhibitions; either effect could lead to injurious indulgences. The movement promoted vegetarianism as crucial to healthful eating habits. Meat was considered a stimulant both to the appetites (including, of course, sexual appetite) and to the organs of the digestive system; it was thus a dual danger, threatening both physical and moral well-being. Scriptural support for this position was drawn from both New Testament injunctions against the cruelty and barbarity of slaughterhouses, and from the book of Genesis which mentioned only fruits and vegetables as the foods of Adam and Eve (Fuller, 1989). The implication of the Old Testament citation in particular associated meat eating with the fall of humanity from divine grace, with imperfection, and with an unruly and sinful human will.

Sexual activity, considered very physically stimulating, was to be tightly curbed, engaged in only occasionally and then for procreative purposes only. Graham contended that 'the Bible doctrine of marriage and sexual continence and purity, is founded on the physiological principles established in the constitutional nature of man' (Graham, 1857: v). Thus, the early health reform movement cemented mind, soul, and body. Morality and physiology were not merely interconnected, but were mutually constitutive: moral living produced physical and mental health; immorality led to disease and insanity; and physiological damage incurred through dangerous stimulations led to mental and moral breakdown. The functional connection between mind and body was clear: it was the duty of the mind, through the exercise of cognition and will-power, to curb the potential excesses of impulse and appetite – which were portrayed as arising in the body in some instinctual or animalistic way (though amplifiable in a vicious cycle by indulgence, an act of weak will).

Following on the heels of these reformers in the next generation was John Harvey Kellogg, who came to health reform through Seventh Day Adventism. In the mid-1870s, Kellogg, an MD, became the chief physician at the Battle Creek Sanitarium, which had been founded in Battle Creek, Michigan a decade before as a place for Adventists to seek health through treatment with natural therapies and instruction in 'the right mode of living' (Numbers, 1976:105). Like the health reformers and popular hygienists who preceded him, Kellogg considered general fitness a requisite to physical and moral health and promoted regular exercise and even strenuous athletic activity as builders and supporters of health. The centerpiece of his attention was diet, however, and Kellogg became a primary progenitor of the early health food movement. His conception of physiology and its relation to disease etiology centered on a theory of auto-intoxication, produced by the release of 'ptomaines' in the intestinal tract by the putrefaction of proteins in the diet. Avoidance of animal protein and reduction of transit time of digestive products through the intestines – promoted through the addition of substantial quantities of fiber to the diet – were Kellogg's keys to health. Like Alcott and Graham before him, he associated physiology with morality, asserting that meat eating and the constipation which was its inevitable result were the cause of the majority of chronic illnesses, as well as of moral and social ills (Kellogg, 1919). Kellogg's philosophy led him to the creation of special health foods produced from unrefined grains (now ironically grown into the sugar- and additive-laden breakfast cereal industry), and 'laid the groundwork for the modern American obsession with bowel regularity' (Whorton, 1988:72).

Echoes of Progressivism and of Victorian era popular health reform resonate in many present day dietary systems of health maintenance and pro-motion, as well as in the consumerist physical fitness movement with its emphasis on the perfectability of the physical form, its equation of high degrees of physical tone and endurance with robust health and clean living, and its 'no pain, no gain' philosophy. Specific religious associations are nowa-days mostly gone from the physical fitness, health foods, and natural healing conceptual systems, replaced by a more secular metaphysics or non-sectarian spirituality (Goldstein, 1999). The secularized frameworks nevertheless keep the moral tone of these and other CAM systems strong, emphasizing as most do the inherent goodness of nature and natural approaches to health; the self-healing and self-regulating nature of the (unpolluted) body; and individual responsibility, through efforts of will, for maintaining health. Many CAM systems continue to conceptualize the body as susceptible to pollution through a buildup of toxins in the intestinal tract, and focus significant preventive and therapeutic attention on bowel health and colon cleansing.[2]

Traditional Chinese Medicine

Traditional Chinese medicine (TCM), with a pedigree of several thousand years, conceptualizes every aspect of the body and its functions radically differently from anything found in Western biomedicine. Reflecting the philosophical orientation of its cultural milieu – as all healing systems, including biomedicine, do – TCM focuses its diagnostic and therapeutic attention on pattern and process rather than linear causality. The human body is conceptualized as a microcosm, linked with, reflecting, and manifesting the same processes as those acting in the physical and social environment and in the cosmos. The cosmos is understood as 'an integral whole, a web of interrelated things and events. Within this web of relationships and change, any entity can be defined only by its function, and has significance only as part of the whole pattern' (Kaptchuk, 1983:15). Physiology in the human microcosm is likewise defined in terms of relationality and function, rather than form. Precise anatomical locations and structures of organs and bodily systems (the central concerns of anatomy in biomedicine) are of relatively little interest or concern by comparison with the functions of and relationships among bodily constituents and systems.

The essential cosmological qualities of *yin* and *yang* characterize all aspects of the body and its subsystems and functions, as they characterize everything in the cosmos. *Yin* and *yang* correspond, respectively, with 'cold, rest, responsiveness, passivity, darkness, downwardness, inwardness, and decrease;' and with 'heat, stimulation, movement, activity, excitement, vigour, light, upwardness, outwardness, and increase,' among other properties (Kaptchuk, 1983:8). *Yin* and *yang* are complementary, rather than oppositional, and are interinfluential, as represented by the curvilinear interface between them in the familiar *yin/yang* symbol. They are mutually generative, each giving rise to the other (represented symbolically by the seed of each that appears within the other); and each can transform into the other, as the shady side of the hill in the morning hours becomes the sunny side in late day, and vice-versa (Beinfield and Korngold, 1991). Having no separable or discrete existence or identities, *yin* and *yang* qualities can only be defined or identified in relation to, or by comparison with, each other.

The human body in TCM is animated, nourished, sustained, and cleansed by five fundamental substances: *qi*, blood, *jing, shen,* and fluids. Only one of these, *blood*, has a correlate in the biomedical model; however, its composition,

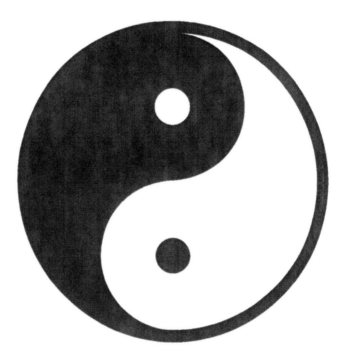

FIGURE 2.1. TRADITIONAL SYMBOLIC REPRESENTATION OF THE ESSENTIAL COSMOLOGICAL QUALITIES OF YIN AND YANG.

properties, behaviour, and functions are far from identical with those assigned to blood in biomedicine. The primary animating substance is *qi*, which is an elemental force of the universe. Being both substantive and ethereal, *qi* can be conceptualized (in rough translation to terms intelligible to Western thought) as 'matter on the verge of becoming energy, or energy at the point of materializing' (Kaptchuk, 1983:35). *Qi* infuses all things in the universe; it is the force that provides both for the 'physical integrity of any entity, and for the changes that entity undergoes' (Kaptchuk, 1983:36). *Jing* is the source of life and the essence that underlies all forms of organic life; it gives rise to processes of organic change such as generativity, growth, development, and decay. *Shen* corresponds approximately to a Western notion of spirit; it is unique to humans, and makes possible human awareness, thought, and personality. *Fluids* are all of the non-blood liquids of the body; their function is to moisten, lubricate, nourish, and cleanse.

Of these fundamental elements, the one which receives the most attention in Anglo-European cultures is *qi*, reconceptualized in these cultures' terms as a variant form of vital energy. *Qi* circulates through the body through a series of channels called (in English) meridians. These are understood to be actual physical channels of conductivity. The fact that they have no corresponding anatomical structures and could not be located on dissection is a non-issue in the Chinese framework, focused as it is on function and relationality, rather than structure, as the crucial aspects of anatomy and physiology. The system of meridians interconnects and unifies all parts of the body, providing the pathways through which the harmonious balance of health is maintained or regained.

Organs are defined and intelligible in terms of their functions and their relationships with each other, with the meridian system, and with the fundamental substances. They are classified as *yin* or *yang* according to their functions, and there are six of each,[3] as well as six 'Curious Organs' (brain, bone, marrow, blood vessels, uterus, and gall bladder). *Yin* organs (heart, lungs, spleen, liver, kidneys, and pericardium) function to 'produce, transform, regulate, and store the Fundamental Substances;' *yang* organs (gall bladder, small intestine, large intestine, bladder, and triple burner) 'receive, break down, and absorb that part of the food that will be transformed into Fundamental Substances, and transport and excrete the unused portion' (Kaptchuk, 1983:53). In this taxonomy, TCM recognizes two organs that do not exist in the biomedical model: the Pericardium (*yin*) and the Triple Burner (*yang*). The Triple Burner is 'the functional relationship [among the] various organs that regulate water in the body' (Kaptchuk, 1983:68); like the meridian system, it is a function without a physical correlate.

The human body is conceptualized as a dynamic and self-regulating complex system, whose characteristics are like those of a landscape (Kaptchuk, 1983), an ecology, or a garden (Beinfield and Korngold, 1991, 1995): the mists and promontories of the high altitudes have different characteristics and give rise to different phenomena than the flowing waters and land forms of the middle altitudes or the boggy marshlands and silts of the low ground, but all are seamlessly interconnected and mutually inter-influential (see illustrations). The condition of the body when functioning optimally is one of fluid and dynamic equipoise. This can be conceptualized in a more Western image as being like the movable balance of a hanging mobile: the parts are inter-connected, and move always in relation to one another. A derangement in one part resonates throughout the entire system, which will, under the proper conditions, eventually return to a new (though not identical) state of balance (C. Hudson, R.Ac., personal communication).

In this system health is defined in terms of harmony and balance among the various aspects and elements of the body (including mental, emotional,[4] and spiritual aspects, among others), seen within its environmental and cosmo-logical contexts. Disease is not an entity, but a pattern of disharmony that eventuates from a confluence of contributing conditions. The therapeutic goal is therefore not eradication of disease *per se*, but modification of perturbing

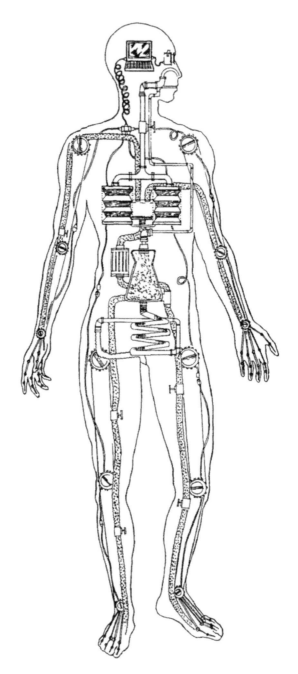

FIGURE 2.2.   METAPHOR OF THE BIOMEDICAL MODEL: THE BODY AS MACHINE. HEALTH IS DEFINED AS ABSENCE
OF DISEASE, AND ABILITY TO FUNCTION WITHIN NORMATIVE PARAMETERS. THERAPEUTIC GOALS ARE TO ERADICATE
SYMPTOMS AND TO MAXIMIZE PERFORMANCE CAPABILITIES. (FROM *BETWEEN HEAVEN AND EARTH* BY HARRIET
BEINFIELD AND EFREM KORNGOLD ILLUSTRATIONS. COPYRIGHT © 1991 BY VAL MINA, SUSANNE PANASIK
AND BRUCE WANG. REPRINTED BY PERMISSION OF BALLANTINE BOOKS, A DIVISION OF RANDOM HOUSE. INC.)

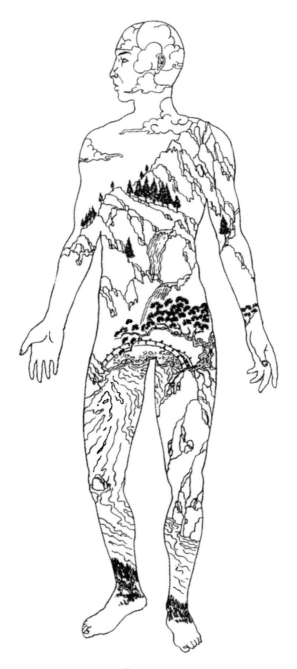

FIGURE 2.3.   METAPHOR OF THE TRADITIONAL CHINESE MEDICAL MODEL: THE BODY AS GARDEN OR ECOLOGY. HEALTH IS DEFINED AS BALANCE, INTEGRITY, ADAPTABILITY, CONTINUITY. THERAPEUTIC GOALS ARE TO RESTORE OR MAINTAIN HARMONIOUS BALANCE AND TO ENHANCE SELF-REGULATORY CAPACITY. (FROM *BETWEEN HEAVEN AND EARTH* BY HARRIET BEINFIELD AND EFREM KORNGOLD ILLUSTRATIONS. COPYRIGHT © 1991 BY VAL MINA, SUSANNE PANASIK AND BRUCE WANG. REPRINTED BY PERMISSION OF BALLANTINE BOOKS, A DIVISION OF RANDOM HOUSE, INC.)

underlying conditions and influences so as to remove imbalance, resulting in a return to the harmonious state which is health:

> ... if you reorganize the existing pattern of disharmony into a harmonious pattern of relationships, the original [health problem] will disappear because the conditions in which it was rooted cease to exist (Beinfield and Korngold, 1991:36).

The models of bodily composition, organization, and function of TCM and Western biomedicine cannot be mapped onto each other in any set of direct correspondences. Part of the present-day appeal of TCM in the United States is precisely its radical difference from Anglo-European conceptualizations of the body – and thus its approaches to health, illness, and care. Any conceptual model, by determining the identification and classification of problems, strongly shapes the kinds of solutions that suggest themselves. Many contemporary Americans whose symptoms are classified as unrelated or 'non-specific' under the biomedical model, find that TCM recognizes their illness experience as a clear diagnostic category with specific corollary treatment options.

Anthroposophical Medicine

Anthroposophy is a philosophical system developed in the early years of the twentieth century by Austrian philosopher Rudolph Steiner. Encompassing many areas of human endeavour – education, agriculture, musical and artistic expression, business, medicine, and others – anthroposophy takes a spiritual and phenomenological view of human beings and their relationship to nature and the cosmos (Cantor and Rosenzweig, 1997). Anthroposophical medicine, though having roots in the conventional biomedical worldview, extends and expands the conventional paradigm to incorporate spiritual and other aspects of persons and their overall well-being that are not reducible to quantifiable measures. Within this framework, physiological processes of the body and developmental, maturational processes of the human being as person and self are seen as analogues, passing in complementary relationships through a series of life cycle stages. For example:

> A principal task of childhood is the development of an independent self. Psychosocially, this is apparent in the necessary but challenging movement from mother's breast to [...] increasingly independent [...] situations. Physiologically it is seen in the development of the immune system, a physical reflection of the self. [...] Common childhood illnesses are key challenges along the way. [...] The physician, like the wise parent [...], must perceive whether or not a particular challenge can be met by a child. Too much interference from a parent whenever a difficulty is encountered will produce a weak-willed child. Similarly, unnecessary intervention on the part of a physician will lead to a disordered, weakened immune system (Cantor and Rosenzweig, 1997:870).

The central guiding principle is *appropriate* intervention: knowing when to intervene directly and when simply to support (without intervention) the innate healing and maturational capacities of the body and self.

In anthroposophical medicine, persons are conceived as having a four-fold nature described in terms of an interacting series of self/bodies; the *physical body* is but one of these. Permeating the physical body and linking it with the self is the *life-'body,'* comprising 'life processes such as metabolism, growth and decay, differentiation, self-regulation, homeostasis, and metamorphosis' (Cantor and Rosenzweig, 1997:874) in both their physiological and their psychological variants. Sentience, the capacity of living organisms to feel and react, operates at the cellular level in terms of 'metabolic reactivity' and neuronal information flow, and at the level of the human psyche in terms of awareness, perception, and subjective experience, constituting the *sentient-'body'* or *soul-'body.'* Self-consciousness, the experience and knowledge of self that makes possible choice, self-determination, and relatedness, constitutes the *self or 'I.'* Each of these aspects or embodiments of persons has its own set of developmental tasks and governing laws. All are interrelated and interactive, and a balance among them creates the conditions for – indeed, constitutes – health. Derangements in physical processes and well being have analogues in the other 'bodies' and their functioning, and all aspects of persons must be addressed for effective healing to occur.

A central organizing principle of diagnostics and therapeutics in anthroposophical medicine is the concept of polarity: a constant tension between opposing systems, qualities, or processes that characterizes the 'spiritual, psychological, and physical organization' of human beings (Cantor and Rosenzweig, 1997:881). The oppositional dualism of divergent poles and their respective pulls and influences is mediated by a third, rhythmic, process. 'Physiologically, three interrelated systems or processes can be described: metabolic system [characterized by movement, fluidity, warmth], nerve-sense system [characterized by static form, dryness, coolness], and rhythmic system' (Cantor and Rosenzweig, 1997:881–882). Rhythmic activity in the body derives from the same source as the rhythms of the natural world and demonstrates the intimate relationship of human beings to nature and the cosmos. Therapeutically conservative, anthroposophical medicine concentrates on qualitatively evaluating each individual person's multidimensional body and self in illness, and on supporting with minimal intervention the innate capacities of the body/self in healing.

A corollary to these views is the belief that pharmaceuticals should be used quite conservatively because their mechanisms of action take over or substitute for inherent protective, recuperative, and homeostatic functions and abilities of the body. By so doing, these agents have the potential to derange or debilitate these bodily functions permanently, creating chronic dysfunction and pharmaco-logic dependence. Anthroposophical medicine shares several tenets that have wide acceptance in the current CAM popular health movement. These include a profound trust in the inherent rightness of natural processes; a holistic view of persons and health that incorporates physical, emotional, mental, and spiritual dimensions; and a preference for natural over synthetic medicaments and for low-technology, minimally invasive interventions.

SHARED CONCEPTS IN COMPLEMENTARY MEDICINE

The three foregoing examples hint at the range of possibilities and complexities of constructions of the body to be found in complementary medicine. They are quite disparate in their central theories and philosophical underpinnings, and are widely removed from one another in historical period and culture of origin. Nevertheless, they share certain broadly defined concepts about the body and its workings – and by extension about the nature and causal conditions of health and illness, and the means to healing and wellness – that give them more common ground with one another than with conventional biomedicine. To name only a few of these: all regard the body as inherently healthy in its natural state and endowed with an ecological capacity for self-regulation and balance. All conceive of the physical body as interconnected with other key aspects of persons such as mind, will, spirit, psyche, or emotions, all of which affect and are affected by health and illness. All recognize humanity's natural state of health to be vulnerable to disruption through a variety of potential challenges, but defensible or recoverable through judicious behaviour and use of therapeutic measures that take account of the interconnections of physical and other elements in both causation and cure.

These and other core concepts – although variously interpreted in their particular details and in their implications within system-specific theoretical frameworks – are found among a large number of healing systems, but are absent in biomedicine. This shared conceptual core is one of the identifying features of the CAM domain, and differentiates it from the domain of conventional medicine. These concepts are tightly integrated and have multiple interconnections that make them mutually reinforcing. For this reason they do not fall neatly into discrete categories, and have therefore been parsed in various ways by different analysts of non-biomedical healing systems (e.g., Hufford, 1988; Fuller, 1989; O'Connor, 1995; Goldstein, 1999).[5] The following brief review of the fundamental concepts of CAM systems focuses particularly on how they portray or implicate the human body:

Interrelation of Body, Mind, and Spirit. Bodies do not (in fact, cannot) 'stand alone'. A complex interconnectedness is posited among body, mind, and spirit;

health and illness incorporate all of these aspects of persons. True healing must likewise take into account all of these aspects and their interconnections with each other and with their wider environments (e.g. society, nature, cosmos).

Health as Harmony or Balance. Health is defined either as, or in terms of, harmony or balance. At a minimum this balance or harmony is internal to the individual, involving the various critical aspects of persons as well as bodily substances and essential qualities (e.g. *yin* and *yang*, hot and cold, etc.). Quite often it also applies to relationships between the individual and external factors such as social, environmental, and cosmological elements.

Vitalism. The human body is animated and sustained by a special type of force, energy, or essence which may in turn be connected with a universal or cosmic source or reservoir. The presence and proper activity of the vital force in the body are essential to life and health. Disruption, obstruction, or depletion of the vital force leads to illness; restoration of its proper embodiment, freedom, and function promotes healing.[6]

Self-healing and Self-regulating Capacity of the Body. The body is an inherently self-regulating system; its vital energy both enables self-regulation and endows the body/mind/spirit with the capacity to heal itself when derangements occur. Much of CAM therapeutics is directed at supporting or promoting the function of the vital energy (vs. suppressing a symptom or eradicating a pathogen), so as to enable the body to heal itself.

Importance of 'Energy.' In addition to the vital force, various other forms and actions of 'energy' play important roles in health, in disease etiology, and in healing. Energy fields in and around human bodies may interact in various ways with the energies of other people and of the surrounding environment. Negative energies may cause illness, and positive energies promote healing.[7]

Attention to Underlying Causes. Identification and treatment of underlying causes of illness is of equal or greater importance than treatment of symptoms or immediate causes. Underlying causes establish the conditions under which sickness may develop and take hold, and often represent some type of fundamental imbalance or disharmony within the body, or between the individual and external elements.[8]

Integrative Moral Tone. CAM systems generally incorporate clear moral elements, such as a presumption of the inherent goodness or correctness of Nature, and a sense of personal responsibility for right behaviour and health-protecting actions. Together with the central importance of harmony and balance, these views underscore the interconnectedness of personal health and the human body, mind, and spirit with the community, the physical environment, and the cosmos.[9]

BODY AND SELF: BEYOND BIOLOGY

An enormous amount of popular press material reveals that complementary medicine is embraced by its proponents on the basis of both personal belief and personal experience. Research findings from a range of professional disciplines also support these contentions (e.g., Hufford, 1988; O'Connor, 1985, 1993, 1995; Busby, 1996; Elder *et al.*, 1997; Kelner and Wellman, 1997; Landmark, 1998; Astin, 1998; Schneirov and Geczik, 1998; Astin, *et al.*, 1999; Goldstein, 1999). CAM systems' constructions of the body, together with the larger conceptual framework of which they form an integral part, play a significant role in the public appeal of complementary medicine.

As embodied beings, we experience life 'in and through the body' (Toombs, 1993; Busby, 1996) long before, as well as after, we develop cognitive and symbolic structures for mapping experience and meaning. The body is both an experiencing subject which is the physical locus of perception and awareness, and an object of its own attentions (Toombs, 1993; Csordas, 1994; Jackson, 1994). In lived experience there is no existential separation between body and self: 'I do not "have" or "possess" a body, I *am* my body' (Toombs, 1993:51). Because 'body and self are [...] contingent on one another' (Saltonstall, 1993:9) the body is 'a focal point of self-construction as well as health construction' (Saltonstall, 1993:7). These interconnections are reflected in many contexts, for example: in the rhetoric of the fitness movement and the healing philosophies of most CAM systems; and in the self-definitional struggles of those whose bodies have been victimized (Scarry, 1985; Winkler, 1994), become disabled or chronically ill (Toombs, 1993; Mairs, 1996), or become the source and locus of chronic pain (Jackson, 1994; Price, 1994).

The strictly material, biological models of the human body and human functioning that inform biomedicine and scientific research are too limited to encompass many aspects of ordinary human experience of the body and the self. Most people who have cultural exposure to medical and scientific knowledge about the body – albeit in laypersons' terms – do accept basic biological knowledge and theory. Significant numbers, however, find biology insufficient to adequately explain their own complex experiences of body and self: 'they do not accept a purely biological conception of their own body. They conceive that there must be an immaterial part in the human body' (Braathen, 1996:152). The immaterial part(s) may be defined as an intelligence or mind; a soul or spirit; a psyche (typically conceived in terms of metaphysical rather than neurochemical functioning (see McGuire, 1988); a vital force or energy that is integral to the human body or to all of nature (Braathen, 1996; Busby, 1996; Davis, 1997; Goldstein, 1999); or as combinations of these or other elements.

However defined, these immaterial elements are believed to be, or experienced as, integral to body and self and thus to wholeness and health. The constituents of the integral body/self are conceived as interacting purposively, reflecting an inherent 'wisdom' of the body (Busby, 1996; Davis, 1997; Kroll-Smith and Floyd, 1997; Weil, 1997; Schneirov and Geczik, 1998). 'All of the cells of the body "know about" the mind, and the mind "knows about" each cell in the body' (Davis, 1997:xl). Part of this body-wisdom is the impulse for preservation of harmonious balance and the innate capacity for self-healing: 'the body has a capacity for awareness of troubles and the mechanisms for repairing tissue' through a dynamic 'healing system' (Weil, 1997:1–2). Nonstructural and immaterial in nature, the innate healing system 'makes use of all of the structural systems [of the body]' as well as of its active 'connections [...] to consciousness' (Weil, 1997:3).

The more holistic models of persons, bodies, and health that characterize CAM systems and modalities are much more closely consonant with these views than the biologically restricted model of conventional medicine. CAM systems encompass a range of preventive and therapeutic practices that address the integrated and multifactorial nature of human beings and their health, and aim to support an innate body-wisdom and self-healing capability. This concordance of CAM theory and practice with popular ontology, or understandings of bodily reality, helps to account for public acceptance and popularity of complementary medicine on grounds of both personal belief and direct personal experience. It is common for individuals to report that one or another CAM modality is in important ways 'more congruent with [their] experience of the body' (Busby, 1996:140) than what they have found in conventional medicine.

SELF-OBSERVATION AND EXPERIENTIAL KNOWLEDGE

Conventional medicine has laid claim to expertise in matters of health and illness, and restricts recognition of authoritative knowledge to only those data generated by professionally trained observers or produced by the controlled and replicable methods of scientific inquiry. Laypersons nevertheless rely a large percentage of the time on their own observations and experiences as sources of authoritative knowledge about health in general and their own health in particular. Ordinary people quite commonly take action on the basis of this type of knowledge without feeling a need for professional ratification. Informally this is played out in such health actions as the routine use of home remedies, over-the-counter medicaments, and myriad other forms of self-care, and in what Yesalis and colleagues (1980) have called 'self-triage.' More formally, this type of self-authorization may coalesce in health-related self-help and support groups (Levin, Katz, and Holst, 1979; Martin, 1992); in social movements like the women's health and alternative therapies movements; or in the agendas of patient activist groups focused on specific conditions or health issues (including 'contested diseases' such as multiple chemical sensitivity or chronic fatigue syndrome).

Common to all of these situations is an acceptance of 'human experience [as] a valid way of knowing' and of 'the body as a source of reliable knowledge' (Kroll-Smith and Floyd, 1997:91, 118). This matter-of-fact lay empiricism stands in sharp contrast to scientific insistence that in the absence of technical expertise and controlled conditions our observations are untrustworthy and potentially misleading (Cassidy, 1995; Davis, 1997). Many lay people no longer accept the 'modernist assumption that personal experiences must be secondary to professional judgment' (Kroll-Smith and Floyd, 1997:112), especially in contested matters of health. Neither the criteria for defining health and illness, nor those for defining valid knowledge, are ceded entirely to licensed professionals (Levin, Katz, and Holst, 1979; O'Connor, 1993; Cant and Sharma 1996). Quite the contrary, personal bodily experience of illness or healing which is unacknowledged by conventional medicine or incongruent with medically accepted facts may trump medical claims, and be considered the ultimate source of authoritative knowledge (O'Connor, 1985, 1993; Kroll-Smith and Floyd, 1997). Personal experience as a source of knowledge *about* the body readily engages with acceptance of an inherent wisdom *of* the body. It is not unusual for users of complementary medicine to say that they 'listen to their bodies' in making health-related decisions, or to assert that 'they know their own body best and trust their own judgment most' (Kelner and Wellman, 1997:210).

Knowledge that originates in the experiences and sensations of the body yields a 'practical epistemology,' or pragmatic knowledge base, whose 'standard of validity [...] can be summed up in the question Does it work? or Is it useful?' (Kroll-Smith and Floyd, 1997:137). The primacy and authority of experience, in both illness states and healing events, lead many people to place the highest value on 'what I feel like, not what [professional experts] tell me I should be feeling or not feeling' (Kroll-Smith and Floyd, 1997:97). Confidence in experientially-derived knowledge is strengthened when people have opportunities to exchange narratives that provide intersubjective validation of experiences (O'Connor, 1985, 1993); exchanges of this type are of course enormously facilitated in the US and other developed nations nowadays by widespread nonprofessional access to the Internet. Failure or refusal of conventional medicine to acknowledge or respond to these personally important and collectively acknowledged experiences readily results in a diminution of trust in medical authority and in the adequacy or comprehensiveness of medical knowledge (Busby, 1996; Kroll-Smith and Floyd, 1997).[10]

Complementary medical systems typically do recognize individual and collectively shared experiences of the body and the self as sources of valid and clinically significant knowledge. In practitioner-based systems[11] information of this type is routinely sought from patients, and is treated as an integral part of the data upon which diagnostic and treatment decisions are based. Complementary systems thus have a high degree of correlation, in practical application as well as in theoretical models, to the ways in which many individuals experience their bodies, their states of health, and their efforts at healing. This ratification of subjective experiences and their meanings makes CAM systems attractive and logical health care venues for people addressing health problems or concerns which have been rejected or gone unacknowledged by the conventional system (see, e.g., Busby, 1996).

IMPLICATIONS FOR HEALTH CARE RESEARCH AND PRACTICE

All cultures of which we have knowledge have given rise to (often plural) health belief systems that address the nature and causes of health and illness, and that incorporate conceptions of the human body encompassing (at least) explanations of its nature, organization, structures, and functions. These conceptions are invariably interconnected with the systems' definitions of health, illness, and disease etiology and with corollary definitions of necessary and appropriate care. Conceptions of the body and of its health, illness, and care are never merely descriptions of 'brute facts' of nature, but always reflect broader cultural worldviews, values, and concerns as well as – indeed as part of – their observations of natural facts. This is as true of biomedicine as it is of any other system of health belief, knowledge, and practice.

Although the immense attention now being paid to complementary medicine by the conventional medical research and practice system is of quite recent vintage, neither the phenomenon of CAM itself nor the ideas and experiences upon which it is founded are new. In the United States (as in all complex societies), the *de facto* resources of health care have always been pluralistic and multifaceted. Conventional biomedicine, the 'official' health care system, has achieved social and political hegemony based in no small part (though not exclusively) on its remarkable therapeutic successes. Nevertheless, it has always operated in parallel with any number of 'unofficial' healing systems – from familial self-care activities, to traditional folk medical systems closely associated with specific cultural heritage groups, to more geographically and demographically widespread and formalized systems such as botanical medicine, chiropractic, and homeopathy.

This is due in large part to the existence of certain needs of sick people that many consider to be better met in other healing systems, as well as to the many satisfactions people find in other diagnostic and therapeutic frameworks (O'Connor, 1993; Astin, 1998). People with health problems strive to multiply their therapeutic options (O'Connor, 1995), and persist in their efforts to obtain what they need. To the extent that conventional medicine (or any system, for that matter) does not meet certain needs in lived experience, other resources are sought to supplement or supplant those already brought to bear. Elder and colleagues (1997), for example, found that a significant percentage of family practice patients using complementary medicine in addition to their conventional care sought these resources to address health concerns other than those for which they sought treatment from conventional medicine. That is, they were using complementary resources at least a percentage of the time to deal with health concerns that conventional medicine either does not recognize or does not address. These commonly include such issues as symptoms considered 'non-specific' or non-significant in the biomedical nosology; felt needs for support of the body's recuperative capacity or vital energy in the wake of debilitating illness or its conventional treatment (Busby, 1996); or desires to promote active wellness rather than only treating sickness (Astin, 1998).

As the conventional medical and research establishments have begun to take complementary medicine seriously, a research agenda has developed based on the presumption that the official system will evaluate CAM systems and modalities using the established tools of scientific research; discover what 'works' (as defined in scientific terms) and incorporate it into the conventional system's therapeutic armamentarium; and dispense with the remainder on grounds of insufficient proof of efficacy (Hufford, 1996). An unspoken accompanying assumption seems to be that those parts of CAM that do not stand up to scientific investigation and explanation can be expected to lose favor with the public as well, and can then be consigned to the dustbin of history. This view precisely parallels the previously long-cherished assumption that as modern medicine and public education became increasingly refined and more universally available over time, 'nonscientific' health beliefs and practices would as a matter of course die out or be eliminated (Hufford, 1988; O'Connor, 1995). The continued vigour of non-biomedical healing systems irrespective of the introduction, availability, and technological advances of biomedicine – and certainly the recent explosion of public interest in and use of complementary medicine – have resoundingly proven this prediction false.

The same fundamental blind spot characterizes the current assumptions shaping the CAM research agenda, namely: a failure to appreciate the robustness of popular epistemologies and ontologies that diverge from the scientific worldview; their profound connections to personally and collectively convincing and meaningful experiences of the body, of health, of illness, and of healing; and the extent to which complementary medical systems incorporate and address these issues. The questions of researchers committed to strictly material models of health and illness, and the questions of people drawing on both theoretical models and personal experiences that incorporate essential immaterial elements, overlap only to a degree. The analytic processes of reductionist investigation raise utterly different kinds of questions than do the wide-reaching syntheses of a holistic view of persons, health, and healing. The scientific criteria of replicability of results and generalizability of findings lead in different investigational directions than does experientially and philosophically derived acceptance of individualization of illness presentation, of indicated treatment, and of therapeutic results. From the point of view of the CAM-using public, 'a beneficial treatment outcome in the moment of care [may be] far more important to health and healing [...] than using only the treatment that matches [a] standard of care for alleviation of symptoms based on a reductionistic world view' (Davis, 1997:xlii). 'What works,' as well as how it works, are likely to be very differently defined by researchers and CAM users.

This by no means suggests that standard scientific investigation of CAM therapeutics is invalid or unimportant, or that people who use complementary modalities have no interest in scientific inquiry into their safety, efficacy, and modes of action: far from it. Such inquiries are very important, and long overdue. Members of the CAM-using public are on the whole delighted to find science taking seriously at last a topic dear to their hearts and minds – though many also consider the inquiries of science necessary but not sufficient to fully explain what they personally want to know. Scholars and researchers from all disciplines need to bear in mind that all the research findings we can muster will not thoroughly or adequately explain public acceptance, support, and use of complementary medicine as long as we fail to understand and address fully the issues and experiences of that public, *as they themselves define them*. These will most certainly include the phenomenology of the lived body/self in its many interconnected dimensions, the ontological and epistemological authority of personal experience, and the lessons of lived experiences of health, illness, and healing.

REFERENCES

Astin, J.A. 1998. 'Why Patients Use Alternative Medicine: Results of a National Study.' *Journal of the American Medical Association* 278:1548–1553.
Astin, J.A., Shapiro, S.L., Lee, R.A. and D. H Shapiro, Jr. 1999. 'The Construct of Control in Mind-Body Medicine: Implications for Health Care.' *Alternative Therapies in Health and Medicine* 5(2):42–47.

Beinfield, H. and E. Korngold. 1991. *Between Heaven and Earth: A Guide to Chinese Medicine*. New York: Ballantine Books.

Beinfield, H. and E. Korngold. 1995. 'Chinese Traditional Medicine: An Overview.' *Alternative Therapies in Health and Medicine* 1(1):44–52.

Braathen, E. 1996. 'Communicating the Individual Body and the Body Politic: The Discourse on Disease Prevention and Health Promotion in Alternative Therapies.' Pp. 151–162 in *Complementary and Alternative Medicines: Knowledge in Practice*, edited by S. Cant and U. Sharma. London: Free Association Books, Ltd.

Busby, H. 1996. 'Alternative Medicines/Alternative Knowledges: Putting Flesh on the Bones (Using Traditional Chinese Approaches to healing).' Pp. 135–150 in *Complementary and Alternative Medicines: Knowledge in Practice*, edited by S. Cant and U. Sharma. London: Free Association Books, Ltd.

Cant, S. and U. Sharma (eds.). 1996. *Complementary and Alternative Medicines: Knowledge in Practice*. London: Free Association Books, Ltd.

Cantor, I.S. and S. Rosenzweig. 1997. 'Anthroposophic Perspectives in Primary Care.' *Primary Care: Clinics in Office Practice* 24(4):867–888.

Cassidy, C. 1995. 'Social Science Theory and Methods in the Study of Alternative and Complementary Medicine.' *Journal of Alternative and Complementary Medicine* 1(1):19–40.

Csordas, T.J. 1994. 'Introduction.' Pp. 1–24 in *Embodiment and Experience: The Existential Ground of Culture and Self*, edited by T. Csordas. Cambridge: Cambridge University Press.

Davis, C.M. 1997. 'Introduction.' Pp. xxix-xiv in *Complementary Therapies in Rehabilitation: Holistic Approaches for Prevention and Wellness*, edited by C.M. Davis. Thorofare, NJ: Slack Incorporated.

Eisenberg, D.M., Kessler, R.C., Foster, C., Norlock, F.E., Calkins, D.R. and T.L. Delbanco. 1993. 'Unconventional Medicine in the United States.' *New England Journal of Medicine* 328(January 28):246–252.

Elder, N.C., Gillcrist, A. and R. Minz. 1997. 'Use of Alternative Health Care by Family Practice Patients.' *Archives of Family Medicine* 6(2):181–184.

Fuller, R.C., 1989. *Alternative Medicine and American Religious Life*. New York: Oxford University Press.

Goldstein, M. 1999. *Alternative Health Care: Medicine, Miracle, or Mirage?* Philadelphia: Temple University Press.

Graham, S. 1857. *Chastity, in a Course of Lectures to Young Men*. New York: Fowler and Wells.

Hufford, D.J. 1988. 'Contemporary Folk Medicine.' pp. 228–264 in *Other Healers: Unorthodox Medicine in America*, edited by N. Gevitz. Baltimore: The Johns Hopkins University Press.

Hufford, D.J. 1996. 'Culturally Grounded Review of Research Assumptions.' *Alternative Therapies in Health and Medicine* 2(4):47–53.

Hufford, D.J. and B.B. O'Connor. Forthcoming. 'American Folk Medicine.' in *Textbook of Complementary Medicine,* edited by W. Jonas and J. Levin. New York: Lippincott Williams & Wilkins.

Jackson, J. 1994. 'Chronic Pain and the Tension Between the Body as Subject and Object.' Pp. 201–228 in *Embodiment and Experience: The Existential Ground of Culture and Self*, edited by T. Csordas. Cambridge: Cambridge University Press.

Kaptchuk, T. 1983. *The Web That Has No Weaver: Understanding Chinese Medicine*. New York: Congdon & Weed.

Kelner, M.J. and B. Wellman. 1997. 'Health Care and Consumer Choice: Medical and Alternative Therapies.' *Social Science and Medicine* 45(2)203–212.

Kellogg, J.H. 1919. *The Itinerary of a Breakfast*. Battle Creek, MI: Funk and Wagnall's.

Kroll-Smith, S. and H. Floyd. 1997. *Bodies in Protest: Environmental Illness and the Struggle Over Medical Knowledge*. New York: New York University Press.

Landmark Healthcare, Inc. 1998. The Landmark Report on Public Perceptions of Alternative Care. Sacramento: Landmark Healthcare Inc.

Levin, L.S., Katz, A.H., and E. Holst. 1979. *Self-Care: Lay Initiatives in Health*. New York: Prodist.

Mairs, N. 1996. *Waist-High in the World: A Life Among the Non-Disabled*. Boston: Beacon Press.

Martin, E. 1992. *The Woman in the Body: A Cultural Analysis of Reproduction* (Second Edition). Boston: Beacon Press.

McGuire, M. 1988. *Ritual Healing in Suburban America*. New Brunswick, NJ: Rutgers University Press.

Morantz, R.M. 1977. 'Nineteenth Century Health Reform and Women: A Program of Self-Help.' Pp. 73–93 in *Medicine Without Doctors: Home Health Care in American History*, edited by G.B. Risse, R.L. Numbers, and J.W. Leavitt. New York: Science History Publications USA.

Numbers, R. 1976. *Prophetess of Health: A Study of Ellen G. White*. New York: Harper and Row.

OAM (Office of Alternative Medicine, NIH) Committee on Definition and Description. 1997. 'Defining and Describing Complementary and Alternative Medicine.' *Alternative Therapies in Health and Medicine* 3(2):49–57.

O'Connor, B.B. 1985. 'The Authority of Experience and Beliefs About Knowing.' Unpublished paper, presented to American Folklore Society annual meeting, Cincinnati, OH.

O'Connor, B.B. 1993. 'The Home Birth Movement in the United States.' *The Journal of Medicine and Philosophy* 18(2):147–174.

O'Connor, B.B. 1995. *Healing Traditions: Alternative Medicine and the Health Professions*. Philadelphia: University of Pennsylvania Press.

Ots, T. 1994. 'The Silenced Body – The Expressive Leib: On the Dialectic of Mind and Life in Chinese Cathartic Healing.' Pp. 116–136 in *Embodiment and Experience: The Existential Ground of Culture and Self*, edited by T. Csordas. Cambridge: Cambridge University Press.

Price, R. 1994. *A Whole New Life*. New York: Atheneum.

Saltonstall, R. 1993. 'Healthy Bodies, Social Bodies: Men's and Women's Concepts and Practices of Health in Everyday Life.' *Social Science and Medicine* 36(1):7–14.

Scarry, E. 1985. *The Body in Pain: The Making and Unmaking of the World*. New York: Oxford University Press.

Schneirov, M.M. and J.D. Geczik. 1998. 'Technologies of the Self and the Aesthetic Project of Alternative Health.' *The Sociological Quarterly* 39(3):435–451.

Toombs, S.K. 1993. *The Meaning of Illness: A Phenomenological Account of the Different Perspectives of Physician and Patient*. Dordrecht: Kluwer Academic Publishers.

Weil, A. 1997. 'Healing Medicine.' *Whole Earth* 91:90–94.

Whorton, J.C. 1988. 'Patient, Heal Thyself: Popular Health Reform Movements as Unorthodox Medicine.' pp. 52–81 in *Other Healers: Unorthodox Medicine in America*, edited by N. Gevitz. Baltimore: The Johns Hopkins University Press.

Winkler, C. 1994. 'Rape Trauma: Contexts of Meaning.' Pp. 248–268 in *Embodiment and Experience: The Existential Ground of Culture and Self*, edited by T. Csordas. Cambridge: Cambridge University Press.

Yesalis, C.E., III, Wallace, R.B., Fisher, Wayne P. and R. Tokheim. 1980. 'Does Chiropractic Utilization Substitute for Less Available Medical Services?' *American Journal of Public Health* 70:415–417.

NOTES

1 Since many CAM systems substantially predate the development of biomedicine, it could be said on historical grounds that it is biomedicine's view of the body that diverges from theirs, rather than vice-versa.

2 Of course not all systems that are defined as CAM in the US and that focus preventive and therapeutic attention on the colon and its cleansing are part of the American historical lineage described in this illustration (e.g., Ayurveda).

3 Kaptchuk identifies five principal *yin* organs, noting that the pericardium is in some interpretations of chinese physiology listed as a sixth *yin* organ. The gall bladder has a dual classification, being simultaneously a *yang* organ, because it performs *yang* functions, but also a Curious Organ 'because it alone contains a pure substance: bile' (Ted Kaptchuk, *The Web That Has No Weaver: Understanding Chinese Medicine*. (Congdon & Weed, 1983), p. 53).

4 Interpretations of what constitutes proper balance are of course themselves culturally determined. Ots points out that Taoist influences in the Chinese worldview conceptualize emotions as damaging to both viscera and 'heart-mind,' leading to negative valuation of emotion and to strong stigmatization of emotionally demonstrative behaviour or demeanour. The ideally balanced Taoist body is 'strong, healthy, [...] and emotion-free' (Thomas Ots, 'The Silenced Body – The Expressive *Leib*: On the Dialectic of Mind and Life in Chinese Cathartic Healing.' In *Embodiment and Experience: The Existential Ground of Culture and Self*, edited by T. Csordas. (Cambridge University Press, 1994), p. 119.

5 Because of the complexity of their interconnections and the implications each has for the others, any listing of CAM core concepts is not only interpretive, but is also necessarily partial: selection and foregrounding of some features in one person's rendering will entail corollary qualities that another writer may highlight as primary features.

6 Plants and other *materia medica* too have vital energy. The vital energy of plants may be a significant part of their therapeutic value, or furnish the entire basis for their healing activity. This view provides a

compelling rationale for preferring natural over synthetic medicaments, since natural products provide vitalistic as well as biochemical benefits. In some cases (e.g. flower essences, and some interpretations of homeopathy) the therapeutic properties of plant materials are predicated entirely on their vitalistic principles, and no standard pharmacologic mode of action is posited at all.

7   Transference of positive energy from healer to patient is a characteristic of systems in which the healer's hands are used therapeutically on or near the patient's body, and the mechanism of action of homeopathic remedies is posited to be energetic, rather than biochemical.

8   This focus of preventive and therapeutic attention on *underlying* causal conditions commonly leads proponents to observe that CAM systems treat the actual causes of disease and ill health, while conventional medicine addresses itself primarily or exclusively to the symptoms.

9   'This perspective integrates the experience of sickness and health within a meaningful view of the world, incorporating the meaning of disease and suffering within the same system that speaks to cause and cure. The moral framework, in turn, furnishes explanations for the pressing questions that seriously sick people have of why (in the moral or metaphysical sense) they are sick, why in this way, and why now' (David Hufford, Bonnie O'Connor, 'American Folk Medicine.' In *Textbook of Complementary Medicine*, edited by W. Jonas and J. Levin. (Williams & Wilkins, forthcoming).

10   Much has been written recently about the growth of an 'anti-science' sentiment among the American public. Many members of the CAM-using public, as well as of activist groups of patients dealing with 'contested diseases' like Environmental Illness (Steve Kroll-Smith and H. Hugh Floyd, *Bodies in Protest: Environmental Illness and the Struggle Over Medical Knowledge*. (New York University Press, 1997) might invert this assertion. Finding compelling and pragmatically useful knowledge in personal experiences which the scientific community dismisses when approached for explanations or assistance, they could logically claim that it is science which is rejecting them, and not the other way around.

11   Pratitioner-based systems account for only about 1/3 of complementary medicine use in the United States (David Eisenberg *et al.*, 'Unconventional Medicine in the United States.' (*New England Journal of Medicine* 328(January 28), 1993), the remainder being in the form of self-care.

CHAPTER 3

Reasons for Using CAM

ADRIAN FURNHAM AND CHARLES VINCENT

INTRODUCTION

The world-wide growth in the interest in, use of, and expansion of complementary and alternative medicine (CAM) has led to an appropriate increase in research. The popular interest in CAM has been matched by a relatively sudden and dramatic increase in the research community on the two central questions in this area: 1. *Does it work?* Is there good evidence from double-blind, placebo-controlled, randomized studies that the therapy 'cures illness' as it says it does. That is, is there any indisputable scientific evidence that documented findings on success are due to anything more than a placebo effect? The answer is either very little or no good evidence is available for the therapeutic success of CAM. 2. *Why choose it?* If the evidence is limited, equivocal and indeed points to lack of efficacy, the central question must by why indeed patients choose (at their own expense) to visit a CAM practitioner. What do they get? Why do they persist?

Here we address the second question, examining speculations and research from a variety of disciplines, including anthropology, economics, medicine, psychology, and sociology. Whilst some speculative hypotheses are difficult to test (for example, interest in CAM is a function of the post-modern era), others have been tested and some supported. Although it is unwise to generalize across different CAM specialities, clear trends are apparent. Most patients are health consumers, sensitive to various social movements (green, patients' rights, self-care and fitness) and few are patients exclusively because of dissatisfaction and disaffection. Also important to patients is the 'pull' of the promise or practice of CAM (Annandale & Hunt, 1998). Wanting to try all health options (shopping for health) is a prominent reason for choosing CAM. To this extent many patients report being 'happy with' both their orthodox medical practitioner (usually a GP) and CAM practitioner (Donnelly et al., 1985). Further, unlike some in the medical profession, few patients are in any way opponents of CAM: they do not believe it to be dangerous or fundamentally wrong. Indeed, there is evidence that medical students (Vincent & Furnham, 1997) and physicians (Ernst, Resch & White, 1995) believe CAM to be moderately effective, though it is not clear whether CAM is seen as a nonspecific or specific powerful placebo, or as an effective psycho-physical therapy. Knipschild *et al.* (1990) noted that Dutch GPs thought manual therapy, yoga, acupuncture, hot baths and homoeopathy most effective. Indeed, there is evidence that older, culture-specific CAM therapies that have a long established history, such as acupuncture and Chinese medicine, appear to be grudgingly accepted by orthodox practitioners and occasionally enthusiastically embraced by them (Boon, 1998; Gursoy, 1996).

The interest in CAM can also be noted by the growth of academic journals aimed at researching issues in all the alternative and complementary medium specialities. Some of the more important are:

1. *Complementary Therapies in Medicine: The Journal for all health care professionals.* Established in 1993. Published in Great Britain by Churchill Livingstone Journals.
2. *The Journal of Alternative and Complementary Medicine: Research on paradigm, practice and policy.* Established 1995. Published in the USA by Mary Ann Liebert, Inc.
3. *Alternative Therapies in Medicine.* Established 1995. Published in the USA by Inno Vision Communications.
4. *Focus on Alternative and Complementary Medicine* Established 1996. Published in Great Britain by the University of Exeter.
5. *Forscherde Komplementarmedizin (Research in Complementary Medicine).* Established 1995. Published in Germany by Karger.
6. *Komplementer Medicine (The Journal of Complementary Medicine).* Established in 1997. Published in Hungary by Tamasi.

Vincent & Furnham (1997) reviewed the use of CAM by patients with specific diseases. Many previous studies showed CAM is generally used for chronic conditions (back problems, pain) or psychological/psychosomatic problems like anxiety, obesity, depression (Eisenberg *et al.*, 1993). Patients with the following diseases have been particularly attracted to CAM: AIDS (Greenblatt *et al.*, 1991), arthritis and rheumatism (Visser *et al.*, 1992; Vecchio, 1994), asthma (Donnelly *et al.*, 1985), gastro-enterology (Verhoef *et al.*, 1990), and cancer (Cassileth, 1986; Downer *et al.*, 1994).

The incredible range of varieties of CAM inevitably means there is a considerable diversity of theories, philosophies and therapies. The arcane diagnostic system of the iridologist stands in dramatic contrast to the osteopath's up-to-date knowledge of human anatomy. Equally, the bizarre explanations of gem therapy bear little or no relationship to that of homoeopathy. Yet there are common themes in the philosophies of CAM. Aakster (1986) believes that they differ from orthodox medicine in terms of five things. Inevitably, these sorts of contrasts exaggerate both the differences and the within-group homogeneity, but they are nonetheless worth considering:

Health: Whereas conventional medicine sees health as an absence of disease, alternative medicine frequently mentions a balance of opposing forces (both external and internal).

Disease: The conventional medicinal interpretation sees disease as a specific, locally defined deviation in organ or tissue structure. CAM practitioners stress many wider signs, such as body language indicating disruptive forces and/or restorative processes.

Diagnosis: Regular medicine stresses morphological classification based on location and etiology, while alternative interpretations often consider problems of functionality to be diagnostically useful.

Therapy: Conventional medicine often aims to destroy, demolish or suppress the sickening forces, while alternative therapies often aim to strengthen the vitalizing, health-promoting forces. CAM therapies seem particularly hostile to chemical therapies and surgery.

Patient: In much conventional medicine the patient is the passive recipient of external solutions, while in CAM the patient is an active participant in regaining health.

Aakster (1986) described what he called three main frames of medical thinking. The first he called the *pharmaceutical* model, which sees disease as a demonstrable deviation of function or structure that can be diagnosed by careful observation. The causes of disease are mainly germ-like and the application of therapeutic technology is all-important. The *integrational* model resulted from technicians attempting to reintegrate the body. Further, this approach is not afraid of allowing for psychological and social causes to be specified in the aetiology of illness. The third model has been labelled *holistic* and does not distinguish between soma, psyche and social. Further, it stresses total therapy and holds up the idea of a natural way of living.

Why do people choose CAM?

This question has been asked by many with rather different motives. For some, the question is why choose CAM over and against conventional medicine? For others it is even more sceptical: what sort of (irrational) people choose such an (ineffective) therapy? Yet others have seen the question almost in terms of branding: why choose the one brand or speciality over another?

Researchers and reviewers from different specialities have come up with various lists of the possible motives of CAM patients. The speculations are most frequently based on their own particular speciality. Thus anthropologists and sociologists have stressed the importance of cultural variables and shifts such as the growth of post modernism Williams & Calnan, 1996). Economists have in part accounted for the rise of interest in CAM as a function of the costs to patients, doctors and health insurance companies. Psychologists and psychiatrists have focused more on interpersonal and intrapsychic explanations for why certain individuals seek out CAM (Vincent & Furnham, 1997). Medical practitioners, too, have speculated about the medical history of particular patients or indeed differences in the average consultation between the CAM practitioner and the GP (Ernst *et al.*, 1995). In this chapter we will first examine speculation, then the empirical evidence.

Speculations about the attractions of CAM

Various writers, mainly sociologists, have proposed explanations for the increasing popularity of CAM. Williams & Calnan (1996) note that people generally live longer and in a more pain-free environment, yet there is increasing ambivalence about modern technological medicine such as transplantation surgery, new reproductive technologies and the use of modern drugs. Medicine is both a fountain of hope and despair because of *reflexivity* – the routine incorporation of new ideas into social relations and practices. Further, growing concern about *risk* (and litigation) encourages a subtle balance between active trust and radical doubt in medical experts. Also, the *media* attempt a demystification role in putting modern medical practices on trial by encouraging the audience to be the jury. Williams and Calnan argue that there is greater critical distance between modern medicine and the lay populace. Lay people are acquiring more sophisticated technical knowledge which makes them more educated and demanding consumers. '... in this world of uncertain times, one thing remains clear: namely that lay people are not simply passive or active, dependent or independent, believers or sceptics, rather they are a complex mixture of all these things (and much more besides). Without wishing to sound too post-modern, reality, in truth, is a mess, and we would do well to remember this as we edge ever closer to the twenty-first century!' (Williams & Calnan, 1996: 1619)

This is an argument about the distrust of, and disillusionment with conventional medicine, rather than an explanation of why people choose CAM. Further, Lupton (1997) found that in the doctor's surgery, patients pursue the 'consumerist' and 'passive patient' position simultaneously and variously depending on context. She believes that the consumerist movement is counter productive as it undermines the faith and trust in conventional medical practitioners that is central to the healing and comfort very ill people desperately seek in the medical encounter.

Cassileth (1998) on the other hand considers the attraction of CAM. She believes that the popularity of a particular therapy is, in part, a function of how well it fits into the sociocultural context of the time. Today, 'metabolic' and 'immuno-enhancing' therapies like diet, self-care, vitamins and internal cleansing reflect the social trends and values of our time. Cassileth believes that there are five underlying social trends of our time that render certain treatments popular. They are:

Various rights movements (including patients' rights)

Consumer movements that shift patients from the dependent role to a partnership/active consumer role

The holistic medicine movement

Self-care and fitness emphases

Disaffection with, and mistrust of, organized medicine

Cassileth suggests that the belief in the power and supremacy of the individual and his/her overriding need to understand and control, leads people to the 'mind has the power to heal' philosophy. Frustration with a lack of ability to cure and control various diseases leads to attempts to achieving control, healing and understanding via less intrusive or toxic therapies. Patients are attracted to alternative therapies whose ideologies fit the current spirit of the times.

McKee (1988) believes the CAM holistic health movement can be accused of promoting both an *individualistic* rather than a social analysis of health, and a *victim-blaming* ideology which serves to transfer the burden of health costs from the state and corporations to the individual. She argues that holistic health serves the interest of capital accumulation, while Western medicine promotes capitalism. Short-term treatment of disease is profitable and medical practice is oriented to crisis intervention and pathology correction, not prevention or health maintenance. She appears to lament the fact that the holistic medicine movement has not helped forge a strong, anti-capitalist peoples' health movement.

Bakx (1991) also provides a socio-political analysis of the popularity of CAM. He believes the crisis of biomedicine, the changes in advanced capitalism and the awareness of green issues are all part of the growth of a postmodern economy and society. Thus social forces have increased dissatisfaction with biomedicine and increased the cultural gap between doctors and patients.

Taylor (1985) focussed on the doctor-patient encounter and the nature of the relationship between practitioner and client which the alternative system offers. Earlier, Hewer (1983) stressed the importance of the nature of the consultation and the relationship between doctor and patient. Taylor (1985) argues that scientific medicine sees the human body as a machine, like any other, which needs servicing. Patients, who are described as cases, should not distract the doctor by their unique personal feelings and experiences. Taylor (1985) argues that the orthodox doctor is teacher and facilitator, while the alternative practitioner is therapist. Too many people have become accustomed to the sort of medicine which 'relies on magic bullets administered by harassed physicians who cannot distinguish us one from another as we flow from waiting room to examination room to billing office' (p,197). Conventional medicine concentrates on sickness and alternative medicine concentrates on wellness. CAM practitioners seem to characterize orthodox medical practices as technological and aggressive and their own as natural and non-invasive. Yet as Taylor notes:

> 'There seems to be little that is "natural" or "non-invasive" about the acupuncturist's technique of sticking needles into various parts of the anatomy. Some kinds of alternative specialists train in schools which do not look very different from medical schools, go into private practice and, when their services are recognised as competitive with mainstream medicine, their prices become competitive too'.

Taylor offers several explanations for the growing popularity of CAM. First a change in the cultural mood. Next, medicine has not changed and still sees itself as 'restoring people to productivity within a certain form of society'. Third, alternatives expand and contract in popularity in proportion to the successes and failures of conventional medicine. Finally, fear of iatrogenic diseases which are problems which stem from medical intervention and drugs which are supposed to cure, but in fact often exacerbate the problem.

But Taylor argues that the failures, costs and uneven distribution of modern medicine alone cannot account for the rise in alternative medicine because they do not explain *recent* interest when cost and access are enduring problems; and consumers indeed have to pay more for alternative medicine which is not covered by the state or by insurance. It is the *simultaneous* dissatisfaction/disaffection with conventional medicine and, the attraction of alternative medicine which seems to have most explanatory power. The rise and fall of different healing systems is contingent in large part on the changing nature of the medical encounter. When medicine can promise neither relief nor cure, the quality of the individual doctor-patient relationship is paramount. The consumer movement, the women's movement and the more general demand for participation all focused on the medical encounter, but traditional medical schools and practising doctors have resisted populist demands and the pressure for democratization and customer service. Not only did medicine resist change, but for many there was a perceptible deterioration of the medical encounter. Malpractice lawsuits have made doctors more cautious; there are fewer generalists and more specialists so a long-term relationship is less likely; and the increase in technological 'break-throughs' has alienated many 'modern' patients. Patients have neither a 'voice option' in the medical encounter, nor an 'exit option' to leave. Changing doctors, getting second opinions, paying for insurance are very difficult for most, hence patients have to confront the many problematic aspects of the relationship with a conventional medical doctor.

What the modern Western patient wants, and appears not to be getting, is to be treated with individual respect; not to have to endure crowded waiting rooms, or being patronised. Being processed as a case is a common complaint among many patients. Patients want to be treated as educated consumers, yet find they are still being met by a wall of clinical autonomy and a refusal to share information. Patients resent being faced by doctors who claim to have nothing to offer and do nothing, either because in their view treatments don't work or because the best policy is judged to be to do nothing. Finally, many patients now want a consumer contract with equal responsibilities. Many patients complain that doctors do not trust them to make appropriate decisions about their health care.

Thus for Taylor, medicine is basically a professional relationship. The fate of CAM is determined not so much by the proven efficacy of its methods, but rather by orthodox practitioners being either unwilling or unable to deliver what the modern patient wants.

For Lynse (1989), there are two reasons why patients choose alternative medicine: push and pull. *Disappointment* with currently available health care and *curiosity*. He uses a historical example to argue three points. First, alternative practitioners use new unaccepted, controversial concepts. It is possible that a new theoretical framework will make it possible to reinterpret pre-scientific explanations. Second, empirical data in support of CAM therapies may be impossible to understand against the background of the prevailing paradigm; that is, effects have not been well recorded or documented, *but are real*. Third, the development of a new paradigm provides the opportunity for reinterpreting pre-scientific terms and data in a new light. For instance, nineteenth-century medicine saw illness in terms of an imbalance of bodily fluids; hence the use of bleeding. It was difficult for doctors to accept the paradigm change to a more modern approach. Lynse argues that theoretical and professional interests conspire against the acceptance of an alternative therapy.

Five studies

To get some idea of the sort of research that has been concerned with the self-reported beliefs and motives of CAM patients, consider the following three studies done in different countries with very different populations and methods, but with very similar results.

Thomas and her medical colleagues in the UK (1991) specifically set out to discover whether CAM patients had turned their backs on conventional medicine. The majority of patients in this sample (64%) reported having received conventional treatment for their main problem from their general practitioner or a hospital specialist before receiving their present CAM treatment; just under a quarter of those who had received conventional treatment continued it while receiving CAM treatment (Table 3.1). The remaining 36% had not received any conventional medical treatment, but they may have received advice on their condition from their general practitioner who may also have suggested CAM therapy. It is also noteworthy that 3% of the patients were recommended to visit their general practitioner by the CAM therapist whom they had been consulting at the time.

They found that the use of prior conventional medical treatment was, not surprisingly, dependent on the type of problem for which patients were seeking help. As the table shows, patients reporting atopic conditions, headaches and arthritis were more likely to report a combination of previous and concurrent conventional treatment, usually drugs. Thomas rejected the view that patients attending CAM therapists do not understand or appreciate the benefits of conventional medicine or that the popularity of complementary medicine represents a 'flight from science'.

'Overall our findings suggest that the patients seeking non-orthodox health care from this group of practitioners have continued to make use of orthodox

TABLE 3.1: USE OF ORTHODOX MEDICAL CARE BY PATIENTS CONSULTING UNITED KINGDOM COMPLEMENTARY PRACTITIONERS

	% of patients with each complaint		
Patient defined problem	No previous or concurrent orthodox care	Previous orthodox care only	Previous and concurrent orthodox care*
Neck	47	46	7
Back	35	50	15
Low back	38	55	6
Arthritis	31	42	27
Fatigue/unwell	32	61	7
Headache/migraine	18	61	21
Anxiety/stress/depression	39	44	17
Atopic conditions	3	44	53
Digestive system disorders	4	86	10
Other	33	49	17
All patients (% of total)	35	50	15

Adapted from Thomas et al. (1991)

medicine; almost a quarter of all patients had visited their general practitioner in the two weeks preceding the surveyed consultation and two thirds had received conventional treatment for their main problem... A substantial minority, however, seems to have sought help directly from a non-orthodox practitioner and most of this group did not report any contact with their general practitioner in the two weeks preceding the survey'.

Thomas and her colleagues go on to suggest that CAM is not deflecting appreciable demand away from the National Health Service, partly because of the limited range of problems treated and the scale on which care is provided, but mainly because the patients concerned have not turned their backs on conventional care. CAM is generally a supplement to rather than a substitute for conventional care. Indeed, this is the finding of nearly all researchers in this area. Thomas did not specifically ask patients why they had turned to CAM, although the chronic conditions they suffered from and the fact that they continued to receive conventional care suggests at least that medicine was not meeting all their needs.

Ernst *et al.* (1995) asked three groups of everyday medical patients (68 Austrians, 89 Britons and 54 Germans) why they thought 'people seek treatment by alternative methods like acupuncture, homoeopathy and chiropractic'. They were offered 9 explanations and asked to tick all that applied.

1.	Because they are disappointed by orthodox medicine.	31.8%
2.	Because it is their last hope.	37.9%
3.	Because they are not really ill.	4.3%
4.	Because they are inclined to unscientific ideas.	8.1%
5.	Because they feel they will be better understood.	28.9%
6.	Because they want to use all possible options in healthcare.	57.8%
7.	Because they previously had a good experience.	37.9%
8.	Because they hope to be cured without side-effects.	47.9%
9.	Because it usually costs extra.	3.8%

They concluded that disenchantment with mainstream medicine is **not** the most prominent reason for choosing CAM. A more positive motivation (e.g. wanting to try all options of health care) may play a prominent role. Second, they noted that few patients are opponents of CAM.

Vincent & Furnham (1996) asked over 250 patients from three CAM practices – acupuncture, osteopathy and homoeopathy – to complete a questionnaire rating 20 potential reasons for seeking complementary treatment. The reasons that were most strongly endorsed were 'because I value the emphasis on treating the whole person'; because I believe complementary therapy will be more effective for my problem than orthodox medicine'; 'because I believe that complementary medicine will enable me to take a more active part in maintaining my health'; and 'because orthodox treatment was not effective for my particular problem'.

Five factors were identified, in order of importance:

1. A positive valuation of complementary treatment.
2. The ineffectiveness of orthodox treatment for their complaint.
3. Concern about the adverse effects of orthodox medicine.
4. Concerns about communication with doctors.
5. The availability of complementary medicine.

Groups were compared, using analysis of co-variance to control for demographic differences between the three patient groups (Table 3.2). Osteopathy patients' reasons indicated they were least concerned about the side-effects of conventional medicine and most influenced by the availability of osteopathy for their complaints. Homoeopathy patients were most strongly influenced by the ineffectiveness of medicine for their complaints, a fact which was largely accounted for by the chronicity of their complaints.

Three of the factors showed significant differences between the three patient groups. Acupuncture and homoeopathy patients seemed 'put off' by the potential side-effects of medicine more than the osteopathy group. This was probably due to the nature of the problems they presented with, and possible use of drugs by their physicians. A second difference between the groups indicated that the osteopathy patients rated the availability of their therapy as more important than the other two groups. The final factor, which referred to the ineffective nature of conventional medicine, was rated most highly by the homoeopathic group, who may have complaints that are particularly resistant to conventional treatment. This would explain why group differences were no longer found after co-variates, including severity of illness, were controlled for.

Hertschel *et al.* (1996) interviewed 419 German patients, half currently using and half not using CAM, through a 168 item questionnaire. They were interested in how the two groups differed on socio-demographic lifestyle, and illness-related data as well as their illness-preventing behaviours, their psychological makeup, doctor-patient relationship and particular doctor preference. Their study was exploratory rather than hypothesis testing, though it yielded some very interesting findings.

CAM patients were more likely to be women. CAM patients were also less likely to smoke and drink and more likely to follow particular (and medical) diets. Many in the CAM group claimed to have been seriously ill, with chronic complaints. They were more likely to change their medical doctor if dissatisfied and to visit their doctor more frequently. CAM patients also spent more on everyday medication and were more willing to do so, if they believe it

TABLE 3.2:   FACTOR SCORES BY PATIENT GROUP

Factor	Acupuncture	Homoeopathy	Osteopathy	Mean	F ratio/sig
Value of complementary medicine	3.92	3.88	3.98	3.90	0.11
Poor doctor communication	2.85	2.95	2.89	2.90	0.19
Side-effects of orthodox medicine	3.05_a	3.01_b	2.67_c	2.91	4.13*
Availability of complementary medicine	2.18_a	2.37_b	2.91_c	3.66	19.2**
Orthodox medicine ineffective	3.51	3.95	3.52		7.00**

Note: letters indicate pairs of groups whose means are significantly different (p < .05) in Scheffé multiple comparisons. *p < .01; **p < .001

worked. Many reported being much more dissatisfied with conventional medicine than patients who were only seeing physicians.

The CAM patients in the study had had more experience of various types of CAM (homoeopathy, natural therapy) as well as psychotherapy than the medical patients. There was no difference in the preventative health measures of either group, however. CAM patients were also more likely to worry about contracting a serious illness and were found to be more prone to boredom, depression, loneliness and alienation. They also tended to be more pessimistic about life. CAM patients who went to both GP and CAM practitioners appeared to expect and receive more empathy from their GP and to have more faith in them than conventional medical patients. Overall patients seemed to seek CAM for migraine, depression, allergies, and skin diseases and medical care for life-threatening conditions like heart attacks, diabetes and cancer.

The authors conclude:

'The present study reveals not only that CAM users adopt a Zeitgeist oriented lifestyle, but also that chronically ill patients are often dissatisfied with conventional medical treatment. In view of the cost and risks of such treatment, the question whether such patients actually benefit from their choice of 'alternative' therapy in the long run needs to be thoroughly investigated in suitable studies.' (p. 149)

Kelner and Wellman (1997) interviewed 300 Canadian patients in total, 60 each of family physicians, chiropractors, acupuncturists, naturopaths and Reiki patients. They were from very different demographic groups.

Overall, the CAM patients, compared to the medical patients, were more likely to be female, educated, working, relatively well off and agnostic. Patients clearly went to the different specialists for different things: the chiropractor for musculoskeletal problems, the GP for cardiovascular problems and the Reiki specialist for emotional issues. Four patients of the CAM practitioners were also very frequent patients of the GPs. Indeed all patients were users of multiple therapies. The patients of chiropractors were most different, consulting for very specific problems. They conclude: 'Alternative therapies are flourishing alongside conventional medicine. What we are seeing here is a pluralistic and complementary system of health care in which patients choose the kind of practitioner they believe will best be able to help their particular problem. What we do not see is an either/or decision about which kind of practitioner is the one to consult for everything pertaining to health care'. (p. 139)

COMPARATIVE STUDIES

A number of empirical studies have been done comparing conventional medicine and CAM groups to attempt to answer specific hypotheses as to why people choose CAM. These studies have, inevitably, a number of problems associated with them, three of which are most critical.

   A. *Sampling*: Many have observed that the demography of the average CAM patient is somewhat different from that of the average GP patient. Often CAM patients are better educated, more middle class, more often female etc. Thus, when comparing the two groups we can never be certain whether differences are a result of these demographic differences, their health histories, and careers, or indeed some other factors that led them to seek out a CAM practitioner. This problem can be dealt with in one of two ways: statistically (i.e. varying out established differences between groups) or attempting to match people, which is extremely difficult and may even be unrealistic. Further, many studies have relatively small, convenience samples, restricted to one geographic region and culture group. Finally and perhaps most critical of all, nearly all CAM patients are also patients of conventional medicines; indeed some subjects recruited at GP surgeries and labelled as medical are also patients of CAM practitioners. It is therefore extremely difficult to obtain 'clean, matched' samples.

   B. *Self-Report*: Nearly all CAM studies of patients rely on self-reported beliefs and behaviours. Whilst acknowledging well established problems with self-report (faking, inability to describe motives etc), there is also the concern that subjects may be particularly biased in these studies. We know for instance that patients frequently do not admit to their GP that they are visiting a CAM practitioner – equally they do not always truthfully report to the latter how many other practitioners they are seeing. Patients may also be inclined to over-exaggerate some answers in order to reduce dissonance. For example, while attending a CAM clinic and confronted with a questionnaire about their experience of conventional medicine and their attitude to 'science', they may emphasis their disillusionment with both.

C. *Cause and Effect*: Finding a difference between groups in a cross-sectional study cannot necessarily tell us about why people chose to visit, or indeed continue visiting, a CAM practitioner. For instance, studying a difference in the mental health (minor psychiatric morbidity) between the two groups may not mean the 'unstable' are attracted to CAM. It could equally be true that chronic illness and pain have led to both psychiatric morbidity and desperate attempts to overcome it; or indeed that experience with a CAM (or medical) practitioner actually led to increased morbidity. Further, why people choose and continue with a CAM (or medical) practitioner may not be for the same reason. If it is true that people 'shop for health', it may be that their choice is as capricious and whimsical as that of a shopper for everyday pharmaceutical products.

HYPOTHESES ABOUT WHY PATIENTS CHOOSE CAM

Both speculators and researchers have provided various lists of possible reasons why people seek out CAM practitioners. These are some of the most frequently mentioned:

1. Mental Health: The psychologically less stable are attracted to the quasi-psychotherapeutic methods and philosophy of CAM (Skrabanek, 1988). Furnham & Smith (1988) and Furnham & Bhagrath (1993), using different instruments, both found evidence for the fact that matched homoeopathic patients were less well adjusted than GP patients.
2. Beliefs about Health: (Prevention of illness, resistance to disease, staying healthy). CAM is as much about prevention as cure and appeals to 'fitness freaks' and the healthy lifestyle groups. Furnham & Smith (1988), Furnham & Bhagrath (1993) and Furnham, Vincent & Wood (1995) found CAM (homoeopath) patients believed more than conventional medical patients that changes in lifestyle (diet, sleep, relaxation) were related to prevention of illness.
3. Health Consciousness: (Interest in health related issues). Those interested in all aspects of health (mental, physical, spiritual) are attracted to CAM (Gray, 1998). Furnham & Bhagrath (1993) found much evidence that CAM patients took a more active interest in health matters.

4. Perceived Susceptibility (vulnerability) to Illness: those who feel they may be particularly vulnerable to specific illnesses (possibly psychosomatic) are attracted to CAM. Furnham & Bhagrath (1993) and Furnham & Smith (1998) found no evidence that CAM patients thought they were more susceptible to a large number of everyday illnesses.

5. Beliefs in the Efficacy of Treatment: CAM patients are naive, uninformed, optimistic or simply gullible because they do not know the lack of acceptable evidence for the efficacy of the treatment (Cassileth, 1980). Furnham & Smith (1988) and Furnham & Bhagrath (1993) found CAM (homeopathy) patients rather more sceptical than medical patients about their treatment. Indeed, CAM patients believe less in the efficacy of their practitioner and the rapid termination of treatment – no doubt because of the chronic nature of their illness and many disappointments in the past.

6. Personal Control over Health: Conventional medical patients are health fatalists and CAM patients health instrumentalists. That is, CAM patients believe they have more personal control over their health than other patients. Although results do not replicate perfectly, there does seem sufficient evidence that CAM patients believe more strongly in self rather than provider control over personal health (Furnham & Bhagrath, 1993; Furnham, Vincent & Wood, 1995; Vincent, Furnham & Willsmore, 1995).

7. Medical History and Career: The particular medical history of patients characterized by chronic, painful and unsuccessfully treated problems (eg back pain) leads them, in desperation, to seek out CAM cures. This is a seriously under-researched area and may well give the greatest clues as to why people seek out CAM practitioners.

8. Beliefs about Scientific (evidence-based) Medicine: Patients are post-modernists (Gray, 1998); they are highly sceptical of the approaches, motives and success rate of conventional biomedicine. Furnham, Vincent & Wood (1995) and Vincent, Furnham & Willsmore (1995) found that CAM patients had not lost their faith in science but compared to medical patients, did indeed believe less in the scientific basis of medical science. Further, CAM patients stressed more than medical patients the role of psychological factors in illness and the many potential harmful side-effects of modern medicine.

9. Attitude to physicians: Deep disenchantment about the style and efficacy of GPs, particularly their bedside manner and poor communication skills. Furnham, Vincent & Wood (1995) found that compared to medical patients, CAM patients were less likely to believe that GPs are sympathetic, have time to listen, are sensitive to emotional issues and are good at explaining the nature of the treatment or why an individual is ill.

CONCLUSION

To talk of patients of CAM practitioners as a homogeneous group is funda-mentally wrong. Patients consulting different types of complementary and alternative practitioners hold different beliefs about their own health, and hold differing levels of scepticism about conventional medicine. Patients differ by degrees in their health beliefs and scepticism about conventional medicine, and do not fall neatly into two distinct groups. It would also seem to be incorrect to talk of patients simply being 'pushed' or 'pulled' toward CAM therapies, as scepticism of the efficacy of GPs and orthodox medicine is combined with greater concern for the planet, healthier lifestyles, greater belief in the import-ance of state of mind, and greater concern with the nature of the consultation. It is this combination, together with their particular medical history, that leads patients to consult CAM practitioners.

Certainly what the research literature appears to indicate is that many CAM patients are more health conscious, take more responsibility for their own health and believe less in fate, luck and chance and appreciate the style and method of CAM practitioners.

It is, however, quite possible that the beliefs and knowledge of those *pulled* or attracted by CAM are quite different, at least initially, to those *pushed* or disenchanted with conventional medicine. It may be hypothesized that com-pared to the more desperate 'pushed' category, the 'pulled' are more likely to be knowledgeable, middle-class adults, with a well-developed consumer-attitude to being a patient.

The growth in both demand and supply of CAM is a phenomenon that has taken both medical practitioners and researchers by surprise. The hubris of post-war medicine based on important and dramatic recoveries has been severely damaged by the sight of thousands of patients seeking 'non-scientific' cures. But patients who pay for CAM are clearly getting something that conventional medicine is not providing (or perhaps cannot or will not). The whole question of pathways to care and cures is certainly one that requires good, multidisciplinary and international research.

Whilst there appear to be very similar findings regarding CAM in developed, Westernized industrial cultures, results may be very different in developing third world cultures. Thus Furnham and Baguma (1999), in a study of health beliefs in East Africa (Uganda), found Ugandans believing that sophisticated, Western, orthodox medicine (that they did not have ready access to) was perhaps the most crucial factor in maintaining their health and preventing illness. In a sense, one can only be disillusioned with something one has had extensive experience of. Whilst developing countries frequently have a thriving 'folk medicine' sector, it may be predicted that they would be far less sceptical of modern biomedicine than people in developed countries. Certainly this is a promising avenue for further research.

REFERENCES

Annandale, E. and Hunt, K. 1998. Accounts of disagreement with doctors. *Social Science and Medicine*, 46:119–129.

Aakster C. 1986. Concepts in alternative Medicine. *Social Science and Medicine*, 22:265–273.

Anderson E, Anderson P. 1987. General practitioners and alternative medicine. *Journal of the Royal College of General Practitioners*, 37(295):52–55.

Astin J. 1988. Why patients use alternative medicine: Results of a national study. *Journal of the American Medical Association*, 279:1548–1953.

Bakx K. 1991. The 'eclipse' of folk medicine in western society. *Sociology of Health and Illness*, 13.

Baum M. 1989. Rationalism versus irrationalism in the care of the sick: science versus the absurd (editorial). *Medical Journal of Australia*, 151(11–12):607–608.

BMA 1993. *Complementary medicine*, Report of the Board of Science and Education.

Boon H. 1998.. Canadian naturopathic practitioners: Holistic and scientific world views. *Social Science and Medicine*, 46:1213–1225.

Budd C., Fisher B., Parruder D. and Price L. 1990. A model of cooperation between complementary and allopathic medicine in a primary care setting. *British Journal of General Practice*, 40(338):376–378.

Bullock M., Pheley A., Kiresuk T., Lenz S. and Culliton P. 1997. Characteristics and complaints of patients seeking therapy at a hospital-based alternative medicine clinic. *Journal of Alternative and Complementary Medicine*, 3:31–37.

Cant S., Calnan M. 1991. On the margins of the medical market place? An exploratory study of alternative practitioners' perceptions. *Sociology of Health and Illness* 13:46–66.

Canter D., Nanke L. 1989. Emerging priorities in complementary medical research. *Complementary Medical Research*, 3:14–21.

Canter D., Nanke L. 1991. Psychological aspects of complementary medicine. Paper presented at University of Keele, January.

Cassileth B.R., Zuphis R.V. Sutton-Smith K., March V. 1980. Information & participation preferences among cancer patients. *Annals & Internal Medicine* 92(6): 832–6.

Cassileth B.R. 1986. 'Unorthodox Cancer Medicine', *Cancer Invetigation* 4(6): 591–8.

Cassileth B. 1988. The social implications of questionable cancer therapies. *Cancer*, 63(7):1247–1250.

Donnelly W., Spykerboer S., and Thong Y. 1985. Are patients who use alternative medicine dissatisfied with orthodox medicine? *Medical Journal of Australia*, 142(10):539–541.

Downer S., Cody M., Mcluskey P., Wilson P., Arnott S., Lister T. and Slevin M. 1994. Pursuit and practice of complementary therapies by cancer patients receiving conventional treatment. *British Medical Journal*, 309:86–89.

Eisenberg D., Kessler R.C. and Foster C. 1993. Unconventional medicine in the United States. *New England Journal of Medicine*, 328:246–252.

Ernst E. 1996. *Complementary medicine: An objective appraisal*. London:Butterworth Heinemann.

Ernst E. and Furnham A. 1998. BMW sales and complementary medicine: Cause or correlation. Unpublished paper.

Ernst E., Resch K-L. and White A. 1995. Complementary medicine: what physicians think of it. *Archives of International Medicine*, 155:2405–2408.

Ernst E., Willoughby M. and Weihmayr T. 1995. Nine possible reasons for choosing complementary medicine. *Perfusion*, 8:356–359.

Finnigan M.1991. The Centre for the Study of Complementary Medicine: An attempt to understand its popularity through psychological, demographic and operational criteria. *Complementary Medical Research* 5:83–88.

Foucault M. 1979. *Discipline and Punishment*, Harmondsworth, Middlesex: Penguin.

Fulder S.J. and Munro R.E. 1985. Complementary medicine in the United Kingdom: patients, practitioners, and consultations. *Lancet* 2(8454):542–545.

Furnham A. 1986. Medical students' beliefs about five different specialities, *British Medical Journal*, 293:1067–1680.

—- 1993. Attitudes to alternative medicine: a study of the perception of those studying orthodox medicine. *Complementary Therapies in Medicine*, 1:120–126.

— 1994. Explaining health and illness. *Social Science and Medicine*, 39:715–725.

— 1997a. Why do people choose and use complementary therapies? in E. Ernst (ed.) *Complementary Medicine: An Objective Approach* (pp. 71–88), London: Butterworth-Heinemann.

— 1997b. Flight from science: alternative medicine, post modernism and relativism. in R. Fuller, P. Walsh and P. Mcginley (eds.) *A Century of Psychology*. pp. 171–191 London: Routledge.

Furnham A., Baguma F. 1999. Cross-cultural differences in explanations for health and illness. *Mental Health, Religion and Culture*. 2, 121–134.

Furnham A., Bhagrath R. 1993. A comparison of health beliefs and behaviours of clients of orthodox and complementary medicine. *British Journal of Clinical Psychology*, 32:237–46.

Furnham A. and Forey J. 1994. The attitudes, behaviours and beliefs of patients of conventional vs complementary (alternative) medicine. *Journal of Clinical Psychology*, 50:458–469.

Furnham A. and Kirkcaldy B. 1995. The health beliefs and behaviours of orthodox and complementary medicine clients. *British Journal of Clinical Psychology*, 25:49–61.

Furnham A. and Smith C. 1988. Choosing alternative medicine: a comparison of the beliefs of patients visiting a GP and a homeopath. *Social Science and Medicine*, 26:685–687.

Furnham A., Hanna D. and Vincent C. 1995. Medical students' attitudes to complementary medical therapies. *Complementary Therapies in Medicine*, 3:212–219.

Furnham A., Vincent C. and Wood R. 1995. The health beliefs and behaviours of three groups of complementary medicine and a general practice group of patients. *Journal of Alternative and Complementary Medicine* 1:347–359.

Gaus W. and Hogel J. 1995. Studies on the efficacy of unconventional therapies:Problems and design. *Drug Research*, 45:88–92.

Gray R. 1998. Four perspectives on unconventional therapies. *Health*, 2:55–74.

Greenblatt R., Hollander H., McMaster J. and Henke C. 1991. Polypharmacy among patients attending an AIDS clinic. *Journal of Acquired Immune Deficiency Syndrome*, 4:136–143.

Gursoy A.1996. Beyond the orthodox: Heresy in medicine and the social sciences from a cross-cultural perspective. *Social Science and Medicine*, 43:577–592.

Harre R. and Krausz M. 1996. *Varieties of Relativism*, Oxford: Blackwell.

Hertschel C., Kohnen R. Hauser G. Lindner M., Haln E. and Ernst E. 1996. Complementary medicine today: Patient decision for physician or magician. *European Journal of Physical Medicine and Rehabilitation*, 6:144–150.

Hewer W. 1983. The relationship between the alternative practitioner and his patient. A review. *Psychotherapy and Psychosomatics*, 40(1–4):172–180.

Kelner, M., and Wellman, B. 1997.. Who seeks alternative care? A profile of the users of five modes of treatment. *Journal of Alternative and Complementary Medicine*, 3, 127–140.

Knipschild P. 1988. Looking for gall bladder disease in the patient's iris. *British Medical Journal*, 297(6663):1578–1581.

Knipschild P., Kleijnen J. and Ter-Riet G. 1990. Belief in the efficacy of alternative medicine among general practitioners in The Netherlands. *Social Science and Medicine*, 31(5):625–626.

Levin J. and Coreil J. 1986. 'New age' healing in the U.S. *Social Science and Medicine*, 23(9):889–897.

Lewith G.T. and Aldridge D.A. 1991. *Complementary medicine and the European Community*. Saffron Walden, Essex: C.W. Daniel.

Lupton D. 1997. Consumerism, reflexivity and the medical encounter. *Social Science and Medicine*, 45:373–381.

Lynse N. 1989. Theoretical and empirical problems in the assessment of alternative medical technologies. *Scandinavian Journal of Social Medicine*, 17:257–263.

McKee J. 1988. Holistic health and the critique of Western medicine. *Social Science and Medicine*, 26:775–785.

Moore J., Phipps K., Marcer D. and Lewith G.T. 1985. Why do people seek treatment by alternative medicine? *British Medical Journal*, 290(6461):28–29.

Murray J, Shepherd S. 1988. Alternative or additional medicine? An exploratory study in general practice. *Social Science and Medicine*, 37:983–988.

Reilly D.T. 1983. Young doctors' views on alternative medicine. *British Medical Journal*, 287(6388):337–339.

Sharma U. 1992. *Complementary medicine today: Practitioners and patients*. London: Routledge.

Skrabanek P. 1988. Paranormal health claims. *Experientia*, 44(4):303–309.

Smith T. 1983. Alternative medicine (editorial). *British Medical Journal*, 287(6388):307–308.

Stalker D. and Glymore L. 1989. (eds) *Examining Holistic Medicine*. Buffalo, NY: Promotheus.

Strong P. 1979. Sociological imperialism and the medical profession. *Social Science and Medicine*, 13:199–211.

Taylor R. 1985. Alternative medicine and the medical encounter in Britain and the United States. In: Salmon J, Warren P, eds. *Alternative Medicine: Prejudice and Policy Perspectives* (pp. 191–221) London: Tavistock.

Thomas K.J., Carr J., Westlake L. and Williams B.T. 1991. Use of non-orthodox and conventional health care in Great Britain. *British Medical Journal*, 302(6770):207–210.

Turner B. 1987. *Medical Power and Social Knowledge*, London: Sage.

Vecchio P. 1994. Attitudes to alternative medicine by rheumatology outpatient attenders. *Journal of Rheumatology*, 21:145–147.

Verhoef M., Sutherland L. and Birkich L. 1990. Use of alternative medicine by patients attending a gastroenterology clinic. *Canadian Medical Association Journal*, 142:121–125.

Vincent C. and Furnham A. 1994. The perceived efficacy of complementary and orthodox medicine. *Complementary Therapies in Medicine*, 2:128–134.

—– 1996. Why do patients turn to complementary medicine? An empirical study. *British Journal of Clinical Psychology*, 35:37–48.

Vincent C., Furnham A. and Willsmore M. 1995. The perceived efficacy of complementary and orthodox medicine in complementary and general practice patients. *Health Education Research*, 10:395–405.

Vincent C. and Furnham A. 1997. *Complementary Medicine: A Research Perspective*. Chichester: Wiley.

Visser E., Peters L. and Rasker J. 1992. Rheumatologists and their patients who seek alternative care: An agreement to disagree. *British Journal of Rheumatology*, 31:488–490.

Wharton R. and Lewith G. 1986. Complementary medicine and the general practitioner. *British Medical Journal*, 292(6534):1498–1500.

Williams S, Calnan M. 1996. The 'limits' of medicalization? Modern medicine and the lay populace on 'late' modernity. *Social Science and Medicine*, 42:1609–1620.

CHAPTER 4

The Therapeutic Relationship Under Fire

MERRIJOY KELNER

The relationship between doctors and their patients is currently receiving a great deal of attention. Plays, films and books are featuring the travails of patients who seek medical care and depicting physicians as emotionally distant, abrupt, pompous, insensitive and even incompetent (Consider for example: *Wit* an off-Broadway hit play by Margaret Elson, *Patch Adams* a film starring Robin Williams, and a recent Canadian book, *Operating in the Dark* by Lisa Priest). Indictments of medicine and the physicians that practice it are cropping up everywhere in North America, the United Kingdom and Europe. The notion that something is seriously lacking in the doctor-patient-relationship seems to have become thoroughly embedded in contemporary Western culture (Pietroni, 1987).

At the same time that patients are criticizing the way their physicians relate to them, we are witnessing a remarkable and widespread surge of interest in complementary & alternative medicine (CAM) and an increasing use of CAM practitioners (Eisenberg *et al.*, 1993, 1998; McGregor and Peay, 1996; Lloyd *et al.*, 1991; Thomas *et al.*, 1991; Mills and Peacock, 1997; Lewith and Aldridge, 1993; CTV/Angus Reid Group, 1997). One of the reasons that has been cited for the current attraction to CAM practitioners is that they are more empathic and collaborative than physicians and take a greater interest in the individual psycho-social aspects of their patients' lives (Bakx, 1991; Oths, 1994). Patients are said to choose CAM practitioners because they seek a more satisfying therapeutic relationship (Brinkhaus *et al.*, 1998). It has also been suggested that the high degree of rapport that exists between the alternative practitioner and his/her patient has a powerful placebo effect and may indeed be the key factor in the ability of these practitioners to help their patients (Ernst, 1995). However, the assumption that CAM patients have more positive and valuable relationships with their practitioners than do patients of family physicians has not yet been subjected to rigorous research

(Mitchell and Cormack, 1998). It is a notion that requires serious examination rather than stereotypical thinking.

This paper will explore the nature of the therapeutic relationship between patients of family physicians and patients of selected alternative practitioners and compare the way these two sets of patients perceive and describe their practitioners. Based on the assumptions noted above, it can be expected that patients of CAM practitioners will be more likely to describe their therapeutic relationships in a positive manner and to depict them as collaborative, empathic and personal.

MODELS

Models of the therapeutic relationship have been developed almost exclusively on the basis of the doctor-patient-relationship. The three most commonly mentioned models are: the paternalistic, the shared decision-making, and the consumerist. This paper looks not only at the doctor-patient-relationship, but also at patient relationships with a range of alternative practitioners, and examines the extent to which the existing models can be applied to them.

The models reflect a variety of therapeutic relationships and assume different degrees of importance depending on what is happening in the society as a whole. As values shift, information explodes, chronic illnesses increase and health care costs keep rising, models that were useful for understanding therapeutic relationships in the past, become less applicable. Now they need to be modified and expanded in order to more accurately reveal the dynamics of these relationships in the current environment.

The Paternalistic model

Beginning in the 1950's, Parsons (1951) posited the relationship between physicians and their patients as the functional interplay between two social roles with inherent duties and responsibilities. The patient assumes a 'sick role' which exempts her/him from the normal obligations of life, but in turn, is obliged to comply with the physician's prescribed treatment and to strive to recover. While the patient always has the option to refuse treatment, s/he is not involved in the process of choosing among treatment options; the physician decides on the preferred option and then presents it to the patient. Parsons later revised his model to acknowledge the patient's participation in decision-making in the context of chronic illness (Parsons, 1975), but he still viewed the relationship as essentially a paternalistic one.

Paternalism, or medical professional dominance as it has been called by some, (Freidson, 1970; Phillips, 1996) means that the physician can override the choices of the patient when he/she judges that it is for the patient's own good. Authority is granted to the physician by the patient because of his/her expert technical knowledge; knowledge that is not available to the patient. The physician 'owns' the technical expertise, while the patient's knowledge of the situation is discounted as irrelevant. Gender, age, educational and ethnic differences usually serve to exacerbate this imbalance of power (Haug, 1979; Emanuel and Emanuel, 1992). In this model of the therapeutic relationship, physician-patient interaction is said to be characterized by limited and didactic communication on the part of the physician, reluctance to give sufficient information to the patient about his/her condition, the use of medical jargon in discussions with the patient, and evasion of direct questions about diagnosis or treatment (Skipper, 1965).

The shared decision-making model

Szasz and Hollender (1956) have termed this the model of mutual participation. In this shared approach, the physician's expertise lies in his/her clinical knowledge, while the patient's expertise stems from knowledge of the contextual facts about his/her own personal situation. The role of the physician is to assist the patient (or the client) to make the treatment choice that is most appropriate through an understanding of how the medical information relates to his/her unique situation. This kind of encounter is particularly suited to the management of most chronic illnesses, where the patient's own experiences provide important clues for therapy. The patient accepts responsibility for carrying out changes in lifestyle recommended by the practitioner as part of the therapy. Such a model requires that there be ongoing dialogue between physician and patient (Katz, 1984). Several authors have delineated variations on the shared decision-making model. Some of the best known are the contractual model outlined by Veatch (1972), Emmanuel and Emmanuel's (1995) deliberative model and the conversation model advanced by Katz (1984).

This model developed as a reaction to medical paternalism, encouraged by concurrent social movements such as the growing emphasis on individual rights, the civil rights movement of 1960's, the feminist movement, and the general rise of consumerism in public life (Light, 1991; Reeder, 1972; Cogswell, 1988). In this model, the basis of the relationship is a collaborative enterprise between physician and patient in which consultation precedes decision-making and information is widely shared.

While there seems to be considerable demand from the public for this more collaborative approach to the doctor-patient-relationship, there is empirical evidence that physicians do not always find it easy to share power and decision-making (McKinlay and Stoeckle, 1988). This lack of congruence between patient expectations of the therapeutic relationship and what doctors are actually able to provide often leads to frustration on the part of physicians and dissatisfaction among patients (Taussig, 1980).

medical care (family physicians) through a popular form of physical manipulation (chiropractors) and mixed holistic care (acupuncture/traditional Chinese medicine and naturopathy) to care characterized mainly by emotional and spiritual healing (Reiki). The choice of alternative practitioners was designed to reflect the spread from the most widely accepted and legitimate (chiropractic) through to one of the least well known and least institutionalized (Reiki). For a description of the methodology used, see Kelner and Wellman, 1997a&b[2].

COMPARING THE SAMPLE OF PATIENTS

Demographic characteristics – A comparison of the demographic characteristics of those who were consulting alternative practitioners with people who were seeing family physicians for their primary health problem, reveals that there are marked differences between the two groups of patients (see Kelner and Wellman, 1997a).

The patients consulting alternative practitioners are more likely to be female, young, married, highly educated, in higher level occupations, more likely to be employed full time and to have high incomes. Patients who consult alternative practitioners are also more likely to report their ethnic origin as Canadian, to have no formal religious affiliation but on the other hand, to consider spirituality an important factor in their lives. This demographic profile of patients of alternative practitioners is consistent with other research in Canada, the United States and in the United Kingdom (Wellman, 1995; CTV/Angus Reid Group, 1997; Blais, 1997; Eisenberg *et al.*, 1993; Thomas *et al.*, 1991; Sharma, 1992; Vincent and Furnham, 1997). The key identifying social characteristics in the work of these scholars are gender, level of education, occupational level, social class and age. The fact that patients of family physicians are not as well educated or as affluent as CAM patients implies that they will adopt a more deferential, less independent stance in their therapeutic relationships.

Primary health problems – There are also differences in the type of health problems reported by the two groups of patients. Patients of family physicians most frequently mentioned life threatening problems such as heart problems, high blood pressure and high cholesterol while none of the alternative patients reported cardiovascular conditions as their main reason for seeking care from their practitioners. Patients consulting alternative practitioners were seeing them for chronic conditions like musculoskeletal problems, headaches and for health maintenance. In a national survey of the health conditions of patients of alternative practitioners in the United States, Eisenberg *et al.* (1993, 1998) confirm that most conditions are minor and chronic, with musculoskeletal problems being the most common presenting problem. Since the health problems of family physician patients are more life threatening and worrisome than the chronic complaints of CAM patients, these health problems may influence patient expectations and their reliance on the expertise and authority of their physicians.

As might be expected, there were also variations between the alternative groups, For example, patients of chiropractors were most likely to seek care for musculoskeletal problems and patients of Reiki practitioners were most apt to be concerned about their emotional health and maintaining and improving their overall well-being. The patients of naturopathic practitioners reported the broadest range of ailments, including colds, flu, allergies, chronic infections and gynaecological troubles

The CAM patients in the study used medical care as a supplement rather than a substitute for their alternative care; 82% of them said they saw their family physician at least once a year for checkups, colds and flu, monitoring of medications and any life-threatening illnesses that might occur. Most of them (88%) said they were happy with their family physicians in general, but that they had been unable to resolve the specific problem for which they were currently seeking help. In the light of these differences of social characteristics and health profiles, this study asks whether there are also differences in the therapeutic relationship that these patients are experiencing with their physicians or CAM practitioners.

COMPARING THE NATURE OF THE THERAPEUTIC RELATIONSHIP

Family physicians and their patients

A typical setting for the doctor patient relationship is formal and often institutional. The physician wears a white coat and practices in a professional office with a receptionist or nurse who sees the patients first. When patients are ushered into their physician's office, the doctor usually sits behind a desk and takes control of the interaction, posing a series of questions to the patient allowing little time for response. If a physical examination is required, patients move to another room, usually removing at least some of their clothing, and then return to the doctor's office to learn their diagnosis and hear the recommended treatment. This kind of setting contributes to social distance and establishes the physician's authority in the healing process.

Despite this portrayal, most of the family physicians' patients in this study reported that they had a positive relationship with their doctors. Most of their relationships developed over a long period of time (mean number of years = 9.7 and the median = 7.0). Close to one fifth (18%) of them had been seeing the same physician for 20 years or more. Over the years, it was quite clear that the patients had built up an association based on shared health experiences and the ease that stems from repeated encounters. These patients did not consult their doctors often, however; as one patient put it: 'He wouldn't make a living on how many times we went to him'. Forty per cent of the patients of family physicians said that in the past, they had seen them only once or twice a year for routine visits or for emergencies, although they were now seeing them more frequently because their current problem was causing them considerable discomfort and anxiety (almost half of them, 48%, were going as often as once a month or more). The family physicians' patients reported that they had been suffering with their problem for a while; the mean number of years was 6.6 and the median was 3.0. Thus, the data show that the typical physician-patient relationship is characterized by repeated visits over long periods of time rather than by frequent encounters in a short period of time.

This group of patients reported good working relationships with their family physicians. Almost all of them (90%) said that their physician had fully met their expectations. The vast majority (88%) reported that their family physicians were always willing to answer their questions and over three quarters of them (78%) said they were given clear and complete explanations about treatments. Most (83%) felt that their physician understood their perspective on their health problem.

When it came to explaining the potential side effects of recommended therapies, satisfaction was not as high; only 58% said that their family physician always did this. Under half (48%) of the patients felt that their physicians were willing to involve them in decision-making about their health care. Nevertheless, an overwhelming majority (92%) said they would recommend their doctor to others with similar problems.

When asked why they thought their physician was helping them, these patients gave several reasons. The most frequently cited (43%) was that they had trust in the doctor's diagnostic knowledge, authority and technical skills as well as in the medications he/she had recommended. One patient put it like this: 'My doctor is a man I trust; he knows what he's doing and he does it well'. The next most often (38%) mentioned reason was that they had a sense of rapport with their doctor. This rapport, they said, was based on their belief that the physician was supportive and interested in learning the facts about their health problems. As one patient said 'My doctor is caring and understanding. He has helped me through my crises '.

Finally, the patients were asked who they thought would be the most helpful with their health problems in general. A majority (70%) of the family physician patients said that they relied primarily on their doctors to help them. These patients can be described as having an external locus of control (Wallston *et al.*, 1976) They feel that their health is beyond their personal control and rely on fate or powerful others, particularly physicians. Just over one quarter (27%) mentioned themselves, or themselves in partnership with their doctors, as the persons they would find most helpful. When asked to explain why they thought their physician was the most helpful person, trust in his/her training and medical expertise was the most frequent response. They also mentioned the fact that doctors can refer patients to the best specialists when they are needed and that their physician has known them for a long time and is thus in a good position to help them.

The surprising finding here is that so many patients of family physicians reported that they had a good sense of rapport with them. In contrast to the studies cited above, where patients complained of a lack of interest and impersonal treatment, this was not the case for the family physicians' patients in this study.

How do these findings compare to the way the CAM patients describe their relationships with their practitioner?

CAM practitioners and their patients

CAM practitioners are not a homogeneous group; their practice patterns differ according to type of modality and also within each modality. Nevertheless, for purposes of analysis, the four types of CAM practitioners are mainly treated here as one group, although from time to time, the more striking differences between them are identified.

In comparison to the settings of the physician-patient encounter, CAM practitioners meet their patients in a less formal and structured environment. The practitioner may practice in an office or at home (chiropractors are more likely than homeopaths or Reiki healers to work in offices), but even in offices, the ambience is informal, with personal touches provided by signs and childrens' drawings on the walls. Most CAM practitioners eschew white coats and present themselves in a more informal manner. Some do not even use a desk, but prefer to sit close to their patients without any barriers between them. History taking, diagnosis and treatment often take place in the same room and the whole interaction seems more like a visit than a consultation.

The CAM patients in the study had been seeing their practitioners for a much shorter length of time than was the case for patients of family physicians (mean = 3.2 and median = 1.0). This difference can be attributed, at least in part, to the recent growth of interest in using alternative health care. A recent Canadian poll (CTV/Angus Reid Group, 1997) reveals that of the 42% of Canadians now using alternatives, just under one half (49%) had started using them within the last five years. Another factor that may explain the shorter duration of the relationship between the CAM patients and their practitioners is that the patients had been trying various kinds of treatments to resolve their chronic problems without receiving much respite and had only recently decided to try this particular type of practitioner. As an acupuncture patient told us 'This whole sequence of events, going from one doctor to another has been going on for about ten years. I've only recently been seeing the acupuncturist, but I've always believed my problem was solvable'. The pattern for CAM patients seems to be that most had suffered with their primary health problems for a considerably longer period of time than the patients of family physicians (mean = 9.2 and median = 5.0). This suggests that they had already tried a number of other kinds of practitioners without finding relief.

What the relationships between CAM patients and their practitioners lacked in duration, they made up for in frequency of contact. CAM patients had not been consulting their practitioners for as long a period of time, but the frequency of their visits was much greater than it is for the patients of family physicians. When CAM patients began their treatments, the frequency of visits tended to be much higher at the beginning, compared to later in the treatment process. The data reflect this pattern by showing that in the past, more than half (52%) of the group of CAM patients in the study saw their practitioners at least once a week. Currently, only 29% were visiting them that frequently, while another quarter (25%) were seeing them a few times a month. The frequency of these visits is related to the type of problem as well as the type of treatment. For example, patients of chiropractors and acupuncture/traditional Chinese doctors see them more often than do patients of naturopaths and Reiki healers, and they typically suffer more from chronic pain. The fact that most kinds of CAM treatments require repeated visits, creates a situation that fosters the development of personal relationships quickly.

The data make it clear that the relationships between doctors and their patients and CAM patients and their practitioners evolve over different time periods and entail different degrees of frequency.

Like the family physician patients, the CAM patients expressed high levels of satisfaction with their current practitioners; 86% of the total group felt that their practitioner was fully meeting their expectations. There were, however, some variations between the CAM groups; more of the patients of chiropractors (90%) and Reiki practitioners (98%) reported that they were fully satisfied than did the other CAM patients.

Most CAM patients (85%) said that their practitioner always was willing to answer their questions; close to three quarters of them (71%) reported that their practitioners always gave them clear explanations about their health problems; just under half of them (47%) found that their practitioner always explained the side effects of their treatments; most (82%) felt that their practitioner understood their perspective very well and 60% reported that their practitioner always involved them in the decisions about their treatment. Almost all (94%) agreed that they would recommend their practitioner to others with similar problems.

Variations between the different groups of CAM patients were evident in these assessments of practitioners. The clients of Reiki healers were most likely to report that their practitioner fully met their expectations and in most cases it was the Reiki practitioners who ranked highest on issues such as answering questions, understanding the patient's perspective and involving patients in decision making. At the other end of the spectrum were the acupuncturists/traditional Chinese doctors who ranked lower on these questions than the rest of the CAM practitioners.

When asked why they thought their practitioner was helping them, the responses of the CAM patients were much more pragmatic than the patients of family physicians. Over half (53%) said it was because they were seeing positive results. As a chiropractic patient said: 'Now I can finally turn my head. He's getting to the root of the problem and not just treating symptoms'. A Reiki client put it this way: 'After the treatment I feel better, looser – as if I have just had a lubrication job in my joints'.

Less than one quarter (22%) of the CAM patients in the study cited trust in the practitioner's skills and knowledge as the principal reason they believed they were being helped; next most often mentioned was rapport (16%), followed by a natural/holistic approach. Differences between the various alternatives were again evident; over three quarters (78%) of the patients of chiropractors mentioned positive results, compared to about one third of the patients of naturopaths (37%) and Reiki healers (30%). The lower ranking of Reiki on the dimension of positive results is particularly interesting in view of the high levels of satisfaction with Reiki practitioners reported above. Clearly, there were other, perhaps more personal reasons for this satisfaction.

The patients of CAM practitioners had more independent and self reliant views than the family physician patients concerning who they believed would be the most helpful with their health problems. Only one fifth (20%) of CAM patients specifically mentioned a physician and only 6% mentioned a practitioner with a natural or holistic approach. The majority (65%) said they would rely most on themselves, or on themselves plus a health care provider of one kind or another. A Reiki patient explained that: 'I left my doctor and went to an alternative because he didn't like the fact that I was a thinker. Most of these doctors don't like people who think and want to take care of themselves. It's that sort of feeling that drove me to find an alternative'.

This belief of patients in their own ability to influence their health has been described as an internal health locus of control (Roter, 1977; Wallston et al., 1976). People who have this kind of orientation perceive their health status as largely under their own personal control. CAM patients reported more confidence in their own ability to influence their health. It was patients of Reiki practitioners who most often expressed this trust in themselves as healer

(58% self, and 22% self plus a practitioner), and they also reported the least faith in doctors as healers (only 8%). Patients of chiropractors showed the least faith in themselves (25%) or themselves plus the practitioner (25%) as resolvers of their health problems.

The CAM patients explained their reliance on themselves in several ways. They believed the primary responsibility for decisions about their own care rested with themselves and that they were the ones who could best practice prevention. They argued that each kind of practitioner has distinctive skills and expertise and that they wanted to select different healing options, depending on their particular situation. They claimed that self-knowledge assists healing and declared that because they knew their own bodies best, they trusted their own judgement more than the judgement of anyone else. This faith in their own instincts and knowledge of their bodies was largely responsible for the tendency to demphasize the place of trust in their relationships with their CAM practitioners.

CAM patients reported that they typically worked as partners with their practitioners in the healing process. Most CAM practitioners employ a holistic approach to treatment which focuses on the emotional and spiritual well-being of their patients, as well as their physical health. They also see each patient as unique, requiring individual assessment and treatment. They rely on input from their patients to keep them informed about changes in lifestyles, moods and attitudes. The CAM patients said their practitioners knew their situations intimately and tried to tailor their advice to fit the patient's life, rather than expecting him/her to adapt to a standard set of recommendations. In turn, CAM patients played their part in the healing process by accepting responsibility for their own care; they were more likely than physician patients to pay attention to their diet, posture, sleep patterns and exercise regimens.

Although both groups of patients expressed satisfaction with their current practitioners, they frequently had negative comments about the relationships they had with the health care providers they had seen in the past (mainly specialist physicians but also some CAM practitioners).

PAST EXPERIENCE

Reasons for dissatisfaction with past therapeutic relations related both to patients' expectations about receiving help and also to the way they were treated. They complained that their previous physicians or CAM practitioners were unable to give them relief from their health problems, or that the help they received was only short-lived. Other complaints, directed primarily at medical specialists, included inadequate or mistaken diagnoses, not being listened to or treated with respect, being rushed, lack of interest in their specific situation and too great a reliance on drugs and surgery instead of trying to get to the root of the problem.

For example, a woman who was currently consulting a Reiki practitioner told us 'I went to see this neurologist; he was supposed to be so good, and I wrote down a list of the symptoms I had and everything. – He didn't even look at it. I was there all of five minutes. – he just handed the list back to me and was writing out a prescription for me, for nerves or something. I tore out of there and I tore up his prescription. He didn't even listen to my problem, you know '.

The fact that the patients expressed considerable dissatisfaction with their previous health care providers is not surprising. If they had received the help they sought and had been able to develop a positive therapeutic relationship they would not have decided to look elsewhere. What we do not know is how the patients will feel in the future about their current physicians or CAM practitioners if they fail to meet their expectations. This research captures patients at only one point in their search for improved health and thus can not reveal the whole story.

DISCUSSION

Physicians and their patients relate to one another within the framework of the biomedical model, whereas CAM practitioners relate to their patients within a more holistic framework. Yet this study shows that in some ways, the relationships between CAM patients and their practitioners do not differ much from the relationships between family physician patients and their doctors. Both groups reported overall satisfaction with their health care providers and said they would recommend them to others. Both groups found care givers who will usually answer their questions, give them explanations, understand their perspective and to a lesser extent, involve them in decisions concerning their health care. It is important to remember that the respondents for this study were recruited in the offices of their health care providers and are thus likely to be satisfied consumers. Unfortunately, we do not know how those who have departed due to dissatisfaction would feel about their caregivers.

Where the two groups of respondents differed most was in the basis for their satisfaction. While only a small percentage of the physician patients were getting positive results from their current treatment, most of them nevertheless expressed trust in the skills and expertise of their doctors and some also mentioned rapport with them as an important element in the healing process. The CAM patients, on the other hand, placed most emphasis on positive results such as less pain and discomfort. Their relationships with their practitioners were largely pragmatic; if the practitioners could help them, they would continue to see them; if not, they would move on to try another practitioner or another kind of therapy.

The other major difference between the groups of patients was the role they saw for themselves in the healing relationship. While almost all respondents expected to have input into decisions about their care, there were differences in emphasis. Most family physician patients believed that their doctors should play the key role. CAM patients, on the other hand, typically believed each patient should have the main responsibility for their own health and decisions about which kind of treatment to pursue. Whereas physicians' patients favoured provider-control and placed their trust in their doctors, CAM patients more often favoured self-control and placed their confidence in themselves, or in themselves in partnership with their practitioners.

These findings indicate that the popularity of CAM practitioners can be attributed in large part to the search for relief from persisting chronic conditions. These patients want a practitioner who can help them cope with their ongoing problems. While physicians have had extraordinary successes with many acute illnesses such as polio, pneumonia and heart conditions, they have not been able to offer much assistance to their patients who suffer with chronic problems. Medicine continues to rely on its existing armamentarium of solutions such as drugs and surgery for conditions which require different and less drastic approaches. Physicians often discourage patients from presenting painful chronic conditions as their primary problems because there is little they can do to help.

The explanation presented at the beginning of this chapter that it is the more intimate and sympathetic style of interaction employed by CAM practitioners that explains their popularity was not upheld by the findings. Instead, they emphasize the continuing search for relief from chronic problems. This finding throws doubt on the claim that it is the response of CAM patients to their practitioners' holistic interest in them that is the chief reason for the ability of CAM to help chronic illness. While there is no question that patients' perceptions of the nature of the therapeutic relationship can have a significant influence on the outcome of their treatments, all kinds of interventions – medical and alternative, have a degree of placebo effect on the healing process (Lewith and Aldridge, 1993; Goldstein, 1999).

When we look at the continuum of care delineated by the three models of the doctor-patient-relationship: (1) paternalistic, (2) shared decision-making and (3) consumerist, we see that each model directs attention to different aspects of how the therapeutic relationship is structured. The paternalistic model was only minimally evident in the reports of the current experiences of all the patients, although one key element of the paternalistic model was still apparent in the relationship between most family physicians and their patients.

It was the physicians who made the decisions about treatments and the patients who trusted in these decisions.

Paternalism was clearly evident, however, when it came to the stories that both groups of patients recounted about their past experiences with medical specialists. In many instances they reported evasion of their questions, limited communication, and complete physician control of decision-making. A distinction was thus apparent in the type of relationship the patients experienced with family physicians, as compared to the more authoritarian and remote medical specialists they had consulted.

It was the mid-point on the continuum, the shared decision-making model, that best reflected the relationships of most patients with their health care providers. Both groups reported that they typically shared clinical information with them, communicated well and proffered emotional support. The model fitted therapeutic relationships with CAM practitioners more closely, however, due to the partnership role they took with patients, particularly around psychosocial issues and recommended lifestyle changes.

At the far end of the continuum, the consumerist model was reflected in the desire of both kinds of patients to find a successful resolution to their chronic problems. This was particularly apparent when patients spoke of their past health care experiences. The pattern was that if the practitioner was found to be unable to help them, or failed to respect them and their opinions about treatment, most decided to act as 'smart consumers' and search for another physician or CAM practitioner who would listen more attentively and make more appropriate, individualized recommendations.

To reiterate, most of the relationships experienced by patients in this study fall somewhere in the middle of the continuum. Paternalism appears to be disappearing for family physicians, who are relating to their patients in more open ways. The authority of the physician over health care decisions is no longer as influential. They are not, however, assuming partnership roles with their patients to the same extent that characterizes therapeutic relationships with CAM practitioners and their patients. An interesting question for the future is whether patients of family physicians will come to expect the same kind of consultative and egalitarian relationship from their doctors that they have been experiencing with their CAM practitioners.

This study demonstrates that models of the practitioner-patient-relationship that were developed solely on the basis of doctors and their patients can be expanded to apply to relationships with patients and CAM practitioners as well. While the models do not fit the realties of health care perfectly, they do direct our attention to salient points concerning the ways in which both physicians and CAM practitioners relate to their patients, and they also enable us to see interesting differences between various types of CAM practitioners.

CONCLUSION

The key finding here is that while there are overarching differences in the nature of the therapeutic relationship that exists in medicine and in alternative care, both kinds of relationships are nevertheless positive and valuable, and not mutually exclusive. The physician relationship is based primarily on trust in expertise, while the CAM relationship is based principally on partnership in healing. The opportunity to take an active role may well be part of the attraction of CAM for patients. The research reported here, however, indicates that their primary motivation is the continuing search for relief from chronic problems. This motivation is not restricted to Canadians who use CAM, but also applies to patients in Britain, the United States and other countries where CAM is currently popular.

Further research on the nature and significance of the therapeutic relationship in CAM is needed to flesh out the picture portrayed here. Rather than rely on patients' accounts of past and present health care experiences, scholars can pursue this topic in depth through use of tape recorders and video cameras during the actual encounters, as Mishler and his colleagues have done for the doctor-patient-relationship (Mishler, 1984). Analysis of the content, the tone and the timing of the consultation between CAM practitioners and their patients can reveal the nuances of the dynamics involved in the healing encounter. Some questions that could be answered using these research methods include: (1) Do different types of CAM practitioners have different kinds of therapeutic relationships with their patients? (2) Do age, gender, and cultural differences generate different kinds of therapeutic relationships with a CAM practitioner? (3) At what point in the treatment process do CAM patients show an interest in the healing philosophy of their practitioners? (4) Do the characteristics of the therapeutic relationship vary according to different societal conditions and contexts? and (5) Will the increasing professionalization of CAM practitioners change the dynamics of the therapeutic encounter in the future? The nature of the relationship between patients and their CAM practitioners has yet to be fully identified.

REFERENCES

Bakx, K. 1991. 'The "Eclipse" of Folk Medicine in Western Society.' *Sociology of Health and Illness* 13:20–38.
Balant, E., M. Courtney, A. Elder, S. Hull, and P. Julian. 1993. *The Doctor, the Patient and the Group.* London: Routledge.
Blais, Regis, Aboubacrine Maiga, and Alarou Aboubacar. 1997. 'How Different Are Users and Non-Users of Alternative Medicine?' *Canadian Journal of Public Health* 88:159–162.

Brinkhaus, B., G. Schindler, M. Linder, A. Malterer, W. Mayer, R. Kohnen, and E.G. Hahn. 1998. 'User Profiles of Patients in Homeopathic and Conventional Medicine.' in *5th Annual Symposium on Complementary Health Care*. Exeter, UK.

Cogswell, Betty E. 1988. 'The Walking Patient and the Revolt of the Client: Impetus to Develop New Models of Physician-Patient Roles.' in *Family and Support Systems Across the Lifespan*, edited by Suzanne Steinmetz. New York: Plenum.

DiMatteo, M.R., S.L. Linn, B.L. Chang, and D.W. Cope. 1985. 'Affect and Neutrality in Physician Behaviour: A Study of Patient's Values and Satisfaction.' *Journal of Behavioural Medicine* 8:397–409.

Eisenberg, David M., Ronald C. Kessler, Cindy Foster, Frances E. Norlock, David R. Calkins, and Thomas L. Delbanco. 1993. 'Unconventional Medicine in the United States: Prevalence, Costs and Patterns of Use.' *New England Journal of Medicine* 328:246–252.

Eisenberg, David M., Roger B. Davis, Susan L. Ettner, Scott Appel, Sonja Wilkey, Maria Van Rompay, and Ronald C. Kessler. 1998. 'Trends in Alternative Medicine Use in the United States, 1990–1997: Results of a Follow-up National Survey.' *The Journal of the American Medical Association* 280:1569–1575.

Emanuel, E.J., and L.L. Emanuel. 1992. 'Four Models of the Physician Patient Relationship.' *Journal of the American Medical Association* 267:2221–2226.

Emmanuel, E.J., and L.L. Emmanuel. 1995. 'Four Models of the Physician-Patient Relationship.' Pp. 163–178 in *Health Care Ethics in Canada*, edited by F. *et al.* Baylis. Toronto: Harcourt Brace.

Ernst, Edzard. 1995. 'Placebos in Medicine.' *Lancet* 345:65.

Felch, William C. 1996. *The Secret(s) of Good Patient Care: Thoughts on Medicine in the 21st Century*: Praeger.

Friedson, Eliot. 1970. *Professional Dominance: The Social Structure of Medical Care*. New York: Atheron Press.

Fulder, Stephen. 1988. *The Handbook of Complementary Medicine*. Oxford: Oxford University Press.

Goldstein, Michael. 1999. *Alternative Health Care: Medicine, Miracle or Mirage?* Philadelphia: Temple Union Press.

Greene, M.G., R.D. Adelman, E. Friedmann, and R. Charon. 1994. 'Older Patient Satisfaction with Communication During an Initial Medical Encounter.' *Social Science and Medicine* 38:1279–1288.

Haug, Marie. 1979. 'Doctor Patient Relationships in the Older Patient.' *Journal of Gerontology* 34:852–860.

Haug, Marie R., and Bebe Lavin. 1981. 'Practitioner or Patient – Who's in Charge?' *Journal of Health and Social Behaviour* 22:212–229.

Haug, Marie R. & Bebe Lavin. 1983. Consumerism in Medicine: Challenging Physician Authority. Beverly Hills: Sage.

Kasteler, J., R. Kane, D. Olsen, and C. Thetford. 1976. 'Issues Underlying Prevalence of "Doctor-Shopping" Behaviour.' *Journal of health and Social Behaviour* 17:328–338.

Katz, Jay. 1984. *The Silent World of Doctor and Patient*. New York: The Free press.

Kelner, Merrijoy, and Beverly Wellman. 1997a. 'Health Care and Consumer Choice: Medical and Alternative Therapies.' *Social Science and Medicine* 45:203–212.

Kronenfeld, Jennie Jacobs, and Eugene Schneller. 1997. 'The Growth of a Buyer Beware and Consumer Protections Model in Health Care: The Impact of Managed Care on Changing Models of the Doctor Patient Relationships.' Presented at the *American Sociological Association Meetings*. Toronto, Canada.

Lewis, J. Rees. 1994. 'Patient Views on Quality Care in General Practice: Literature Review.' *Social Science and Medicine* 39:655–670.

Lewith, George T., and David Aldridge (Eds.). 1993. *Clinical Research Methodology for Complementary Therapies*. London: Hodder & Stoughton.

Light, D. 1991. 'Professionalism as Countervailing Power.' *Journal of Health and Public and Political Law* 16.

Linn, M.W., B.S. Linn, and S.R. Stein. 1982. 'Satisfaction with Ambulatory Care and Compliance in Older Patients.' *Medical Care* 20:606–614.

Llyod, P., D. Lupton, and C. Donaldson. 1991. 'Consumerism in the Health Care Setting: An Examploratory Study of Factors Underlying the Selection and Evaluation of Primary Medical Services.' *Australian Journal of Public Health* 15:194–201.

Lupton, Deborah (Ed.). 1996. *Your Life in their Hands: Trust in the Medical Encounter*. Cambridge: Blackwell Publishers.

Lupton, D., C. Donaldson, and P. Llyod. 1991. 'Caveat Emptor or Blissful Ignorance? Patients Ad the Consumerist Ethos.' *Social Science and Medicine* 33:559–568.

Marquis, M.S., A.R. Davis, and J.E. Ware. 1983. 'Patient Satisfaction and Change in Medical Care Provider: A Longitudinal Study.' *Medical Care* 21:821–829.

McGregor, Katherine J., and Edmund R. Peay. 1996. 'The Choice of Alternative Therapy for Health Care: Testing Some Propositions.' *Social Science and Medicine* 43:1317–132.

McGuire, Meredith. 1988. *Ritual Healing in Suburban America*. New Brunswick: Rutgers University Press.

McKinlay, J., and J. Stoeckle. 1988. 'Corporatisation and the Social Transformation of Doctoring.' *International Journal of Health Services* 18(2):191–205.

Mills, S., and W. Peacock. 1997. 'Professional Organization of Complementary and Alternative Medicine in the United Kingdom.'. Exeter: Centre for Complementary Health Studies, Department of Health, University of Exeter.

Mishler, E.G. 1984. *The Discourse of Medicine: Dialetics of Medical Interviews*. Norwood: Ablex Publishing Company.

Mitchell, Annie, and Maggie Cormack. 1998. *The Therapeutic Relationship in Complementary Health Care*. London: Churchill Livingstone.

O'Connor, Bonnie Blair. 1995. *Healing Traditions: Alternative Medicine and the Health Professions*. Philadelphia: University of Pennsylvania Press.

Oths, K. 1994. 'Communication in a Chiropractic Clinic: How a D.C. Treats his Patients.' *Cultural Medical Psychiatry* 18(1):83–103.

Parsons, Talcott (Ed.). 1951. *The Social System*. Glencoe, IL: Free Press.

Parsons, Talcott. 1975. 'The Sick Role and the Role of the Physician Reconsidered.' *Millbank Memorial Fund Quarterly* 53:257–278.

Phillips, Daphne. 1996. 'Medical Professional Dominance and Client Dissatisfaction.' *Social Science and Medicine* 42:1419–1425.

Pietroni, P. 1987. 'Holistic Medicine: New Lessons to be Learned.' *The Practitioner* 231:1386–1390.

Reid, Angus. 1997. 'User Profile, Reasons for Using Alternative Medicines and Practices, Health Care Responsibility.'. Toronto: CTV/Angus Reid Group Poll.

Reeder, Leo. 1972. 'The Patient –Client as a Consumer: Some Observations on the Changing Professional-Client Relationship. Journal of Health & Social Behaviour. 13(4): 406–12.

Roter, D.L. 1977. 'Patient Participation in the Patient-Provider Interaction: The Effects of Patient Question Asking on the Quality of Interaction, Satisfaction and Compliance.' *Health Education Monograph* 5:281–315.

Sharma, Ursula. 1992. *Complementary Medicine Today: Practitioners and Patients*. London: Routledge.

Skipper, J. 1965. 'Communication and the Hospitalized Patient.' Pp. 61–82(21) in *Social Interaction and Patient Care*, edited by J. Skipper and R. Leonard. London: Pitman Medical.

Sutherland, L.R. and Verhoef, M.J. 1994. 'Why do Patients Seek a Second Opinion orAlternative Medicine?' *Journal of Clinical Gastroenterology* 19(3):194–197.

Szasz, Thomas S., and Marc H. Hollender. 1956. 'A Contribution to the Philosophy of Medicine: The Basic Models of the Doctor-Patient Relationship.' *American Medical Association: Archives of Internal Medicine* 97:585–592.

Taussig, M. 1980. 'Reification and Consciousness of the Patient.' *Social Science and Medicine* 14B:3–13.

Thomas, Kate J., Jane Carr, Linda Westlake, and Brain T. Williams. 1991. 'Use of Non-orthodox and Conventional Health Care in Great Britain.' *British Medical Journal* 302:207–210.

Veatch, R.M. 1972. 'Models for Ethical Medicine in a Revolutionary age.': Hastings Centre Report.

Vincent, Charles, and Adrian Furnham. 1997. *Complementary Medicine: A Research Perspective*. Chichester, England: John Wiley & Sons.

Wallston, B., K. Wallston, G. Kaplan, and S. Maides. 1976. 'Development and Validation of Health Locus of Control Scale.' *Journal of Consultation of Clinical Psychology* 44:580–585.

Ware, J.E., and A. Ross-Davies. 1983. 'Effects of the Doctor-Patient relationship on Subsequent Patient Behaviours.' in *American Public Health Association*. Dallas, TX.

Wellman, Beverly. 1995. 'Lay Referral Networks: Using Conventional Medicine and Alternative Therapies for Low Back Pain.' pp. 213–238 in *Research in the Sociology of Health Care*, Volume 12 edited by Jannie J. Kronenfeld. Greenwich: Conn: JAI Press.

Williams, G.H. 1993. 'The Movement of Independent living: An Evaluation and Critique.' *Social Science and Medicine* 17:1003–1009.

ENDNOTE

1. In the Canadian national health insurance scheme, all medical services are covered by government insurance. Alternative care, on the other hand, is paid for by patients out of their own pockets, with the partial exception of chiropractic.

2. It is important to recognize that there is some overlap between the groups being analysed here. Several investigators have shown that individuals do not abandon conventional medicine when they use alternative therapies (Lewith *et al.*, 1996; Kelner and Wellman, 1997a; Eisenberg *et al.*, 1993, 1998; Vincent and Furnham, 1997). Many use both, either sequentially or at the same time. Moreover, some patients may simultaneously consult more than one alternative practitioner for their current complaint. It is also true that many alternative practitioners and even some family physicians are qualified in more than one discipline and may utilize a mixture of therapeutic practices in treating an individual patient. In spite of these complications, for purposes of analysis the patient groups in this study have been defined according to the type of practitioner in whose office they were first contacted.

Section 2:
Use and Availability of CAM

It used to be thought, in spite of a lack of good data, that CAM patients were more likely to come from low socioeconomic groups (Wardwell, 1952; Naegele, 1970; White and Skipper, 1971). However, just a decade later, rigorous studies threw doubts on the validity of this profile of users (Coulter, 1985; Kelner *et al.*, 1980) and showed that they did not differ from the general population of medical patients. Current research paints a picture of well educated, affluent and sophisticated clienteles.

This more contemporary view fits with social scientists' longstanding interest in the relationship between social status and culture. Erickson (1996) and DiMaggio (1987) contend that higher social status is accompanied by a taste for a greater variety of forms of culture. In this case, we can equate alternative forms of health care with cultural variety and thereby explain the greater use by high status patients. While adequate financial resources play a part in people's ability to choose CAM, the broader social networks typical of high status individuals also encourage the use of a range of health care strategies (Peterson, 1992). In this section, the book moves to appraisal of who uses CAM therapies and how they find their way to the practitioners. These additional considerations add depth and breadth to the analyses in the previous section.

Coulter, Ian D. 1985. 'The Chiropractic Patient: A Social Profile.' *Journal of the Canadian Chiropractic Association* 29:25–28.

DiMaggio, Paul. 1987 'Classification in Art.' *American Sociological Review* 52:440–455.

Erickson, Bonnie. 1996. 'Culture, Class, and Connections.' *American Journal of Sociology* 102:217–251.

Kelner, Merrijoy, Oswald Hall, and Ian Coulter. 1980. *Chiropractors, Do They Help?* Toronto: Fitzhenry and Whiteside.

Naegele, K.O. 1970. *Health and Healing.* San Francisco: Jossey-Boas Inc.

Peterson, Richard A. 1992. 'Understanding Audience Segmentation: From Elite and Mass to Omnivore and Univore.' *Poetics* 21:243–258.

Wardwell, W. 1952. 'A Marginal Professional Role: The Chiropractor.' *Social Forces* 30:335–48.

White, M., and J.K. Skipper. 1971. 'The Chiropractic Physician: A Study of Career Contingencies.' *Journal of Health and Social Behaviour* 12:300–6.

CHAPTER 5

The Characteristics of CAM Users: A Complex Picture

JOHN A. ASTIN

This chapter offers some explanations for the current popularity of complementary and alternative medicine (CAM) in North America and Western Europe. In this chapter, I build on my previously published findings (Astin, 1998b) to further explore the question of why people use CAM and link these findings to the data on the characteristics of CAM users. The significance of the findings for both future research and public policy are highlighted.

WHY PEOPLE USE CAM

Three primary explanations have been proposed to explain why people use CAM (Astin, 1998b): 1) dissatisfaction with conventional medicine; 2) desire for personal control; and, 3) philosophical or value congruence. Here, I examine the evidence to support these explanations.

Explanation #1: Dissatisfaction with conventional medicine

This section discusses the findings of a number of investigators who have explored negative attitudes toward and experiences with conventional biomedicine as a motivating factor in peoples' decision to utilize CAM. 'Dissatisfaction' is a complex construct that includes: disenchantment with conventional medical care, dissatisfaction with specific treatment approaches or practitioners, and lack of symptom relief. Taylor (1984) has provided historical evidence showing a decreasing level of trust and confidence in the medical profession as a whole, beginning in the late 1960s and early 70s. It seems reasonable to suggest that the rising interest in various health care alternatives over the past two decades stems, in part, from negative experiences or perceptions of conventional medicine. More recently, Murray and Rubel (1992) have suggested that an important reason people seek treatment from CAM practitioners is because they have experienced some past or present disappointment with conventional treatment, such as its being too impersonal, technologically oriented, or costly. Some research also suggests that the therapeutic relationship is a significantly more satisfying and positive experience for a number of individuals being treated by CAM providers (Oths 94), and that poor communication between conventional doctors and their patients may drive the latter to seek treatment outside of orthodox medicine (Marquis, Davies and Ware, 1983).

Parker and Tupling (1977) found that dissatisfaction with conventional medicine was higher in a group of patients using a variety of natural therapies (chiropractic, acupuncture, and naturopathy) as compared to those patients being treated by general practitioners. This dissatisfaction included feelings that the conventional treatment they received was not successful, objections to the use of drugs, and personal dissatisfaction with conventional doctors' expressive or interpersonal skills.

In a study of cancer patients' use of CAM (Cassileth *et al.*, 1984), the most frequently stated reason for use was the natural (non-toxic qualities) of alternative regimens, while some explained their decision in terms of their terminal diagnoses and the willingness to try anything that might help. The medical profession was viewed in decreasingly positive terms, according to whether people received conventional treatments only, both conventional and alternative, or solely alternative therapies.

In a questionnaire study in Norway of over 400 patients with atopic dermatitis and psoriasis (Jensen, 1990), the absence of satisfactory long-term effects of conventional, physician-provided therapy was the primary reason for use of CAM. In a study from Canada (Sutherland and Verhoef, 1994), investigators examined determinants of CAM use by patients being treated for gastrointestinal problems. Greater skepticism toward conventional medicine as well as dissatisfaction with conventional physicians were both predictive of CAM use.

A recent investigation of German patients by Furnham and Kirkaldy (1996) suggests that those who select CAM approaches may do so less from disenchantment or bad experiences with conventional medical techniques than from a deep-seated belief in the effectiveness of CAM. Vincent and Furnham (1996) note that future research may need to separate out reasons for first trying CAM, from reasons for continuing to use it. They suggest that the initial movement toward CAM may be driven more by dissatisfaction with mainstream medicine, whereas continued involvement with CAM may reflect more positive attitudes toward and beliefs about these therapies.

In her examination of non-traditional healing groups among middle-class suburbanites, McGuire (1988) found substantial criticism of conventional medicine and practitioners. This included the perception that conventional medicine tended to address symptoms rather than causes and relied excessively on, or prematurely used surgery and drugs. Among these alternative healing group participants, the conventional doctor was seen primarily as a diagnostician-technician, rather than a care-giver who addressed patients' ways of thinking about self and the world.

However, McGuire's study did not support the idea that CAM adherents are more dissatisfied than non-adherents. In fact, she found the greatest degree of dissatisfaction with conventional medicine and practitioners among non-users of CAM as well as people who used CAM treatments that were practitioner-based (rather than based on self -care or lay healing groups).

Explanation #2: Desire for control

Several lines of work (Montbriand and Laing, 1991) suggest that individuals seek out CAM in order to gain a sense of personal control and empowerment. For example, Murray and Rubel (1992) suggest that users of CAM are attracted to promises of greater freedom of choice and clearer explanations of disease, as well as being influenced by a contemporary holistic health move-ment that stresses treating the whole person and taking charge of one's own health.

Riessman (1994) has similarly suggested that the rising interest in CAM practices can be understood in terms of their fit with individuals' desire to feel more empowered, particularly as consumers. This is reflected in the large number of CAM therapies (e.g. relaxation, use of herbals and supplements, guided imagery, and a plethora of self-help groups) that do not rely so much on professional authority, and thereby appeal to individuals who desire greater autonomy and personal control over their health care decisions.

Duggan (1995) sees the growing involvement in various forms of CAM as representing a shift from authoritarian medical intervention to authoritative self-care. For example, McGuire (1988) found that CAM adherents were less inclined to accept their doctors' authority without question. Instead, they saw themselves as 'contractors of their own health care', viewing doctors as one among many possible sources of information, advice, and help. They reported trusting their *own* knowledge regarding when, if, and what type of healing to seek out. McGuire notes that in this model, patients exert far greater power and control over their own health care decisions. Doctors are seen as 'knowl-edgeable resource persons for self-aware patients (p. 201).' Among this group, many interviewees stated that they valued *part* of their doctors' help – primarily their diagnostic abilities in order to rule out the possibility of some-thing more serious – but were unwilling to surrender personal control regarding treatment options.

Several studies have also examined how patients using CAM score on the Health Locus of Control Scale, a measure that assesses the sources from which people gain a sense of control regarding their health (Wallston *et al.,* 1976). Furnham and Bhagrath (1993) found that patients seeing a homeopath believed less that a powerful other (e.g., doctor) could exercise control over their health status. Sutherland and Verhoef (1994) also observed a trend (though statistically non-significant) suggesting that CAM users are less likely to believe in the control of a powerful other over their health.

Explanation #3: Philosophical/Value congruence

Researchers have also hypothesized that people are drawn to CAM therapies because they perceive these approaches to be more congruent (i.e., consistent) with their own world-view, their spiritual or religious philosophy, and/or distinctive beliefs regarding the nature of health and illness. As Charlton (1993) notes the current vogue for alternative therapies may be taken as evidence that there is a hunger among at least some of the public for a more broadly spiritual dimension to medicine – a holistic approach which relates therapy to the patient's overall purpose in life. Charlton identifies three distinct models of the health care practitioner: 1) benevolent Father Figure 2) Shopkeeper (e.g., the doctor as mechanic or technician); and 3) Priest (e.g., CAM practitioners who view and treat illness within the larger context of spirituality and life meaning).

A number of writers have pointed to the similarity between the philosophy and theory underlying many forms of CAM (e.g., chiropractic, homeopathy, acupuncture) and certain metaphysical beliefs and practices (Fuller, 1989). For example, many CAM therapies hold as a central tenet, the belief in a universal life force or healing energy that is present in and around the human body and mind. Also, as Fuller (1989) notes, one can see historically a strong relationship between the development of certain forms of holistic health and a number of new religious and spiritual movements (e.g., New Thought, Christian Science).

Levin and Coreil (1986) argue that in contemporary American society there is an emergent subculture that can be broadly defined in terms of involvement in various forms of esoteric, spiritual pursuits (e.g., meditation, eastern and western mystical traditions). They further note that these interests are often coupled with the belief in and use of various forms of holistic healthcare and alternative medical approaches. As McGuire (1988) reports, many of these people see health and physical well-being within the larger context of personal (psychological) or spiritual growth and development. Her findings also suggest that interest in CAM may be a reaction to and a way to counter what people experience as an overly rationalized life experience (of the self, body, and emotions).

In the following section, the results of a national survey are used to assess the strength of these three explanations and to identify the characteristics of CAM users in the United States.

WHY PEOPLE USE CAM: RESULTS OF A NATIONAL STUDY

Methods

Drawing from a national sample of U.S. adults surveyed in 1994 (N = 1,035), multivariate analysis was carried out to examine the relative predictive power of the three major explanations (dissatisfaction, desire for control, and philosophical congruence) (Astin, 1998b). In addition, health status and demographic factors (age, gender, income, education, ethnicity) were examined as potentially important predictors of CAM use. Participants completed an extensive mail survey, originally developed by Ray (1995), that gathered information on use of CAM, perceived benefits and risks of these therapies, health beliefs and attitudes, views toward and experiences with conventional medicine, political beliefs, values, and world-view.

Following Eisenberg (1993a; 1998), CAM utilization was defined in this study as use within the previous year of any of the following treatments: acupuncture, homeopathy, herbal therapies, chiropractic, massage, exercise/movement, high dose megavitamins, spiritual healing, lifestyle diet, relaxation, imagery, energy healing, folk remedies, biofeedback, hypnosis, psychotherapy, and art or music therapy. Several of the these treatments, however, were deemed not to be alternative or unconventional if they were used to treat particular health-related problems: (1) *exercise* for lung problems, high blood pressure, heart problems, obesity, muscle strains, or back problems; (2) *psychotherapy* for depression or anxiety, and, (3) *self-help groups* for depression or anxiety. In other words, CAM was defined so as to exclude those practices that are already part of standard medical care and recommendations such as exercise to treat hypertension or psychotherapy to treat depression (Astin, 1998b).

Results

As noted above, prior studies have been equivocal regarding the extent to which use of CAM can be explained by peoples' dissatisfaction with or distrust of conventional medicine and practitioners. Contrary to a number of previous findings (Cassileth *et al.*, 1984; Dimmock, Troughton and Bird, 1996; Furnham and Bhagrath, 1993; Furnham and Forey, 1994; Furnham and Smith, 1988; Jensen, 1990; Marquis, Davies and Ware, 1983; Oths, 1994; Sutherland and Verhoef, 1994), this national study found that negative attitudes toward or experiences with conventional medicine were *not* predictive of CAM utilization. Among those who reported being highly satisfied with their conventional practitioners, 39% used CAM while only 40% of those reporting high levels of dissatisfaction were users of CAM. In other words, the degree of satisfaction with conventional medicine could not distinguish CAM users from non-users, suggesting that dissatisfaction is *not* a sufficient condition to lead people to try CAM.

It has been posited (Baldwin, 1998) that pragmatic concerns (i.e., conventional care has not been effective) are an important motivating factor in CAM use. Baldwin suggests that perceptions that CAM has been more efficacious as well as feelings that it fits more closely with peoples' philosophical beliefs both imply some degree of dissatisfaction with conventional medicine. Satisfaction, however, may be closely tied to patients' level of expectation. For example, people who treat their colds with an herbal remedy such as echinacea may at the same time be very satisfied with their physicians, simply because they do not expect that conventional medicine will be able to offer much in the way of preventing or treating such health-related problems (Astin, 1998a).

The findings of the national survey also showed that contrary to Explanation #2, having a greater desire for control could not distinguish CAM users from non-users. For example, 19.2% of CAM users reported wanting to keep control of health care-related decisions in their own hands, as compared with 17.2% of non-users. Similarly, differences were not significant in terms of those who wished to leave decisions in their doctor's hands, with 6.0% of CAM users and 6.8% of non-users endorsing this position.

The vast majority of respondents in this study expressed a desire either to keep control in their own hands, (17.9%) or have an equal partnership with their doctors (75.5%). This finding suggests that most Americans no longer view the doctor as the ultimate authority figure or controlling force with respect to health care decisions. Individuals who exclusively use conventional forms of health care are just as likely to hold these attitudes as are CAM adherents.

Results from this study did, however, lend support to Explanation #3, the association between one's spiritual or philosophical orientation toward life and interest in CAM. First, having a holistic belief in the importance of body, mind and spirit in treating health-related matters was a significant predictor of CAM utilization. Sixty-one percent of CAM users endorsed this holistic health orientation as compared with 47% of non-users. There are a number of possible explanations for this association. People who have been involved with CAM may have come to modify their health beliefs through contact with these therapeutic systems and the philosophies that underlie them. Second, people who hold a holistic philosophical orientation toward health may be attracted to various CAM practices because they perceive a greater acknowledgment of and appreciation for the role of non-physical factors (mind/spirit) in creating health and illness. Lastly, belief in the importance of body, mind, and spirit *and* use of CAM may represent a proxy for some higher-order construct such as a general open mindedness to new ideas and concepts.

Another significant predictor of CAM use was belonging to a particular subculture that can be described as 'Cultural Creatives'. As discussed by Ray (1997, 1995), the Cultural Creatives (CCs) are identifiable by a distinct constellation of values. These include: 1) globalism – e.g., love of the foreign and exotic and concern for planetary ecology; 2) feminism – e.g., concerns about rights of women and children, desire to improve neighborhoods, relationships as well as concerns about family; 3) focus on the inner life – e.g., interests in spirituality, altruism, self-actualization, personal growth psychology; and, 4) social conscience – e.g., desire to heal and rebuild society as well as heal themselves physically and spiritually. Ray (1995) suggests that these individuals are at the leading edge of cultural change; coming up, he says, with the most new ideas in American culture. The CCs tend to be upper-middle class, are 60% women, and are highly educated. Ray contrasts the Cultural Creatives with the Moderns, who represent the current cultural mainstream (materialist and consumer oriented), and Heartlanders, a subculture of traditional and conservative values and beliefs. It is not surprising, then, that those categorized as Cultural Creatives were significantly more likely to utilize CAM (55%) than those not classified in this cultural group (35%).

The attraction of CAM for this group of people becomes clear when we observe some of the specific values typically subscribed to by the Cultural Creatives. For example, among those who placed great importance on putting time into psychological development, 59% used CAM therapies as compared with 31% who felt this was not an important or valued activity. We find a similar pattern in response to the question of how important it is to find ways to create social change, with 55% of those saying it is extremely important using CAM, as contrasted with 30% who felt it was not important.

A third finding that lends support to the philosophical and value congruence explanation is that among a list of 19 items examining spiritual or religious experiences, the statement 'I have had a transformational experience that causes me to see the world differently than before' emerged as a significant predictor of CAM use (Astin, 1998b). Of those who answered yes, 53% reported use of CAM, as compared with 37% of those who responded no or not sure. This finding further implies that interest in and involvement with CAM may, in part, be reflective of shifting cultural paradigms regarding beliefs about the nature of life, spirituality and the world in general. It should be noted, however, that what respondents meant by a transformational experience may have differed depending on their religious or spiritual orientation. For example, a majority (59%) of those who endorsed this item strongly agreed with the statement 'I have been born again in Jesus.' Among this group, 49% used CAM. On the other hand, among those who tended to reject more traditional or fundamentalist religion and also reported having had a transformational experience, 68% used CAM

To summarize, while findings from this study failed to show support for either the dissatisfaction or desire for control hypotheses, they did lend support to the notion that people seek out CAM because they find these therapies to be more congruent or consistent with their philosophical orientation to health and life. In addition to a distinctive set of beliefs, users of CAM have also been distinguished by their demographic characteristics and their health status.

Demographic characteristics, health status and use of CAM

Consistent with the findings of several earlier studies (Bernstein and Shuval, 1997; Fairfield *et al.*, 1998; Kelner and Wellman, 1997a), education emerged in this study as the one sociodemographic variable that predicted use of CAM. Thirty-one percent of those with high school education or less reported use of CAM, as compared with 50% of those with graduate degrees. Racial or ethnic differences did not predict use of CAM and no significant differences were found with respect to gender with 41% of females and 39% of males reporting using CAM. Contrary to most findings (Millar, 1997; Ostrow *et al.*, 1997), higher income also did not predict use of CAM. Finally, whereas previous studies had suggested that age was an important determinant of CAM utilization (Eisenberg *et al.*, 1993b), here it did not emerge as a characteristic that could distinguish users from non-users.

There are several possible explanations for the role of education in influencing people to use CAM. Being more educated may make it more likely that people will: 1) be exposed to various non-traditional forms of health care (e.g., through reading of popular or academic books on the subject); 2) educate themselves about their illnesses and the variety of treatments available to them (both conventional and non conventional); 3) question the authority of conventional practitioners (i.e., they are less likely to simply accept the doctor's knowledge and expertise on faith); and, 4) have access to more financial resources enabling them to afford CAM treatments frequently not covered by insurance. This latter explanation is unlikely, however, given income's failure to predict CAM utilization.

Those who reported poorer overall health status were also significantly more likely to use CAM in this study. There are several possible explanations for this finding. First, those who report poor health have, by definition, had less success in treating their health-related problems, and as a result of their continued pain, suffering, and discomfort are more likely to be open to seeking out alternatives. Second, a significant number of those who report poor health, pain, disability, and physical symptoms, may be somatizers. Somatization, a psychiatric term, has been defined as the propensity to experience and report somatic symptoms that have no pathophysiological explanation, to misattribute them to disease, and to seek medical attention for them (Barsky and Borus, 1995). Research on somatization suggests that these individuals are disproportionately high users of medical services; they get more medical tests, and tend to experiment with (shop around for) different health care providers. Given these findings, it seems reasonable that somatizers would be more likely to seek out various health care alternatives.

While not a direct test of the somatization hypothesis, Furnham and Beard (1995) found no differences between and users and non-users of acupuncture in coping styles – that is, acupuncture patients were no more likely to be categorized as monitors (those who tend to seek out threat-relevant information and are more attentive to internal bodily symptoms). In that study, CAM users could also not be distinguished from non-users on a scale of minor psychiatric disturbances (using a measure of psychosomatic complaints known to be related to psychological distress). Secondary analyses of these data do suggest that somatization may be an important factor to examine in future research. Those respondents who reported an array of symptoms that closely resembles the psychiatric diagnostic criteria for somatization were significantly more likely to be CAM users and this effect could not be accounted for by their health status.

Along with poor overall health status, several specific health-related problems were associated with CAM utilization. These were: anxiety, back problems, obesity, depression, insomnia, urinary tract problems, and chronic pain. It is not the case that these particular ailments were necessarily the most likely to be treated by unconventional means, but rather, that if respondents experienced one of these health-related problems, they were more likely to utilize CAM in general. These types of symptoms are frequently found in those characterized as somatizers or the worried well, and these individuals may, in turn, be more likely to seek out various health care alternatives (Lipowski, 1988). It is also probably the case that conventional medicine has had less success in treating these types of health problems and that in the process of experimenting with various CAM therapies, individuals discover the vast array of health care alternatives that exist to treat other health-related problems as well.

SUMMARY: PROFILE OF THE CAM USER

Based on the results of the national study reviewed here, this chapter has outlined several ways in which people who use CAM are distinctive. They are more likely to be educated. They tend to have a philosophical orientation toward health that can be described as holistic (i.e., they believe in the importance of body, mind and spirit in health). They are more likely to have had some type of transformational spiritual or religious experience that has changed their world-view in some significant way. They tend to be classified in a subculture (the Cultural Creatives) identifiable by a commitment to environmentalism, feminism, involvement with esoteric forms of spirituality and personal growth psychology, and love of the foreign and exotic. They are also more likely to report poorer health overall. Contrary to our hypothesis and the findings of other researchers, CAM users in this study do not appear to be any more or less dissatisfied with their conventional medical care, nor are they any more desirous of maintaining control over their health care.

It is important, however, to point out that this profile of the CAM user represents a rather crude approximation or generalization. In point of fact, there are individuals who use CAM who are extremely dissatisfied with conventional forms of health care, as well as those who report high levels of satisfaction and trust. There are also CAM users who report being in excellent health and users who have relatively low levels of education. There are large numbers of users who subscribe to traditional religious values and are involved in fundamentalist religions (e.g., the Religious Right), and there are users who are involved in very nontraditional spiritual practices such as yoga and meditation, and who hold very liberal/progressive political views. While there are those CAM users who desire to keep control of health care decisions in their own hands, there are also significant numbers of users who desire to give control over to their health care practitioners.

The pattern becomes even more complex when we consider that CAM is by no means a homogenous phenomenon, and that the factors predicting use of CAM may vary as a function of the specific type(s) of therapy (Fairfield *et al.*, 1998; Kelner and Wellman, 1997b). For example, while users of spiritual healing tend to be non-white and believe in the power of religious faith to heal, users of massage tend to be more educated, desire to keep control in their hands, be Cultural Creatives, and not believe in the healing power of religious faith. And yet having 'a transformational experience which changed my world-view' is associated with use of both these therapies.

What is clear from the above summary is that while particular personal, social, and cultural characteristics may predict use of CAM, there is con-siderable diversity among CAM users with respect to their beliefs, demo-graphics, attitudes, health status, and personalities. No matter which way we characterize people who use complementary/alternative care, the reasons why they make such choices are complex.

FUTURE DIRECTIONS FOR RESEARCH

The findings reviewed here suggest a number of areas for future research.

1. Most studies to date have relied on retrospective accounts to understand why people use CAM. The use of prospective research designs would enable us to examine healthy individuals and their health care decision-making over an extended period of time, exploring factors that influence their choice of health care approach for preventive care or wellness, and for addressing specific illnesses or medical problems.

2. Since CAM is not a homogeneous set of therapies, research should move away from studying CAM use in general, and focus on examining specific CAM therapies instead (Astin *et al.,* 1998). Research suggests that predictors of CAM use may vary according to the specific type of therapy and also that determinants of CAM use may vary with the specific types of health problems people are facing (Hilsden, Scott and Verhoef, 1998; Kelner and Wellman, 1997a).

3. Future research might examine whether people rely on intuitive decision-making strategies (Agor, 1986) or employ various decision-making short cuts (heuristics). For example, an individual's choice to experiment with some CAM therapy may be the result of an availability bias – that is, they may have been influenced by a single case example of someone being healed by a CAM therapy (Tversky and Kahneman, 1974). Other personal characteristics of interest might include: somatization; openness to novelty and experimentation; conformity; and curiosity.

4. In arguing for the use of in-depth interviews as a research tool, a colleague once shared with me that 'surveys are a mile wide and a millimeter thick.' Using qualitative methods can bring a richness and depth to our understanding of the psychological, social, and cultural factors underlying the use of CAM (McGuire, 1988; Sharma, 1992; Verhoef, Scott and Hilsden, 1998). To take but one example, to better understand the nature of the relationship between people's spiritual beliefs and experiences and use of CAM, in-depth interviews could be used to explore questions such as:

   a. When individuals report that spirit (along with body and mind) is important in treating health-related matters, what do they mean by this term, and *why* do they feel this way (i.e., what are the mechanisms through which spiritual factors are believed to influence health outcomes)?

   b. How do individuals perceive that spiritual practices such as prayer and meditation affect their health? What are the variety of ways (techniques, strategies, and contexts) in which people use such practices to address their health-related problems?

    c. To what extent do people experience CAM therapies as more supportive of, or sensitive to spiritual issues (e.g., acknowledging their potentially important role in health-related matters)? Related to this, do various CAM therapies provide people with something (e.g., a sense of meaning or purpose) above and beyond symptom relief?

    d. Following Wilber's suggestion (1998, 1999), are there certain individuals among those categorized as Cultural Creatives or New-Agers for whom interest in CAM and spirituality may reflect regressive, anti-scientific or anti-rational tendencies rather than some positive personal and/or cultural transformation or paradigm shift?

5. Finally, the use of larger sample sizes that include non-English speaking populations would allow for more detailed testing of differences in patterns and predictors of CAM use among various racial and ethnic groups.

POLICY IMPLICATIONS

The studies reviewed here examining psychological, social, and cultural predictors of CAM utilization, have the potential to make a number of important theoretical and practical contributions. First, they can provide useful information to conventional practitioners and physicians about the health beliefs and practices of many of their patients as well as delineate areas where they and the existing health care system may be failing to address or meet peoples' health care needs adequately.

Second, such studies can help to identify and clarify prevailing cultural attitudes and conceptions about health and illness. As well, they can examine the degree to which the growing interest in and involvement with various forms of CAM represents a type of paradigm shift (Kuhn, 1970) regarding health beliefs and practices (e.g., the nature of mind/body interactions, the role of spiritual beliefs in health, recognition of the limits of technological, biomedical approaches to treat an array of health problems).

Finally, the information derived from these studies can serve as a useful adjunct to the carefully controlled studies now underway on the clinical efficacy of CAM. These combined research efforts have the potential to change some of the ways conventional biomedicine is practiced. These studies might also serve to create further dialogue between the biomedical community, governmental agencies, and private insurance companies regarding the potential value of including CAM treatments among services they cover (Pelletier *et al.*, 1997).

REFERENCES

Agor, W.H. 1986. *The logic of intuitive decision-making: a research based approach for top management.* New York: Quorum Books.

Astin, J.A. 1998a. 'Why patients use alternative medicine.' *JAMA (letter in reply)* 280:1661.

Astin, J.A. 1998b. 'Why patients use alternative medicine: results of a national study.' *JAMA* 279:1548–53.

Astin, J.A., A. Marie, K.R. Pelletier, E. Hansen, and W.L. Haskell. 1998. 'A review of the incorporation of complementary and alternative medicine by mainstream physicians.' *Arch Intern Med* 158:2303–10.

Baldwin, L. 1998. 'Why patients use alternative medicine.' *JAMA (letter)* 280:1659.

Barsky, A.J., and J.F. Borus. 1995. 'Somatization and medicalization in the era of managed care.' *JAMA* 274:1931–4.

Bernstein, J.H., and J.T. Shuval. 1997. 'Nonconventional medicine in Israel: consultation patterns of the Israeli population and attitudes of primary care physicians.' *Soc Sci Med* 44:1341–8.

Cassileth, B.R., E.J. Lusk, T.B. Strouse, and B.J. Bodenheimer. 1984. 'Contemporary unorthodox treatments in cancer medicine. A study of patients, treatments, and practitioners.' *Ann Intern Med* 101:105–12.

Charlton, B.G. 1993. 'The doctor's aim in a pluralistic society: a response to "healing and medicine" [editorial].' *J R Soc Med* 86:125–6.

Dimmock, S., P.R. Troughton, and H.A. Bird. 1996. 'Factors predisposing to the resort of complementary therapies in patients with fibromyalgia.' *Clin Rheumatol* 15:478–82.

Duggan, R.M. 1995. 'Complementary medicine: transforming influence or footnote to history?' *Altern Ther Health Med* 1:28–33.

Eisenberg, D.M., R.B. Davis, S.L. Ettner, S. Appel, S. Wilkey, M. Van Rompay, and R.C. Kessler. 1998. 'Trends in alternative medicine use in the United States, 1990–1997: results of a follow-up national survey.' *JAMA* 280:1569–75.

Eisenberg, D.M., T.L. Delbanco, C.S. Berkey, T.J. Kaptchuk, B. Kupelnick, J. Kuhl, and T.C. Chalmers. 1993a. 'Cognitive behavioral techniques for hypertension: are they effective? [see comments].' *Ann Intern Med* 118:964–72.

Eisenberg, D.M., R.C. Kessler, C. Foster, F.E. Norlock, D.R. Calkins, and T.L. Delbanco. 1993b. 'Unconventional medicine in the United States. Prevalence, costs, and patterns of use.' *N Engl J Med* 328:246–52.

Fairfield, K.M., D.M. Eisenberg, R.B. Davis, H. Libman, and R.S. Phillips. 1998. 'Patterns of use, expenditures, and perceived efficacy of complementary and alternative therapies in HIV-infected patients.' *Arch Intern Med* 158:2257–64.

Fuller, R.C. 1989. *Alternative medicine and American religious life.* New York: Oxford.

Furnham, A., and R. Beard. 1995. 'Health, just world beliefs and coping style preferences in patients of complementary and orthodox medicine.' *Soc Sci Med* 40:1425–32.

Furnham, A., and R. Bhagrath. 1993. 'A comparison of health beliefs and behaviours of clients of orthodox and complementary medicine.' *Br J Clin Psychol* 32:237–46.

Furnham, A., and J. Forey. 1994. 'The attitudes, behaviors and beliefs of patients of conventional vs. complementary (alternative) medicine.' *J Clin Psychol* 50:458–69.

Furnham, A. and B., Kirkcaldy. 1996. 'The Health Beliefs and Behaviours of Orthodox and Complementary Medicine Clients'. *British Journal of Clinical Psychology.* 35:49–61.

Furnham, A., and C. Smith. 1988. 'Choosing alternative medicine: a comparison of the beliefs of patients visiting a general practitioner and a homoeopath.' *Soc Sci Med* 26:685–9.

Hilsden, R.J., C.M. Scott, and M.J. Verhoef. 1998. 'Complementary medicine use by patients with inflammatory bowel disease [see comments].' *Am J Gastroenterol* 93:697–701.

Jensen, P. 1990. 'Use of alternative medicine by patients with atopic dermatitis and psoriasis.' *Acta Derm Venereol* 70:421–4.

Kelner, M., and B. Wellman. 1997a. 'Health care and consumer choice: medical and alternative therapies.' *Soc Sci Med* 45:203–12.

Kelner, M., and B. Wellman. 1997b. 'Who seeks alternative health care? A profile of the users of five modes of treatment.' *J Altern Complement Med* 3:127–40.

Kuhn, T. 1970. *The structure of scientific revolutions.* Chicago: University of Chicago Press.

Levin, J.S., and J. Coreil. 1986. '"New age" healing in the U.S.' *Soc Sci Med* 23:889–97.

Lipowski, Z.J. 1988. 'Somatization: the concept and its clinical application.' *Am J Psychiatry* 145:1358–68.

Marquis, M.S., A.R. Davies, and J.E. Ware, Jr. 1983. 'Patient satisfaction and change in medical care provider: a longitudinal study.' *Med Care* 21:821–9.

McGuire, M.B. 1988. *Ritual healing in suburban America.* New Brunswick: Rutgers University Press.

Millar, W.J. 1997. 'Use of alternative health care practitioners by Canadians' *Can J Public Health* 88:154–8.

Montbriand, M.J., and G.P. Laing. 1991. 'Alternative health care as a control strategy.' *J Adv Nurs* 16:325–32.

Murray, R.H., and A.J. Rubel. 1992. 'Physicians and healers – unwitting partners in health care.' *N Engl J Med* 326:61–4.

Ostrow, M.J., P.G. Cornelisse, K.V. Heath, K.J. Craib, M.T. Schechter, M. O'Shaughnessy, J.S. Montaner, and R.S. Hogg. 1997. 'Determinants of complementary therapy use in HIV-infected individuals receiving antiretroviral or anti-opportunistic agents.' *J Acquir Immune Defic Syndr Hum Retrovirol* 15:115–20.

Oths, K. 1994. 'Communication in a chiropractic clinic: how a D.C. treats his patients.' *Cult Med Psychiatry* 18:83–113.

Parker, G., and H. Tupling. 1977. 'Consumer evaluation of natural therapists and general practitioners.' *Medical Journal of Australia* 1:619–622.

Pelletier, K.R., A. Marie, M Krasner, E. Hansen, and W.L. Haskell. 1997. 'Current trends in the integration and reimbursement of complementary and alternative medicine by managed care, insurance carriers, and hospital providers.' *American Journal of Health Promotion* 12:112–122.

Ray, P. 1995. *The integral culture survey: a study of values subcultures and the use of alternative health care in America. Report to the The Fetzer Institute and The Institute of Noetic Sciences.* Sausalito: Institute of Noetic Sciences.

Ray, P. 1997. 'The emerging culture.' *American Demographics* February: http://www.demographics.com.

Riesmann, F. 1994. 'Alternative health movements.' *Social Policy*:53–57.

Sharma, U. 1992. *Complementary medicine today: Practitioners and patients.* London: Routledge.

Sutherland, L.R., and M.J. Verhoef. 1994. 'Why do patients seek a second opinion or alternative medicine?' *J Clin Gastroenterol* 19:194–7.

Taylor, R.C.R. 1984. 'Alternative medicine and the medical encounter in Britain and the United States.' in *Alternative medicine: popular and policy perspectives,* edited by J.W. Salmon. New York: Tavistock.

Tversky, A., and D. Kahneman. 1974. 'Judgement under uncertainty.' *Science* 185:1124–1131.

Verhoef, M.J., C.M. Scott, and R.J. Hilsden. 1998. 'A multimethod research study on the use of complementary therapies among patients with inflammatory bowel disease.' *Altern Ther Health Med* 4:68–71.

Vincent, C. and A. Furnham. 1996. 'Why Do Patients Turn to Complementary Medicine? An Empirical Study'. *British Journal of Clinical Psychology.* 35:37–48.

Wallston, B.S., K.A. Wallston, G.D. Kaplan, and S.A. Maides. 1976. 'Development and validation of the Health Locus of Control (HLC) Scale.' *Journal of Consulting and Clinical Psychology* 44:580–585.

Wilber, K. 1998. *The marriage of sense and soul: integrating science and religion.* New York: Random House.

Wilber, K. 1999. *One Taste: the journals of Ken Wilber.* Boston: Shambhala.

CHAPTER 6

Changes in Characteristics of CAM Users Over Time

RÉGIS BLAIS

INTRODUCTION

The popularity of complementary and alternative medicine (CAM) in industrialised countries is now well documented (Buckle, 1994; Eisenberg *et al.*, 1998; Ernst, 1996; Fulder and Munro, 1985; Goldbeck-Wood *et al.*, 1996; Fisher and Ward, 1994; Millar 1997; Northcott and Bachynsky, 1993; Thomas *et al.*, 1991; Verhoef *et al.*, 1990; 1994). The demographic characteristics that distinguish users and non-users of alternative medicine have also been studied. Although there may be differences across jurisdictions, the consistent finding is that the former are generally more educated and well off than the latter (Eisenberg *et al.*, 1993, 1998; Kelner and Wellman, 1997b; Le Groupe MultiRéso, 1992; McGuire, 1988; Vincent and Furnham, 1997). Research also indicates that while users of CAM still use medical care, they make fewer visits to physicians (Blais, Maïga and Aboubacar, 1997). Most of these studies, however, have been cross-sectional in nature, thus providing a picture of CAM users at only one given point in time. As alternative therapies become better known to the public and used by a larger proportion of the population, it is possible that the profile of users may change over time. To illustrate this point, let us take an example drawn from a profession that, in Canada, has long been considered alternative to main stream medicine, i.e. the practice of midwifery.

Before the beginning of the nineties, midwifery was not regulated in Canada. Moreover, the services of midwives were not covered by universal health insurance, and clients had to pay out of their own pockets. Under these conditions, midwives were considered 'alternative' in a way that is similar to CAM, and the profile of their clients was difficult to document. Nevertheless, in the province of Quebec, a small survey showed that midwives' clients were better educated than the general population, more critical of conventional medicine, and were interested in demedicalizing the process of birth (Saillant, O'Neil and Desjardins, 1987). Starting in 1993, pilot projects of midwifery practice were implemented and funded by the Quebec government. Evaluation of these pilot projects indicated that the clientele of midwives changed over a period of four years (Blais *et al.*, 1997). The initial clients of midwives were similar to their clientele prior to the pilot projects: they seemed to be critical of the official health care system, wanted to have a say in the care they received and were looking for care that is more human and less medicalised. As the clientele has grown, however, more recent clients do not seem to have such distinctive characteristics and appear to be more like the population in general. It seems that without public funding, there would not have been such a change in the profile of women using midwifery. We do not know whether such a 'rapprochement' between users and non-users of CAM is also occurring or, whether, on the contrary, users of CAM are becoming more different from non users.

This chapter reports the findings of a follow-up study which partially fills this gap by comparing users and non-users over time. Its purpose was to examine whether socio-economic characteristics, health profile and health care use of CAM have changed between 1987 and 1993 in the province of Quebec (population 7 million), in comparison with non-users of CAM.

METHODS

Where Did the Data Come from?

Data came from two sources: the Quebec Health Surveys conducted in 1987 (QHS87) and in 1993 (QHS93). The two surveys were conducted essentially the same way. A representative sample of 11,323 households across the province were surveyed in 1987 and 13,266 in 1993 (Bellerose *et al.*, 1995; Courtemanche and Tarte, 1987). One respondent from each household was identified and interviewed in person about the demographic characteristics and general health status of every household member. Household members 15 years of age or over were asked to fill out a more detailed questionnaire to be sent back by mail (response rate: 81% in 1987 and 85% in 1993). In 1987, interview data were available for 31,995 non-institutionalised persons and self-adminis-tered data were available for 19,724 of them (Santé Québec, 1988). The corre-sponding figures for 1993 are 34,848 and 23,564.

As this book makes clear, the concept of CAM includes various types of health practices (Wardwell, 1994). The question of who is a user of CAM and who is not can be the object of long debates. For the purposes of this research, a user of alternative medicine was operationally defined as a person who reported seeing a practitioner of a non-medical therapy at his or her last professional health care consultation during the two weeks prior to the survey. The CAM therapies studied included: chiropractic, acupuncture, massage, homeopathy, herbal medicine, hypnosis, healing, naturopathy, osteopathy, midwifery and natural nutrition. A non-user was defined as someone who saw a conventional health professional at the last consultation (mainly physician, but also physiotherapist, nurse, dentist, dietician, etc.) and who had not seen a CAM practitioner in the last two weeks prior to the date when respondents were surveyed. The health problems that prompted the last consultation were noted in the surveys for everyone[1]. Each survey was analysed separately.

People usually consult CAM practitioners and physicians for different health reasons. But it was not on the basis of these differences that we wanted to distinguish users and non-users of CAM. Moreover, we did not want limited access to medical care to be a reason for using CAM. That is why we attempted to control for two essential determinants of health care utilisation that are often overlooked in studies comparing users and non-users of CAM. These two factors were: need (i.e. the health condition or problem that brought a person to seek help) and access to health care facilities (Andersen, 1995; Hulka and Wheat, 1985). In other words, given the same health problem and without particular barriers to health care, we wanted to know how users and non-users of CAM differed. To do so, we proceeded as follows.

All users of CAM were first identified in the surveys. The file was then searched for non-users of CAM having the same health problem, as indicated by the diagnosis code, and residing in the same geographic area (we used the standard 32 community health districts of the QHS87 and the 30 homogeneous areas of the QHS93). The latter was considered a substitute or proxy variable for access to health care facilities: while access may vary across areas, it was assumed that it would be more or less the same for everyone living in the same small area. It is also important to mention that in Quebec, as in the other Canadian provinces, economic access is guaranteed to all residents by a universal health system that provides conventional medical services free of charge at the point of consumption. Users of CAM were matched with non-users by diagnosis and district of residence. When two or more non-users had the profile corresponding to one user of CAM, one non-user was randomly selected. In 1987, 421 persons visited a CAM practitioner in the two weeks prior to the survey, and 355 did so at their last consultation. In 1993, the corresponding numbers were 805 and 676, representing an increase of 91% over 1987. The process of matching resulted in the selection of 200 users and 200 non-users of CAM in 1987 (total sample: 400) and 353 users and 353 non-users in 1993 (total sample: 706).

What was measured?

For both surveys, the two groups were compared on the following demographic characteristics: age, sex, education, activity, marital status and household income. Health profile was defined by four variables: number of good health habits (from

1 to 5: no alcohol consumption, no smoking, exercise, no overweight and adequate sleep), self-rated health, measured on a scale from 1 to 5 (1: excellent, 2: very good, 3: good, 4: fair, 5: poor), a 14-item indicator of psychological distress adapted from the Psychological Symptom Index (Ilfeld 1978; Préville *et al.*, 1992) and limitations on activities because of a health problem or a chronic condition (compared to others of the same age and in good health). Data on self-rated health and psychological distress were available only for those 15 years of age and older, since it came from the self-administered questionnaire. Measures of health care consumption covered three aspects: whether the person had visited a general practitioner or a specialist physician in the last two weeks and the number of medications currently being taken. Data analysis was performed using appropriate statistical techniques[2].

RESULTS

In both Quebec surveys, chiropractors were the main CAM practitioners people were consulting: they were visited by 72% of the study population in 1987, but only 52% in 1993. In 1987, the only other therapy used by more than 4% of the sample was acupuncture (11%). In 1993, the picture was somewhat different; practitioners of both acupuncture and homeopathy were consulted by 9% of the respondents and naturopathy and massage therapy by 6% and 7% of them respectively.

Reasons for consulting CAM practitioners

The reasons for which patients consulted CAM practitioners were varied (Table 6.1). While musculoskeletal problems were the predominant diagnoses in both surveys, fewer patients presented these problems in the later survey (58% vs. 46%). In addition, the other main change over time was that many more patients consulted CAM practitioners for general or special 'medical' examinations (26% vs. 7%).

Demographic characteristics of CAM users and non-users in 1987 and 1993

The differences in demographic characteristics between users and non-users of CAM were generally the same in both 1987 and 1993 (Table 6.2). While the two study groups were no different in terms of gender and marital status over time, they differed significantly, however, on the four other dimensions examined. CAM was more popular among the 30 to 44 year-olds, and less so among older adults and the elderly. This was true in both surveys. One change that can be seen between 1987 and 1993 is that the proportion of CAM users among children and young adults (0–29 year-old) was lower than that of non-users in 1987, while it was higher in 1993. In both surveys, users of CAM

Table 6.1:   Reasons for which Patients Consulted Practitioners of Alternative Medicine

Class of diagnoses (ICD-9)	1987 (n = 200) %	1993 (n = 353) %
Musculoskeletal system and connective tissue	58	46
Respiratory system	5	8
Nervous system and sense organs	3	5
Ill-defined conditions	7	4
Other diseases	15	9
General or special medical examinations	7	26
Other factors influencing health status and contact with health services	6	3

were also more likely to have a higher education, to be working, and to live in a household whose income was higher.

Health profiles and consumption of health services for users and non-users of CAM

Since users and non-users of CAM differed on several demographic characteristics, such as age, education and household income, comparisons between the two groups on their health profiles and consequently in their consumption of health services had to take those differences into account[3].

In 1987, there were no significant differences between users and non-users of CAM on the four health dimensions studied: good health habits, self-rated health, limitation of activity and psychological distress (Table 6.3). However, in 1993 users of CAM had significantly more good health habits than non-users and fewer reported limitations of activity because of a health problem. Differences in the same direction could be perceived in the earlier 1987 survey, but they were not statistically significant. Users and non-users of CAM rated themselves similarly on dimensions of health and psychological distress.

Finally, the pattern of health services utilisation was similar in both surveys. Fewer users of CAM than non-users visited either a general practitioner or a specialist in the two weeks before the surveys (Table 6.4). Yet, there were no differences between the two groups as to the number of medications taken in the last two days.

DISCUSSION

This research confirms the findings of a number of previous studies concerning the profile of people who use CAM: they are more likely to be well off, better educated and middle-aged or young adults (Drivdahl and Miser, 1998;

TABLE 6.2: DEMOGRAPHIC CHARACTERISTICS OF USERS AND NON-USERS OF ALTERNATIVE MEDICINE

Variable	Quebec Health Survey 1987					Quebec Health Survey 1993				
	Users of alternative medicine n	%	Non-users of alternative medicine n	%	p (chi-square)	Users of alternative medicine n	%	Non-users of alternative medicine n	%	p (chi-square)
Age (yr)					0.002					0.001
0–29	48	24	62	31		109	31	93	26	
30–44	83	42	47	24		133	38	103	29	
45–64	50	25	61	31		90	25	101	29	
65 and over	19	10	30	15		21	6	56	16	
Sex					N.S.					N.S.
Female	121	60	102	51		204	58	212	60	
Male	79	40	98	49		149	42	141	40	
Education (yr)					0.001					0.001
0–7	31	20	42	28		21	8	51	19	
8–12	50	32	68	46		73	27	103	38	
13 and over	75	48	38	26		181	66	117	43	
Activity					0.001					0.001
Working	100	52	64	33		177	50	128	36	
Student	12	6	12	6		58	16	39	11	
Homemaker	36	19	46	24		39	11	61	17	
Unemployed	14	7	36	19		32	9	53	15	
Retired	20	10	26	14		22	6	48	14	
Other	9	5	8	4		25	7	24	7	

TABLE 6.2: *CONTINUED*

Variable	Quebec Health Survey 1987						Quebec Health Survey 1993					
	Users of alternative medicine		Non-users of alternative medicine		p (chi-square)		Users of alternative medicine		Non-users of alternative medicine		p (chi-square)	
	n	%	n	%			n	%	n	%		
Marital status					N.S.						N.S.	
Married	99	64	88	61			153	56	148	54		
Widow, divorced, separated	20	13	22	15			40	15	51	19		
Never married	37	21	35	24			82	30	73	27		
Household income					0.001						0.001	
<$20,000	37	21	71	40			36	12	101	34		
$20,000–$29,999	49	28	38	21			50	17	30	10		
$30,000–$39,999	29	16	24	14			42	14	38	13		
$40,000 and over	63	35	44	25			171	57	126	43		

TABLE 6.3: HEALTH PROFILE OF USERS AND NON-USERS OF ALTERNATIVE MEDICINE

Variable	Quebec Health Survey 1987					Quebec Health Survey 1993				
	Users of alternative medicine		Non-users of alternative medicine		p (Cochran-Mantel-Haenszel)[1]	Users of alternative medicine		Non-users of alternative medicine		p (Cochran-Mantel-Haenszel)[1]
	n	%	n	%		n	%	n	%	
Good health habits (no.)					N.S.					0.002
1–2	31	20	43	29		61	22	109	41	
3	48	31	47	32		89	33	82	30	
4	50	33	42	29		86	31	56	21	
5	25	16	15	10		39	14	22	8	
Self-rated health					N.S.					N.S.
Excellent	14	9	17	11		35	13	29	11	
Very good	65	41	54	36		86	32	59	22	
Good	51	33	42	28		111	41	108	40	
Fair/poor	27	17	37	25		41	15	76	28	
Limitation of activity due to health problem or chronic disease					N.S.					0.001
Yes	25	13	54	27		46	13	113	32	
No	175	88	146	73		307	87	240	68	
Psychological distress					N.S.					N.S.
Low-medium	118	77	97	68		193	71	176	66	
High	35	23	45	32		80	29	91	34	

[1] Adjusted for age, education and income

TABLE 6.4: HEALTH SERVICES UTILIZATION BY USERS AND NON-USERS OF ALTERNATIVE MEDICINE

Health service	Quebec Health Survey 1987					Quebec Health Survey 1993				
	Users of alternative medicine		Non-users of alternative medicine		p (Cochran-Mantel-Haenszel)[1]	Users of alternative medicine		Non-users of alternative medicine		p (Cochran-Mantel-Haenszel)[1]
	n	%	n	%		n	%	n	%	
Visit to general practitioner physician (2 wks before survey)					0.001					0.001
Yes	20	10	146	73		45	13	229	65	
No	179	90	54	27		308	87	124	35	
Visit to specialist physician (2 wks before survey)					0.001					0.001
Yes	5	3	40	20		16	5	88	25	
No	195	98	158	80		337	95	265	75	
Medication taken in last 2 days (no.)					N.S.					N.S.
None	55	28	67	34		105	30	81	23	
1 or 2	111	56	89	45		162	46	151	43	
3 or more	34	17	44	22		86	24	117	34	

[1] Adjusted for age, education and income

Eisenberg *et al.*, 1993; Kelner and Wellman, 1997b; Le Groupe Multi Réso, 1992; MacLennan *et al.*, 1996; Schar *et al.*, 1994; Sharma, 1992; Shekelle *et al.*, 1991, 1995; Vincent and Furnham, 1997). Other comparisons are more difficult to make because many of the variables examined here have rarely been looked at in previous studies. But what is more original and important is the analysis of the use of CAM over time.

Although the QHS87 and QHS93 were performed on two different samples, it seems clear that CAM is becoming more popular. Between 1987 and 1993, there has been an increase of more than 75% in the proportion of respondents who reported having consulted CAM practitioners. A similar trend has also been shown elsewhere (Eisenberg *et al.*, 1998). This cannot simply be accounted for by a general increase in health care consumption in Quebec, since use of medical services among non-users of CAM appears to have decreased slightly for general practitioners and increased slightly for specialists in the six-year period.

Besides this apparent increase in the popularity of CAM, there seemed to be a change in the nature of the use: the 1993 clientele concentrated less on one major therapy (chiropractor) and visited others to a larger extent than before. Another change is in the reasons for consultation. People did not go to CAM practitioners only to treat a problem that had been diagnosed but not helped by conventional medicine. In the later survey, they consulted CAM practitioners somewhat more for purposes of examination. Whether this replaces or adds to conventional medicine diagnostic assessment cannot be inferred from this study. If people visit CAM practitioners for 'diagnosis' in addition to conventional professionals, this could represent extra cost to them and/or society. If they consult the former instead of the latter, some medical conditions may be overlooked. Another possibility is that they resort to CAM after conventional medicine has been unable to give them satisfaction for their health problems. Indeed, some studies have shown that users of CAM complained that conventional medicine was too focused on treating symptoms rather than seeking the underlying causes of their conditions (Murray and Shepherd 1993; Sharma, 1992). (See also Section I in this book.) Either way, these findings show that conventional medicine is being challenged in its capacity to understand, explain and treat some 'difficult' health problems.

As mentioned, differences in demographic characteristics between users and non-users of CAM remained essentially the same from 1987 to 1993. However, three comments are worth making. First, it is not clear whether the increased popularity of these therapies among children and young adults represents a real trend for the future. It may be that as CAM gains in popularity among adults, these adults bring their children to CAM practitioners and encourage young adults in their families to consult them too. This study did not examine this hypothesis and more data would be needed to test it. However, some researchers who looked at a paediatric clientele found that parents of children who used CAM were more likely to use it themselves (Spigelblatt *et al.*, 1994).

Second, both surveys indicated that women represent a larger proportion of users of CAM than men. This pattern is supported by previous studies (e.g. Millar, 1997). However, women also generally consume more conventional health care than men (Hulka and Wheat 1985). This underlines the usefulness of comparing users to non-users in order to identify the unique characteristics of the former.

Third, as shown elsewhere, this study revealed that use of CAM was more popular among better educated persons. Several explanations can be proposed for this finding. An obvious one is that those with a higher level of education also often have higher incomes, allowing them to pay for CAM services which are not covered by health insurance. Another explanation may be that better educated persons tend to be more critical of conventional medicine and want to make their own choices concerning health and health care. In this sense, they may more easily try therapies other than those prescribed by physicians and conventional providers in general. Yet another reason could be that better educated persons are more knowledgeable about CAM than those with lower education. Another recent survey on the use of CAM in Quebec, Canada showed that knowing other persons who use CAM is significantly associated with education: about half of the persons with 13 years of schooling and over know at least one CAM user, while less than one third of persons with lower education do (Baril and Laplante, 1997).

In terms of health profile, the main finding is that those who consulted CAM practitioners appeared to be in somewhat better health than those who did not in 1993, while there was no difference between the two groups in 1987. The available data cannot tell us whether being healthier is a characteristic of patients prior to visiting CAM practitioners or a consequence of such consultations. Both phenomena may be operating at once. To test the first hypothesis, a longitudinal design with data collected from the same persons at different points in time would be needed. To examine the second hypothesis, evaluation studies would be required.

Other studies have shown that a substantial proportion (up to 83–88%) of clients of CAM also used conventional medical services (Eisenberg *et al.*, 1993; Verhoef *et al.*, 1994). From the data available in the Quebec surveys analyzed here, it was not possible to determine whether CAM users also visited physicians for the same health problem. As an imperfect proxy estimation of this possibility, we measured whether medical visits were made in the two week period during which a CAM practitioner was consulted. The results indicated that very few CAM users (no more than 13% vs. up to 73% of non-users of CAM) saw a physician during those two weeks. The very short time frame on which this finding is based may explain, at least in part, why it seems so different from other studies.

If much fewer CAM users made medical visits than non-users, does this mean large cost savings? Not necessarily. One must take into account the cost of CAM, whether paid for by clients themselves or by private or public insurance. Also, about the same proportion of persons in both groups report taking medication. As prescription drugs are becoming an increasingly expensive item in the overall health care budget, over time this finding will tend to reduce the differences in costs between CAM users and non-users. Yet another aspect must be taken into consideration. Although users and non-users of CAM rate their health similarly, their differential demographic and health profiles, especially in 1993, suggest that the later group is likely to have greater health needs and, consequently, require more medical care. This means that if CAM users do not see physicians as often as non-users because they have fewer health needs, the potential savings are not due to CAM itself. However, it is possible that some medical visits were avoided and savings made by consulting less expensive non-conventional practitioners. Further research is needed to clarify this issue.

So, does this study indicate that users and non-users of CAM are becoming more similar or are they moving apart over time? Overall, the results show that CAM continues to attract a particular clientele (i.e. middle-aged and young adults, better educated, well-off, less physically sick) that is different from the public as a whole. Since these therapies remain largely paid for by the clients themselves, and to a lesser extent, by private insurance, they are available mainly to a particular class of affluent people. It is likely that the clientele for CAM will only change substantially when these services are covered by public health care insurance and thus become essentially free of charge. Only then are we likely to see a change in the profile of the clientele, similar to the pattern that evolved with the services of midwives in Quebec when they became available to the general public.

LIMITATIONS OF THE STUDY

This study has a number of limitations. First, the study sample in the QHS93 is larger than in the QHS87, making differences more easily statistically significant in the first case. However, the differences between users and non-users of CAM are large enough to be only slightly affected by this. Second, while the two surveys were conducted in the same manner, they were not identical. To permit comparisons between them, some interesting variables that were present in only one of the two surveys could not be used (e.g. an indicator of overall health was calculated only in the QHS87). Third, measures of health care utilisation were rather crude and did not provide a detailed picture (e.g. What type of specific medical services were used? What specialists were consulted? What type of medication was taken? For what health conditions?). Fourth, it would have been interesting to document whether peoples' expectations toward CAM have changed over time. There was some hint about that in the changing reasons for consultation, but more details are needed to understand the motivations of CAM users. Fifth, just two points of observation (1987 and 1993) cannot provide conclusive indications regarding the trend of CAM utilisation. These limitations emphasize the fact that continuing assessment of the phenomenon, and in particular of specific therapies, is essential.

CONCLUSION

Using a follow-up technique which analysed two surveys conducted six years apart, it was possible to obtain a better picture of users and non-users of CAM than with the usual single cross-sectional studies. The trend seems to be that users will remain a particular subgroup of people as long as CAM is not integrated into the official health care system. In recent years, prompted by the public demand for CAM and the benefits it brings to many users, a number of authors have described opportunities and attempts to integrate CAM into conventional medical practices (Baldwin, 1996; Spiegel et al., 1998) or have spoken in favour of such an integration (Jacobs, 1995). Whether it would be good public health policy for the government to recognise these therapies and reimburse their cost (although the two issues are separate) depends on the answer to two fundamental questions.

The first question is: In these times of resource constraints, do those practices 'buy' the same (or more) health benefits for less money than conventional, currently insured therapies? More rigorous outcomes research is needed to answer this vitally important question (Bullock et al., 1997; Ernst et al., 1997). (See also Section 3 of this book.) The second question, which may be even more complex, is: What professional and organisational arrangements (e.g. level of professional autonomy of CAM practitioners, relationships between them and conventional health care providers, reference patterns, reimbursement mechanisms, liability insurance, hospital privileges) are needed so that CAM and conventional medicine can each play their role in the health care system and contribute the most to the health of the population? Analysing natural partnership experiences and implementing pilot projects may bring insights to this issue. Given the increasing demand for CAM, answering those two questions should become a health policy priority.

REFERENCES

Andersen, Ronald M. 1995. 'Revisiting the behavioral model and access to medical care: does it matter?' *Journal of Health and Social Behavior* 36:1–10.

Baldwin, Fred D. 1996. 'Unconventional therapy in Pennsylvania practices.' *Pennsylvania Medicine* 99(11):9–11.

Baril, Gérald and Benoît Laplante. 1997. *Enquête sur la culture scientifique et les choix reliés à la santé. Rapport de recherche.* Montréal: Institut national de la recherche scientifique – Culture et Société.

Bellerose, Carmen *et al.* 'Chapitre 1: méthodes.' 1995 pp. 1–11 in *Santé Québec – Et la santé, c[,]ja va en 1992–1993?* Montréal: ministère de la Santé et des Services sociaux, Gouvernement du Québec.

Blais, Régis, Aboubacrine Maïga and Alarou Aboubacar. 1997. 'How different are users and non users of alternative medicine?' *Canadian Journal of Public Health* 88:159–162.

Blais, Régis *et al.* 1997. *Évaluation des projets-pilotes de la pratique des sages-femmes au Québec. Rapport de recherche R97-08.* Montréal: Groupe de recherche interdisciplinaire en santé, Université de Montréal.

Buckle, Jane 1994. 'The status of complementary/alternative medicine in the United Kingdom.' *Nurse Practitioner Forum* 5:118–20.

Bullock, Milton L., Alfred M. Pheley, Thomas J. Kiresuk, Scott K. Lenz and Patricia D. Culliton. 1997. 'Characteristics and complaints of patients seeking therapy at a hospital-based alternative medicine clinic.' *Journal of Alternative & Complementary Medicine* 3(1):31–7.

Courtemanche, Robert and Franc[,]lois Tarte. 1987. *Plan de sondage de l'Enquête Santé Québec. Cahier technique 87-02.* Québec: Enquête Santé Québec.

Drivdahl, Christine E. and William F. Miser. 1998. 'The use of alternative health care by a family practice population.' *Journal of the American Board of Family Practice* 11:193–9.

Eisenberg, David M., Ronald C. Kessler, Cindy Foster *et al.* 1993. 'Unconventional Medicine in the United States. Prevalence, Costs, and Patterns of Use.' *New England Journal of Medicine* 328:246–52.

Eisenberg, David M., Roger B. Davis, Susan L. Ettner *et al.* 1998. 'Trends in alternative medicine use in the United States, 1990–1997: results of a follow-up national survey.' *Journal of the American Medical Association* 280:1569–75.

Ernst, Edzard (ed.). 1996. *Complementary medicine: an objective appraisal.* Oxford: Butterworth Heineman.

Ernst, Edzard, I. Siev-Ner and D. Gamus. 1997. 'Complementary medicine – a critical review.' *Israel Journal of Medical Sciences* 33:808–15.

Fisher, Peter and Adam Ward. 1994. 'Complementary medicine in Europe.' *British Medical Journal* 309:107–11.

Fulder, Stephen J. and Robin E. Munro. 1985. 'Complementary Medicine in the United Kingdom: patients, practitioners and consultations.' *Lancet* 2 (8454):542–5.

Goldbeck-Wood, Sandra, Alexander Dorozinsky, and Liv G.Lie. 1996. 'Complementary medicine is booming worldwide.' *British Medical Journal* 313:131–3.

Hulka, Barbara S. and John R. Wheat. 1985. 'Patterns of utilization: the patient perspective.' *Medical Care* 23:438–60.

Ilfeld, Frederic W. 1978. 'Psychological status of community residents along major demographic dimensions.' *Archives of General Psychiatry* 35:716–24.

Jacobs, Jennifer. 1995. 'Homeopathy should be integrated into mainstream medicine.' *Alternative Therapies in Health and Medicine* 1(4):48–53.

Kelner, Merrijoy and Beverly Wellman. 1997a. 'Health care and consumer choice: medical and alternative therapies.' *Social Science & Medicine* 45:203–12.

Kelner, Merrijoy and Beverly Wellman. 1997b. 'Who seeks alternative health care? A profile of the users of five modes of treatment.' *Journal of Alternative & Complementary Medicine* 3(2):127–140.

Le Groupe MultiRéso. 1992. *Enquête sur les thérapies alternatives pour le ministère de la Santé et des Services sociaux.* Montréal: Author.

MacLennan, Alastair H., David H. Wilson and Anne W. Taylor. 1996. 'Prevalence and cost of alternative medicine in Australia.' *Lancet* 347(9001):569–73.

McGuire, Meredith B. 1988. *Ritual healing in suburban America.* New Brunswick, N.J.: Rutgers University Press.

Millar, Wayne J. 1997. 'Use of alternative health care practitioners by Canadians.' *Canadian Journal of Public Health* 88:154–8.

Murray, Joanna and Simon Shepherd. 1993. 'Alternative or additional medicine? An exploratory study in general practice.' *Social Science & Medicine* 37:983–8.

Northcott, Herbert C. and John A. Bachynsky. 1993. 'Concurrent utilization of chiropractic, prescription medicines, nonprescription medicines and alternative health care.' *Social Science & Medicine* 37:431–5.

Préville, Michel. 1992. *La détresse psychologique: détermination de la fiabilité et de la validité de la mesure utilisée dans l'enquête Santé Québec, Enquête Santé Québec 87, Les cahiers de recherche, no 7.* Québec: Ministère de la Santé et des Services sociaux.

Saillant, Francine, Michel O'Neill and Danièle Desjardins. 1987. 'Entre le coeur et la raison: portrait de la clentèle d'une nouvelle sage-femme québécoise.' Pp. 295–315 in *Accoucher autrement*, edited by Francine Saillant and Michel O'Neill. Montréal: Editions Saint-Martin.

Santé Québec. 1988. *Et la santé, c[,]a va? Rapport de l'Enquête Santé Québec, tome 1.* Québec: Author.

Schar, A., V. Messerli-Rohrbach and P. Schubarth. 1994. 'Conventional or complementary medicine: what criteria for choosing do patients use?' *Schweizerische Medizinische Wochenschrift – Supplementum* 62:18–27.

Sharma, Ursula. 1992. *Complementary medicine today: practitioners and patients.* London: Routledge.

Shekelle, Paul G. and Robert H. Brook. 1991. 'A community-based study of the use of chiropractic services.' *American Journal of Public Health* 81:439–42.

Shekelle, Paul G., Martin Markovich and Rachel Louie. 1995. 'Factors associated with choosing a chiropractor for episodes of back pain care.' *Medical Care* 33:842–50.

Spigel, David, Penny Stroud and Ann Fyfe. 1998. 'Complementary medicine.' *Western Journal of Medicine* 168:241–7.

Spigelblatt, Linda S., Gisèle Laîné-Ammara, I. Barry Pless and Adrian Guyver. 1994. 'The use of alternative medicine by children.' *Pediatrics* 94:811–4.

Thomas, Kate J., Jane Carr, Linda Westlake and Brian T. Williams. 1991. 'Use of non-orthodox and conventional health care in Great Britain.' *British Medical Journal* 302:207–10.

Verhoef, Marja J., Margaret L. Russell and Edgar J. Love. 1994. 'Alternative medicine use in rural Alberta.' *Canadian Journal of Public Health* 85:308–9.

Verhoef, Marja J., Loyd R. Sutherland and Lawrence Brkich. 1990. 'Use of alternative medicine by patients attending a gastroenterology clinic.' *Canadian Medical Association Journal* 142:121–5.

Vincent, Charles and Adrian Furnham.. 1997. *Complementary medicine: a research perspective.* Chichester, England: Wiley.

Wardwell, Walter I. 1994. 'Alternative medicine in the United States.' *Social Science & Medicine* 38:1061–8.

World Health Organization. 1977. *International classification of diseases, 9th revision,* Geneva: Author.

ENDNOTES

1   A diagnosis code corresponding to each health problem was attributed using the International Classification of Diseases, version 9: ICD-9 (WHO 1977).

2   To test differences between users and non-users of CAM, analyses were made using the chi-square test for demographic variables and the Cochran-Mantel-Haenszel test for health profile and health care consumption, adjusting for appropriate demographic variables if needed.

3   The Cochran-Mantel-Haenszel test was used, and adjustment for age, education and income was made. Although there was also a significant difference between the two groups in terms of activity, we did not adjust for this variable since it was highly correlated with household income.

CHAPTER 7

Social Networks and Mass Media: the 'Diffusion' of CAM

THOMAS W. VALENTE

This chapter takes a diffusion network perspective to investigate the factors that influence access to and use of complementary and alternative medicine (CAM). The primary focus is on how social networks channel peoples' use of therapies or constrain their access to them. The diffusion network perspective provides a set of guidelines useful for understanding CAM use and the factors likely to affect who will use CAM and when. Here I treat the use of CAM as an innovation on the part of the person who seeks it out. An *innovation* is any idea or practice perceived as new by the user (Rogers, 1995). While many CAM therapies are in fact very old technologies or ideas, their current adoption and use are innovations in today's health care system. Indeed, many CAM therapies are unknown to most physicians, but may be more familiar to other groups in contemporary society.

PHYSICIAN AND PATIENT USE OF CAM

When studying the potential or actual diffusion of CAM in society, an important distinction needs to be made between diffusion within the provider or physician community and within the lay or patient population. Medical innovations often must diffuse through these two populations simultaneously to be widely accepted. Since many medical therapies are prescribed by physicians, these medical innovations often have to diffuse through the physician community before they can be widely adopted by patients. Thus, the physicians serve a gatekeeping function in some ways designed to slow diffusion. This pattern has been clear in the case of CAM; until recently very few physicians were aware of the nature of CAM therapies and were reluctant to recognize or recommend them.

On the other hand, many people have become extremely well-educated about the available therapies for a particular illness. In such situations, the patient population may be more informed than the physicians they see for that illness, and the patients may in fact put pressure on them for certain therapies such as acupuncture or reflexology. Thus, there may be a dynamic push-pull process in which physicians are seen as pushing certain therapies while patients are pulling for certain other therapies. There can be tension between physicians and patients when deciding which therapies to prescribe for an illness. This tension is sometimes alleviated and sometimes exacerbated by the complex process of patient education. Patient education is sometimes facilitated by healthcare institutions, but oftentimes occurs outside of such institutions, in support groups, in ad-hoc patient organizations, and importantly in the case of CAM, through the mass media.

The point is that there are both supply and demand factors that interact with one another in a complex dynamic process that influences the diffusion of CAM in mainstream medical treatment. In the last decade, a market for alternative health care providers emerged to address the needs of people who wanted alternatives, but could not get them through mainstream healthcare services. As the numbers and types of these providers grew, and the testimonials of satisfied users spread, the market for alternatives broadened to the point where traditional service providers could no longer ignore it.

In this chapter I will focus on the factors that influence *patients'* knowledge and use of CAM. In particular I will focus on specific factors expected to influence their transitions as they seek information about CAM in the process of trying to find appropriate care for an illness. Part of the framework I follow is a traditional staged model of behavior change in which patients are expected to move through the various knowledge, attitude, and practice stages of behavioural transition (Rogers, 1995; Valente Paredes and Poppe, 1998).

STAGES OF BEHAVIOR CHANGE

A key element in the diffusion of innovations is that individuals do not immediately adopt an innovation, but instead pass through stages of change that determine the timing of behavioral transition (Chaffee and Roser, 1986; Prochaska DiClemente and Norcross, 1992; Rogers, 1995; Valente and Rogers, 1995; Valente Merritt and Poppe, 1996). Specifically, individuals first become aware of a new idea or practice such as chiropractic, before they develop a positive attitude toward that practice and then actually try it. After a trial period in which individuals evaluate the technology for themselves, they may decide to adopt it and make it a regular part of their lifestyle or they may ignore it. In the final stage of adoption, the person becomes an advocate for the new technology (i.e., chiropractic care) (Figure 7.1).

FIGURE 7.1: ADOPTION STAGES (FROM VALENTE ET AL., 1996)

Diffusion of Innovations (Rogers, 1995)	Steps to Behaviour Change (SBC) (Piotrow, et al., 1997)	Complementary & Alternative Medicine Definitions
Awareness	Knowledge • Recalls message • Understands topic • Can name source of supply	Knows that various new therapies are available for a variety of conditions.
Persuasion	Approval • Likes message • Discusses with others • Thinks others approve • Approves him/herself	Believes that CAM can alleviate certain conditions more effectively than traditional therapies.
Decision	Intention • New behaviour fills need • Intends to get info. • Intends to practice	Decides to consider CAM treatments when confronted with conditions.
Implementation	Practice • Gets info./services • Gets product • Continues use	Uses CAM therapies to treat some or many conditions.
Confirmation	Advocacy • Knows benefits of new practice • Advocates to others • Supports further use	Understands advantages of CAM therapies, advocates their use to others and supports continued CAM research.

Progress through these stages may seem slower for earlier adopters than for later ones because the earlier adopters face more risk and uncertainty in their adoption and because few other people in their community have tried the innovation. The lack of other prior users means that individuals do not have a base of users to consult and so are making adoption decisions with little social support (Wellman and Wortley, 1990). Consequently, earlier adopters may be more cautious in their adoption behaviour. In some cases, however, earlier adopters may move through these stages quickly because they can not delay adoption due to severe pain. They hope that a new technology like chiropractic will give them relief and consequently do not wait for social support.

Figure 7.1 also depicts definitions of each adoption stage in the CAM context. Individuals who know that various CAM therapies are available to treat certain conditions are in the 'awareness' stage. Once those individuals believe that these CAM therapies can alleviate certain conditions more effectively than other treatments they are in the 'persuasion' stage. Deciding to consider CAM use and actually trying CAM therapies constitute the 'decision' and 'implementation' stages, respectively, while advocating CAM use to others constitutes the 'confirmation' stage.

Of course, there are individuals and situations that deviate from this staged model of behaviour change (Valente, Poppe and Paredes, 1998). For example, some innovations are so advantageous that little time is spent passing from awareness of the innovation to its adoption. This may be true for certain: (1) innovations, (2) individuals, and (3) situations. Some innovations are clearly better than those that preceded them and as a consequence are quickly adopted with little evaluation (e.g., color TV was quickly substituted for black and white). Some individuals are keen to be the first to try new ideas and techniques when they become available (technology buffs often fall into this category). Finally, there are certain critical situations when individuals do not have the luxury of slow and deliberate evaluation of therapies to decide on their use but feel they must take a chance that the new technique will help them. For example, this may be the case for cancer patients who are pronounced terminal and feel that they have little recourse but to use CAM therapies in the hope that they can stave off the disease's progression.

STAGES OF DIFFUSION

Generally, innovations spread throughout a population over a substantial period of time. For example, a profitable and attractive innovation such as hybrid seed corn took 14 years to diffuse to all farmers in two counties of Iowa (Ryan and Gross, 1943). In some cases, innovations diffuse quite rapidly, while in others they diffuse more slowly. The factors that influence the spread of innovation are numerous (Rogers, 1995) and a full enumeration of them is clearly beyond this chapter. The following factors have been identified as being associated with more rapid diffusion of innovations:

1) Less radical innovations spread more rapidly (Robertson, 1973);
2) Innovations perceived as more advantageous, more compatible, trialable, observable, and less complex spread more rapidly (Fliegel and Kivlin, 1966);
3) Less expensive innovations spread more rapidly (Griliches, 1957);
4) The presence of 'innovation champions' speeds diffusion (Valente, 1995).

As innovations spread, different groups of people adopt them. Figure 7.2 shows a typical diffusion curve. Four types of adopters have been identified based on their time of adoption (Rogers, 1995):

1) early adopters[1] (16%);
2) early majority (34%);
3) late majority (34%); and
4) laggards (16 %);

The percentages for each stage can be calculated from data on time of adoption. (Early adopters are those who adopted one standard deviation earlier than the average time of adoption, while the early majority are those who adopted before the average time of adoption and so on.) The following labels can be used to further describe the adoption types:

1) early adopters – pioneers or trend setters;
2) early majority – market development;
3) late majority – spread; and
4) laggards – maturation.

Early adopters. Early adopters of CAM were generally influenced to use CAM for three reasons:

1) the therapy was easy to use and presented little risk;
2) the individual was in the habit of trying these new techniques; and/or
3) the individual faced chronic or acute illness and was desperate for some treatment.

These early adopters followed a relatively short information seeking and decision-making process because they had compelling reasons to adopt the new techniques. Many early CAM users adopted technology that was patently advantageous and presented little risk. For example, meditation has obvious advantages and poses little risk to the user. The benefits of such behavioural adoption would be apparent to the users almost immediately. In

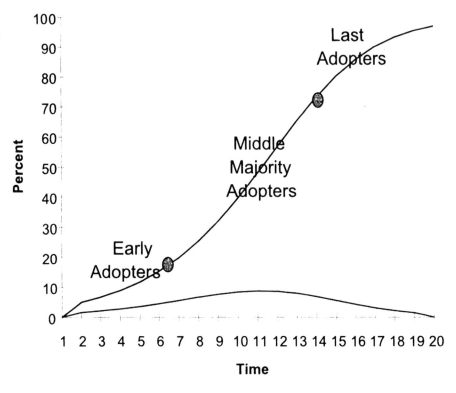

FIGURE 7.2:   GRAPH OF DIFFUSION STAGES

addition, the technology might be compatible with the person's prior beliefs and attitudes.

Some early adopters are in the habit of trying new techniques in this area when they become available. Such individuals are natural risk-takers and often delight in being the first in their group to experience new technologies such as St. John's Wort. These early adopters may be perceived as being slightly marginal in their social milieux, given their propensity to continually adopt new technologies. Finally, some early adopters of CAM did so because they had no choice. For example, many persons infected with AIDS had few treatments that they could use with any hope of success and thus resorted to CAM therapies in large numbers.

Middle Majority Adopters. The middle (early and late) majority adopters are the next groups to adopt CAM after the early adopters. The early majority adopters take up innovations faster than the average adoption time, and hence these adopters are considered innovative, but not radically so. Early majority adopters have demographic and psychographic characteristics more-or-less consistent with the general population. As alternate therapies make their way into mainstream society they will diffuse to these middle majority groups. Currently, it is estimated that over 40% of the U.S. population use CAM (Eisenberg, Davis, Ettner *et al.*, 1998). Thus we see that the diffusion of CAM is passing from the early to late majority stages at the end of the 20th century in the United States.

Given this level of market maturity, there is a substantial time-lag between the point when new users of CAM first became aware of these innovative therapies and the point at which they actually use them for the first time. During the time period when individuals pass through the adoption stages, they will engage in considerable information seeking, as well as purposive evaluation of the techniques being considered.

As the innovation diffuses to the second half of the population, that is late majority adopters, there will be considerably less risk to adoption. In fact, many individuals may have more than a few friends or acquaintances who have tried the alternative medical therapy and thus will feel less risk and uncertainty in their adoption decision. Moreover, they can turn to these prior adopters for advice and comfort as they try the innovation.

The middle majority represents the group that will make the most extensive evaluation of the innovation. Their appraisals of it may greatly influence the diffusion of the new therapy. Early adopters will spend less time evaluating the specifics of each alternative therapy, while the middle majority will actually discuss the attributes of the innovation more extensively with others in their network, in a process of information seeking and exchange.

INFORMATION NEEDS OF POTENTIAL CAM AUDIENCES

After individuals become aware of a new alternative, they will want to learn more about it. For example, if an individual is told by a physician about a possible CAM therapy such as Reiki, that may be appropriate for his/her condition, the patient is likely to seek out some information that describes the therapy. Patients may discuss this with their family members, close friends and other confidants. These network ties are likely to have a strong influence on whether they consider adopting Reiki. A key factor in this process is whether people have someone in their network who has tried the therapy or knows someone else who has tried it (see Wellman, 1988 for a description of networks).

Finding prior users is an important step in the process of adoption since prior users provide important sources of support and information that ease adoption decisions (Valente, 1995). If the prior users are similar to the patient contemplating adoption, he/she is likely to be reassured that the new technology is appropriate and this makes it easier to adopt (Burt, 1987, 1995). The characteristics of the person's information environment strongly influences his/her ability to decide to use CAM and policymakers should be attuned to the informational needs of potential CAM audiences.

After patients become aware of new alternatives, they typically first consult their network of family, friends and associates. The network's ability to provide them with information, influence and support will be directly linked to their decision to try or not try the alternative. The more developed patients' networks, the more extensive and diverse (Valente, 1995), the more rapid and conclusive the decision-making will be. Individuals without such network support face a more uncertain adoption environment in which they are forced to make decisions about adopting CAM with less information and less assurance that support will be forthcoming during their trial stage.

It is also possible that in addition to their networks, some patients will turn to other sources of information to help them make their decisions. First, they may be more attuned to information in the mass media, now that they are aware of certain CAM therapies. Second, increasing numbers of patients are likely to turn to the Internet or their local library to seek more specific information about the alternative that interests them. Increasingly, this type of information search is likely to provide a rich trove of information that people can use to make their adoption decisions. As CAM therapies become more widely used, more information about their effects and applications will be available on the Internet and other electronic media.

The information search eventually leads to a decision to try or not try CAM. If individuals decide *not* to try the alternative, they may simply be postponing the decision and, in effect, deciding to decide later on, or they may be deciding definitively not to try the alternative. If they are postponing, then the information they have collected may be stored and used to inform a decision at a later date. For most people, reappraisal of their adoption decision will only occur if some cue-to-action triggers a reconsideration of the therapy.

If individuals decide to go ahead and adopt the alternative medical therapy, then they have now embarked on the most critical stage of the behavior change process. The decision to try the innovation may occur soon after they learn about the alternative, or may take a considerable amount of time. Regardless, once they initiate trial of the innovation they become a new adopter of a CAM therapy. Here individuals begin to rely heavily on their own impressions, interpretations, and experiences with the therapy. If they feel better, or the therapy addresses the problem it was designed to address, then they are likely to begin feeling positively about CAM and pass that information on. Positive impressions generally result in continued adoption, and over time, individuals come to feel that CAM represents a new component of their healthcare repertoire.

In contrast, should the CAM therapy produce side effects, unanticipated effects, or prove to be non-effective, then individuals will likely disadopt or discontinue the therapy. They may spend some initial efforts communicating these reactions to their caretakers and their social networks, however, they are at high risk of disadoption at this stage. Follow-up with new adopters is absolutely essential to insuring that new adopters stay adopters.

Some users will be satisfied with the therapy they have adopted and become continuing and confirmed users of CAM. There are three primary consequences to this behavior. New acceptors:

1) become models that others may witness using CAM;
2) can become advocates for CAM; and
3) may more readily adopt other CAM therapies.

Creating this pool of CAM users is quite obviously fundamental to establishing a mature market of CAM therapies, for multiple reasons. Chief among them, however, is that this pool becomes the main influence on adoption and the spread of CAM therapies to other users. The interaction between users and non-users represents the key to understanding how diffusion spreads through networks.

NETWORK CHARACTERISTICS

Individuals become aware of and evaluate innovations in the larger context of the behavior of the rest of the population. As I have argued, the diffusion stage is an important component in understanding how individuals can be expected to adopt CAM. Early adopters are considered distinct from the middle majority, and in all likelihood, the middle majorities will have some exposure to CAM through their networks of friends, family and acquaintances. These contacts will often provide a first source of awareness of CAM or provide the first reaction to the individual's mention of it.

Figure 7.3 displays a hypothetical personal network for an individual contemplating adoption of a CAM therapy. Individuals will turn to others for advice, information, support and reactions concerning the new therapy. If they have friends who use the alternative, the risk and uncertainty to adoption are diminished, thus facilitating trial and continued use. If there are no users in their network, individuals will seek out impersonal sources of information such as newspapers, magazines, television, the web and so on, which are often not satisfactory or sufficient for adoption.

Individuals who decide to adopt CAM are often influenced by friends, family and associates who have already adopted it for their own use. As the proportion or volume of CAM users increases, it is more likely that a person

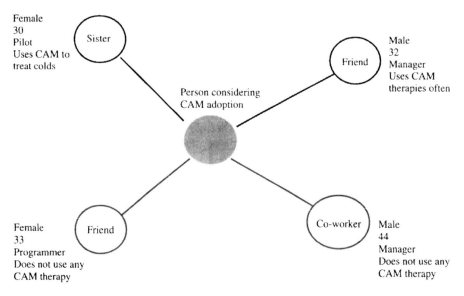

Female
30
Pilot
Uses CAM to
treat colds

Sister

Friend

Male
32
Manager
Uses CAM
therapies often

Person considering
CAM adoption

Female
33
Programmer
Does not use any
CAM therapy

Friend

Co-worker

Male
44
Manager
Does not use any
CAM therapy

FIGURE 7.3:   HYPOTHETICAL PERSONAL NETWORK OF ONE PERSON.

will try a new therapy. Although there is probably a direct correlation between the presence of other CAM users in an individual's network and use by that person, there is research suggesting that some people try new ideas and practices even though they have few adopters in their personal network (Valente, 1995, 1996). These 'low threshold' adopters can serve as local opinion leaders in their networks and provide the impetus needed for innovations to reach a critical mass of acceptors (Valente, 1995, Valente and Davis, 1999).

Local leaders and low threshold adopters have been found to have higher socio-economic status than their peers and to rely on impersonal sources of information such as magazines, journals, mass media and so on (Valente, 1995). For the middle majority, the presence of others in their networks who have already adopted provides an important sounding board for innovation. Nevertheless, individual information-seeking-and-exchange characteristics as well as decision-making style can intervene to predispose some leaders to adopt CAM earlier than most of the people in their networks.

As an innovation like CAM moves through its diffusion stages, the role of networks in the adoption process changes. Early adopters are accustomed to making adoption decisions independent of their network of friends, family and associates. The middle majority, however, will be more strongly influenced by the interaction they have with their networks, and some will be able to adopt CAM in spite of their networks' hesitation, while others will demonstrate increased resistance and wait still longer before adopting.

THE INFLUENCE OF THE MASS MEDIA

Different media channels and messages have been shown to be appropriate at different diffusion stages (McGuire, 1989, Rice and Atkin, 1989). For example, early in the diffusion process, targeted media should be created to assist early adopters with their adoption of CAM. Since early adopters have no peers to rely on for information and since the risk and uncertainty are high, specific media with detailed information about an innovation like CAM should be disseminated to these users and made available (Valente, 1995). These early adopters will then become the major source of referral for the middle majority, particularly since these early adopters will have the most experience with CAM and their opinion is likely to be valued.

As diffusion spreads to the middle majority, mass media or more widespread campaigns may be appropriate to facilitate broader discussion and diffusion of CAM. The low threshold adopters at this stage may be more widely dispersed throughout society and so should be reached through mass media type channels. Also, testimonials from earlier adopters of CAM may be incorporated into messages since a pool of early users is now available.

CONCLUSIONS

This chapter has sketched a broad outline of how social networks and mass media factors might influence the diffusion of CAM. The main point is that the network influences are likely to be dependent on the stage of the innovations' diffusion. For early adopters, network influences on adoption may be minimal, since adoption decisions are often based on personal or situational factors not amenable to prolonged decision-making. For the middle majority, network influences on adoption may be extensive, since decisions to adopt are based on a protracted process of information seeking and exchange.

Promotional programs seeking to accelerate CAM diffusion should focus on the informational environment of potential users. In most cases, individuals will rely on the opinions and attitudes of their family, friends and associates to inform their adoption decision. Promotional materials should be attuned to providing information that will facilitate this collective decision-making. As CAM use spreads and the world wide web proliferates, electronic sources of information will increasingly be used in many different countries to initiate and validate the use of CAM for health care problems.

ENDNOTE

1.   Diffusion theory divides the early adopters into innovators (2.5%) and the early majority (13.5%), but here we collapse them into one group.

REFERENCES

Burt, Ronald S. 1987. Social contagion and innovation: Cohesion versus structural equivalence. *American Journal of Sociology*, 92:1287–1335.

Burt, Ronald S. 1995. *Structural holes: The Social Structure of competition*. New York: Belknap.

Chaffee, S.H., and Roser. (1986). Involvement and the consistency of knowledge, attitudes, and behaviours. *Communication Research*, 13, 373–399.

Eisenberg, David M., Roger B., Davis, Susan L. Ettner, Scott Appel, Sonja Wilkey, Maria Van Rompay, & Ronald C. Kessler. 1998. 'Trends in Alternative Medicine Use in the United States, 1990–1997: Results of a Follow-up National Survey. *The Journal of the American Medical Association* 280: 1569–1575.

Fliegel, Frederick C. and Joseph E. Kivlin. 1966. Attributes of innovations as factors in diffusion. *American Journal of Sociology*, 72:235–248.

Griliches, Zvi. 1957. Hybrid corn: An exploration in the economics of technical change. *Econometrica*, 25:501–522.

Mcguire, William J. 1989. Theoretical foundations of campaigns. In *Public communication campaigns* edited by Ronald E. Rice and Charles K. Atkin. Newbury Park, CA: Sage.

Prochaska, James O., Carlo C. DiClemente and John C. Norcross. 1992. In search of how people change: Applications to addictive behaviors. *American Psychologist*, 47:1102–1114.

Rice, Ronald E. and Charles K. Atkin. 1989. *Public communication campaigns*. Newbury Park, CA: Sage.

Robertson, Thomas S. 1973. *Innovative behavior and communication*. New York: Holt, Rinehart and Winston.

Rogers, Everett M. 1995. *Diffusion of innovations (4th ed.)*. New York: The Free Press.

Ryan, Bryce, and Gross, Neal C. (1943). The diffusion of hybrid seed corn in two Iowa communities. *Rural Sociology*, 8(1):15–24.

Valente, Thomas W. 1996. Social network thresholds in the diffusion of innovations. *Social Networks*, 18:69–89.

Valente, Thomas W. 1995. *Network models of the diffusion of innovations*. Cresskill, NJ: Hampton Press.

Valente, Thomas W. and Rebecca L. Davis. 1999. Accelerating diffusion of innovations using opinion leaders. *The Annals of the American Academy of the Political and Social Sciences*.

Valente, Thomas W., Patricia Paredes and Patricia R. Poppe. 1998. Matching the message to the process: The relative ordering of knowledge, attitudes and practices in behavior change research. *Human Communication Research*, 24:366–385.

Valente, Thomas W., Patricia R. Poppe and Alice Payne Merritt. 1996. Mass media generated interpersonal communication as sources of information about family planning. *Journal of Health Communication*, 1:259–273.

Valente, Thomas W. and Everett M. Rogers. 1995. The origins and development of the diffusion of innovations paradigm as an example of scientific growth. *Science Communication: An Interdisciplinary Social Science Journal*, 16:238–269.

Valente, Thomas W. and Walter Saba. 1998. Mass media and interpersonal influence in a reproductive health communication campaign in Bolivia. *Communication Research*, 25:96–124.

Valente, Thomas W,. Susan C. Watkins, Miriam N. Jato, Ariane Van der Straten and Louis-Philippe M. Tsitsol. 1997. Social network associations with contraceptive use among Cameroonian women in voluntary associations. *Social Science and Medicine*, 45:677–687.

Wellman, Barry. 1988. Chapters 1 and 2. In *Social structures: A network approach* edited by Barry Wellman and Steve D. Berkowitz. Cambridge, UK: Cambridge University Press.

Wellman, Barry and Scott Wortley. 1990. Different strokes from different folks: Community ties and social support. *American Journal of Sociology*, 96:558–588.

CHAPTER 8

Partners in Illness: Who Helps When You Are Sick?

BEVERLY WELLMAN

IDENTIFYING HEALTH CARE SUPPORTERS IN THE COMMUNITY

Since the 1960s, sociologists and anthropologists have been interested in the association between the use of medical services and the influence of family, friends and others on health care choices (Mechanic, 1968; Suchman, 1965; Kleinman, 1980; Ryan, 1998). Kadushin (1966) found that the use of psychiatric services was associated with membership in an informal social circle that was supportive of psychotherapy. Patients who belonged to such a circle were more likely to receive support, advice and encouragement, compared to the clinic patients who were not members of a psychiatrically oriented informal group.

While some researchers have argued that the presence of everyday symptoms of illness is not necessarily sufficient to bring a person to medical care (Alonzo, 1979; Coe et al., 1984; Levanthal and Hirschman, 1982), others have noted the important influence of family, friends and others on the process of seeking care (McKinlay, 1972; Salloway and Dillon, 1973; Pescosolido, 1986, 1992). Such scholars have discovered empirically that who one talks to influences what one does, and particularly, what course of action is taken to resolve health problems (Pescosolido et al., 1998). For example, McKinlay (1975) found that those people whose social networks were composed primarily of family tended to be underutilizers of health care, while those whose social networks were composed primarily of friends tended to be heavy utilizers of medical care.

On a more general level, Friedson (1960) identified the importance of the 'lay referral system'; Kleinman (1980) and Kleinman, Eisenberg and Good (1978) described how the 'popular sphere' (members of one's community) influenced health, and Chrisman and Kleinman (1983) expounded upon the interrelationship between the use of the popular sphere, the 'professional' sector (Western medicine) and the 'folk' sector (complementary and alternative therapies) in the quest for health care. Yet despite these documented overlaps and linkage between the popular, professional and folk sectors, most scholars have tended to analyse the use of a single sector, the professional sphere. In chapter ten, Pescosolido discusses the Network Episode Model which takes a broad perspective on how people find their way into various treatments. It focuses on the social influences exerted by community members on the dynamic process of dealing with emotional and physical health problems. Adopting a network analytic approach has made it possible to broaden the focus and ask patients from a variety of modes of treatment to tell us who were the people they depended on for support and information for their health concerns, and ultimately their health care choices. This is the model used in the research reported here.

The key question posed was: To whom do patients involved in various treatment modalities turn when they have a health problem? The research looked at the patients of four different kinds of alternative practitioners (chiropractors, acupuncturists/traditional Chinese medicine doctors, naturopaths and Reiki healers) as well as the patients of family physicians (called general practitioner in the UK and primary care givers in the USA). It examined the ties that provided three major kinds of health support: 1) talking about health (i.e., health confidants), 2) giving general information about health, and 3) giving specific information about alternative therapies and practitioners. The main objective was to explore the support and information that patients received from family and friends, as well as from practitioners. In this connection, scholars have shown that not all network members are supportive, and that among those network members who are supportive, different members provide different kinds of support (Wellman and Wellman, 1992). Although ties with healthcare professionals (physicians) are included in the analysis, previous research (Eisenberg *et al.*, 1993, Wellman, 1995) has shown that patients are not learning about alternatives to conventional medical care from their physicians. Using a network approach and not pre-defining who the health information providers would be, made it possible to discover and describe how health support flowed to patients in this study from their social networks, and subsequently to identify how some patients found their way to complementary and alternative medicine (CAM) practitioners. For example, while spouses provide a wide range of support compared to network members outside the household (Wellman and Wellman, 1992), friends and family members each tend to provide different kinds of support (Wellman and Wortley, 1989, 1990).

Interviewing patients from five treatment groups, made it possible to examine the linkages between 300 Toronto-area patients and their 1344 health ties (See Kelner and Wellman, 1997a and 1997b for detailed information on sample selection.). The fundamental problem was to disentangle what types of ties were associated with which kinds of health support for patients in each of the five treatment groups. A secondary goal, but nonetheless germane to the study, was to assess the importance of:

- The *strength of ties,* from very close intimates to acquaintances. 'Strong ties' were measured by asking patients to tell us how close they felt to the person giving them support. The scale ranged from 1 (extremely close) to 5 (acquaintance only, not close at all). Given the research objectives and large data set, the five categories were collapsed into three: very close, close and acquaintance.
- The *basis of the relationship,* be it kinship, friendship, family physician, or alternative practitioner. In response to the original question, 'Who do patients turn to when they have a health problem?', all of the relational responses to the health support questions were grouped into four categories that reflected the informal, professional and folk sectors: kin, friends,[2] physicians and alternative practitioners
- The *access* that patient and network members have to each other. Access or frequency of contact was measured by: frequency of face-to-face contact, frequency of phone contact and residential distance from one another. Frequency of face-to-face and phone contact were measured on a scale ranging from 182 ('a few times per week') through 52 ('weekly'), 12 ('monthly'), 2 ('2 times per year') to 0 ('never'), with gradations in between. Distance was measured in minutes from 0 ('same residence') to 400 ('more than 5 hours away'), with meaningful time distances in-between.

In essence, we asked if the patients of family physicians had more family members and fewer alternative practitioners in their networks than the patients of CAM practitioners? By examining the relationships of supportive health networks for each treatment group, it was possible to reach a conclusion to this question,

THE STRENGTH OF TIES

Granovetter (1973) provides a useful way of understanding how some patients moved from informal to conventional medical care to alternative care. He argues that it is weak ties – not strong ties[3] – that are important for the diffusion of information. Whereas strong ties tend to be found between persons who are members of the same social circle, weak ties tend to be found between socially dissimilar persons, which gives them access to more diverse social circles. Hence, Granovetter argues, weak ties transmit a greater range of information.

In support of Granovetter's weak ties argument, Weimann (1982, p. 769), in his study of communication flows, notes the importance of 'marginals' as 'bridges' or 'importers' of new information. Nevertheless, strong ties are often more supportive and persuasive (Wellman and Wortley, 1990; Wellman, 1992). For example, Lee (1969) and Badgley, Fortin-Caron and Powell (1987) found that many women used ties with close friends and family as key sources of information for locating (then illegal) abortionists.

Therefore, we examined the relationship between the strength of a tie, the type of treatment a patient was in, and the type of support given. For example, did people who have strong ties become health confidants for family physicians? Did people who have weak ties provide information about alternative practitioners? We expected that weak ties would predominate in providing information about alternative practitioners – because information about them is not widely known – while strong ties would predominate in providing support and information about the more established treatments of family physicians and chiropractors. For example, the prediction for Reiki clients would be that they would have the largest networks of all five groups of patients, and by extension, a larger proportion of their networks would be comprised of acquaintances (weak ties). Furthermore, given that Reiki therapy is relatively unknown, not popular, and not reimbursable from the state or private insurance, one should expect to find support for Granovetter and Weimann's arguments about weak ties as bridges to Reiki and Reiki practitioners.[4]

BASIS OF RELATIONSHIP

Where did a majority of supportive information come from; the popular, medical and/or folk (CAM) sectors? Many health care professionals are aware that much of the health information their patients acquire; comes from the lay public, including the Internet. In this study, we differentiate between family and friends. Research has shown that family – especially close family – tend to be supportive (Pratt, 1976). People have a normative claim on their relatives' help in dealing with taxing health situations, and densely-knit kin networks are structurally connected so that members can learn about health problems and mobilize collective support (Wellman, 1990). Yet friends may tap into more diverse social circles and hence, be more apt to know about alternative forms of health care.

To recognize the importance of family and friends in health networks is not to downplay the importance of health care practitioners in such networks. They can serve as confidants, sources of information, and sources of referral to other practitioners. But the situation is not symmetric for physicians and alternative practitioners. For one thing, alternative practitioners (except for chiropractors) have no officially recognized status, and their fees are not covered by the government's health insurance plan. Moreover, many physicians have a low regard for alternative therapies, while CAM therapists have been shown to have more mixed and more accepting opinions about physician-based medicine (Wellman, 1995; Kelner, Hall and Coulter, 1980). This suggests, on the one hand, that family physicians will be substantial participants in the networks of their patients, but CAM practitioners will not be members of these networks. On the other hand, we predict that both family physicians and CAM practitioners will be substantial participants in the networks of patients who use CAM therapies.

ACCESS

Information, advice and support about health can only be provided if the giver and the recipient are in communication with each other. Such communication is also the principal means by which network members learn about each other's health problems. In addition, the more that people are in contact, the more likely they are to empathize with each other (Homans, 1961). Wellman and Wortley (1990) have found that the supportiveness of such contact is independent of the strength of the tie and the basis of the relationship. In other words, the more contact that network members have, the more health support they can be expected to provide.

The physical proximity of network members may also matter, despite the communication facilitated by the telephone and the Internet (Wellman and Tindall, 1993). It has been demonstrated that communication media are never a total substitute for the full range of communication that face-to-face contact provides (Wellman and Gulia, 1999). This is an especially important consideration when people are communicating about delicate matters of health. Moreover, physical proximity means that network members can more easily provide concrete health care.

GATHERING A HEALTH NETWORK SAMPLE

The information on health ties comes from the patients' responses to the following four questions:

(1) Who do you talk to when you have problems with your health?
(2) Who, if anyone, gives you information about health in general?
(3) Who, if anyone, gives you information about alternative health care practitioners?
(4) Who, if anyone, gives you information about alternative therapies?

For each question, patients were asked to name a maximum of three persons. The responses to the questions on information about therapies and practitioners were combined in order to simplify the complex management of data and also because the responses to the two alternative support questions tell a similar story. In total, three hundred patients spoke about 1,344 people who were important to their health histories.[5]

STUDYING HEALTH TIES IN METROPOLITAN TORONTO

The patients came from all parts of Metropolitan Toronto, a city with a population of more than three million people. While most of the patients in this study were Canadian and European, the city is ethnically diverse and multi-cultural. 'Institutionally complete' ethnic communities tend to take care of their members' health needs by using physicians and other health care practitioners who come from their own ethnic group (Breton, 1964). This means that a variety of alternative therapies and therapists which are particular to certain ethnic communities are available to everyone else in the city. The patients we interviewed reflected the cosmopolitan nature of Toronto. They came from a variety of backgrounds and displayed a variety of patterns for obtaining help for their health problems. Had English not been a requirement, the percentage of foreign born would have been higher.

Patient characteristics

The three hundred patients in this study exhibited different kinds of social characteristics, depending on the type of health care they were currently using. The characteristics highlighted here are the ones that are relevant to their health network behaviour. In the case of gender, women were in the majority in all five of the treatment groups. Their percentage was highest among patients who were using acupuncture/traditional Chinese medicine (70%), naturopathy and Reiki (85%) and lowest among patients of chiropractors (58%). In terms of age, the highest mean age was found among the patients of family physicians (m = 56, md = 60 and the lowest mean age was found among the patients of chiropractors (m = 40, md = 37). Echoing the research of scholars here and in other countries (Astin, 1998, Eisenberg et al., 1998; Furnham and Smith, 1988; Sharma, 1995), the data here show that CAM patients were well educated. In fact, they were better educated than the patients of family physicians, and Reiki patients had achieved the highest educational level of any of the groups (88% had university degrees). In addition, these CAM patients were also more affluent than family physician patients; Reiki patients earned the highest income of all (51% earned at least $65,000 per year).

Health Problems

CAM patients reported more about chronic problems than did the patients of family physicians, who said they saw their doctors for more acute kinds of problems such as cardiovascular conditions as well as diagnosis and monitoring. Not surprisingly, chiropractic patients consulted their practitioners almost entirely for musculoskeletal problems. Other differences between groups were minimal, although more patients used Reiki for emotional problems than any other patients.

Patients' Health Ties

CAM patients had more health ties to members of their social community than did patients of family physicians (Table 8.1). In other words, these patients had more people in their social networks with whom they could discuss health issues. Of all the CAM groups, Reiki patients had the highest number of health ties (mean = 5.2) compared to family physician patients (mean = 3.9). It is worth noting that more than half of the health ties for each of the treatment groups were female (family physician ties = 55%, chiropractic ties = 52%, acupuncture/tcm ties = 62%, naturopathy = 59%, and Reiki = 71%).

A majority of the health ties were the people who are referred to here as 'health confidants' (i.e., the people with whom patients talked when they had a health problem). For all groups of patients in the study, health confidants constituted approximately half of their total health ties. When patients were asked who gave them general advice and information about health, the percentages were slightly lower. About one third of all health ties in all treatment groups provided such information. Information about CAM practitioners and CAM therapies was provided even less frequently by any of the patients' health ties. Less than one fifth of family physician patient ties provided any information in this regard as compared to less than a quarter for chiropractic patients, and about one quarter for the other CAM patients.

Tie Strength

Most people that these patients talked to about their health were people that they felt close to, and with whom they had strong ties. This was especially true of the family physician patients (Table 8.2). CAM patients also reported many strong ties among the people they talked with about their health, but acquaintances played a somewhat stronger role in this than they did for the family physician patients. The pattern varied modestly with the type of health support provided, although in almost all cases strong ties predominated. For general health information, the picture did not vary by treatment group (Table 8.3), The patients were getting it from people to whom they felt close. Even when it came to receiving information about specific alternative practitioners and therapies, most of the patients still relied on their close ties (Table 8.4). In fact, family physician patients and Reiki patients received no information of this kind from acquaintances, while the other three groups received only a small amount of this kind of information from acquaintances

Relational basis of support

Health ties were mainly with family and friends (Table 8.1). In the case of patients of family physicians, family members comprised almost half (46%) of the health ties who provided some type of health support, while friends comprised almost one third of ties (30%). Similarly, family also played an important role for CAM patients, but friends generally provided an even larger amount of support and information. For example, in the case of naturopathy, friends and other lay persons comprised 42% of their health ties, for acupuncture/tcm it was 38% and for Reiki 34%. Indeed, friends comprised at least one third of the health ties for all CAM patients, regardless of treatment group.

When examining health ties from the professional sector, the findings were that all treatment groups had health networks comprised of medical doctors. Major differences existed, however, between the patients of family physicians and all CAM patients. Almost one quarter (22%) of the health ties of family physician patients were with medical doctors, whereas they constituted only about 10% for all other CAM groups. By comparison, CAM patients reported health ties with other alternative practitioners but not to the same extent as family physician patients with their doctors. Once again Reiki patients provided an exception to the other CAM patients. They had health ties with several different types of alternative practitioners as well as with family physicians.

Moreover, the different kinds of relationships provided varying types and amounts of support. When looking at the people who were health confidants, it was apparent that very close family and friends constituted most of these networks (Table 8.2). For family physician patients, health confidants were drawn primarily from family (54%), particularly close family members (48%) whereas for CAM patients, friends played at least as great a role if not more so. What is distinctive about the Reiki patients in this respect is that their close friends included alternative practitioners (17%) who served as health confidants. .

The patterns were fairly similar, but the percentages were slightly lower for people who provided general health information. Most of it came from very close family and friends too (Table 8.3); only in the case of Reiki are alternative practitioners mentioned often in this respect. For chiropractic patients, just over one third (36%) of their health information came from

TABLE 8.1: HEALTH TIES OF 300 PATIENTS ACROSS FIVE TREATMENT GROUPS

Network Composition	Family G.P. n = 236	Chiropractor n = 264	Acupuncture/tcm n = 272	Naturopath n = 259	Reiki n = 313	Total n = 1344
Mean # of Ties	3.9	4.4	4.5	4.3	5.2	4.5
% Immediate Kin	43	28	32	25	21	29
% Extended Kin	3	5	3	5	2	4
% Friends	23	32	31	34	29	30
% Co-Workers	2	2	4	4	3	3
% Other Non-Related	5	1	3	4	2	3
% Family GP & Other Medical	22	12	10	10	10	12
% Chiropractors	4	12	2	1	3	4
% Acupuncturists/tcm	–	–	7	1	1	2
% Naturopaths	–	–	–	7	2	2
% Reiki	–	–	–	–	13	3
% Other Alternative	–	3	2	2	6	3

TABLE 8.2: BASIS OF RELATIONSHIP BY TIE STRENGTH 'HEALTH CONFIDANTS'

Basis of relationship

Family physician patients

Tie Strength	%Kin	%Friend	%Family g.p	%Alt. Pract.	Row %	Total#
Very Close	48	20	14	0	82	99
Close	5	3	7	0	15	18
Acquaintance	1	2	1	0	3	4
Column %	54	24	22	0	100	–
Column N	65	29	27	0	–	121

Acupuncture/tcm patients

Tie Strength	%Kin	%Friend	%Family g.p	%Alt. Pract.	Row %	Total#
Very Close	38	24	1	3	66	83
Close	6	12	6	5	28	36
Acquaintance	0	3	2	1	6	7
Column %	44	38	8	9	100	–
Column N	56	49	10	11	–	126

Reiki clients

Tie Strength	%Kin	%Friend	%Family g.p	%Alt. Pract.	Row %	Total#
Very Close	31	25	1	17	75	112
Close	1	4	3	9	16	24
Acquaintance	1	1	3	4	9	14
Column %	33	30	7	29	100	–
Column N	50	30	7	29	–	150

Chiropractic patients

Tie Strength	%Kin	%Friend	%Family g.p	%Alt. Pract.	Row %	Total#
Very Close	42	28	2	3	75	103
Close	1	5	4	6	17	23
Acquaintance	1	1	5	0	8	11
Column %	45	34	11	9	100	–
Column N	62	47	15	13	–	137

Naturopathic patients

Tie Strength	%Kin	%Friend	%Family g.p	%Alt. Pract.	Row %	Total#
Very Close	34	32	5	5	75	97
Close	2	9	5	5	21	27
Acquaintance	2	1	0	0	4	5
Column %	39	43	8	10	100	–
Column N	50	55	11	13	–	129

TABLE 8.3: BASIS OF RELATIONSHIP BY TIE STRENGTH GENERAL HEALTH INFORMATION

Basis of relationship

Family physician patients

Tie Strength	% Kin	% Friend	%Family g.p	%Alt. Pract.	Row %	Total#
Very Close	28	23	21	0	73	51
Close	0	3	13	1	17	12
Acquaintance	1	7	1	0	10	7
Column %	30	33	36	1	100	–
Column N	21	23	25	1	–	70

Chiropractic patients

Tie Strength	% Kin	% Friend	%Family g.p	%Alt. Pract.	Row %	Total#
Very Close	29	23	21	0	73	51
Close	0	3	13	1	17	12
Acquaintance	1	71	0	0	10	7
Column %	30	33	36	1	100	–
Column N	21	23	25	1	–	70

Acupuncture/tcm patients

Tie Strength	% Kin	% Friend	%Family g.p	%Alt. Pract.	Row %	Total#
Very Close	30	22	0	1	54	38
Close	3	17	6	10	35	25
Acquaintance	3	1	6	1	11	8
Column %	35	41	11	13	100	–
Column N	25	29	8	9	–	71

Naturopathic patients

Tie Strength	% Kin	% Friend	%Family g.p	%Alt. Pract.	Row %	Total#
Very Close	19	32	4	9	64	58
Close	4	12	6	6	28	25
Acquaintance	2	4	1	0	8	7
Column %	25	49	11	14	100	–
Column N	23	44	10	13	–	90

Reiki clients

Tie Strength	% Kin	% Friend	%Family g.p	%Alt. Pract.	Row %	Total#
Very Close	21	24	0	21	66	56
Close	2	6	6	9	24	20
Acquaintance	0	2	3	5	10	9
Column %	24	32	9	35	100	–
Column N	20	27	8	30	–	85

family physicians. The rest of the CAM patients also reported receiving health information from family physicians, but to a considerably lesser extent.

Information to patients about alternative practitioners and therapies came from a small subset of their patients' social networks. In fact, among family physician patients, almost no information about CAM came from any member of their network. The only CAM therapy that they mentioned was chiropractic and the information about this stemmed from very close or close family and friends. For the CAM patients, this kind of information was also provided by the people they knew and trusted (Table 8.4). This is true for all CAM groups, but in the case of Reiki, the sources of information included other close/very close alternative practitioners as well as family and friends.

Frequency of contact

It is not surprising that the health ties of these patients were people with whom they were in contact on a fairly regular basis. They tended to see them frequently, talk to them often on the telephone and live within close proximity (Table 8.5). Once again, family physician patients were different from the CAM groups, in that they had more frequent contacts with their health ties. The profile for all CAM groups looked fairly similar; approximately two-thirds of these patients saw or spoke to their health ties frequently and about three-quarters of them lived in the same residential area and some even lived in the same house.

DISCUSSION

Someone to talk to

The patients in this study did not lack for people to talk to about their health, nor did they lack health informants. Almost everybody mentioned someone; in only two cases did patients say they did not speak with anyone about their health. A typical network contained two family members, one or two friends, and one practitioner (physician or alternative). Yet, there was one major difference between patients of family physicians and patients of CAM practitioners: the size of the networks. Family physician patients had the least number of ties available for support, compared to the clients of Reiki who had the greatest number of health ties. The number of patients ties of people who used chiropractors, acupuncturists/traditional Chinese medicine doctors and naturopaths fell in between these two extremes.

Beyond that, a similar pattern was evident for the five treatment groups. Most of their ties were made up of health confidants: people with whom patients discussed their health problems. Fewer ties served as sources of health information, and even fewer provided advice and information about CAM

TABLE 8.4: BASIS OF RELATIONSHIP BY TIE STRENGTH INFORMATION ABOUT ALTERNATIVE THERAPIES AND PRACTITIONERS

Basis of relationship

Family physician patients

Tie Strength	% Kin	% Friend	%Family g.p	%Alt. Pract.	Row %	Total#
Very Close	32	35	16	0	84	26
Close	3	3	10	0	16	5
Acquaintance	0	0	0	0	0	0
Column %	35	39	26	0	100	–
Column N	11	12	8	2	–	31

Chiropractic patients

Tie Strength	% Kin	% Friend	%Family g.p	%Alt. Pract.	Row %	Total#
Very Close	18	26	0	11	56	15
Close	0	11	4	15	30	8
Acquaintance	4	7	0	4	15	4
Column %	22	44	4	30	100	–
Column N	6	12	1	8	–	27

Acupuncture/tcm patients

Tie Strength	% Kin	% Friend	%Family g.p	%Alt. Pract.	Row %	Total#
Very Close	20	23	0	0	43	13
Close	10	23	0	7	40	12
Acquaintance	0	13	3	0	17	5
Column %	30	60	3	7	100	–
Column N	9	18	1	2	–	30

Naturopathic patients

Tie Strength	% Kin	% Friend	%Family g.p	%Alt. Pract.	Row %	Total#
Very Close	26	19	3	10	58	18
Close	0	16	3	3	22	7
Acquaintance	0	19	0	0	19	6
Column %	26	55	6	13	100	–
Column N	8	17	2	4	–	31

Reiki practitioner

Tie Strength	% Kin	% Friend	%Family g.p	%Alt. Pract.	Row %	Total#
Very Close	12	25	4	27	69	35
Close	2	12	0	18	31	16
Acquaintance	0	0	0	0	0	0
Column %	14	37	4	45	100	–
Column N	7	19	2	23	–	50

TABLE 8.5: ACCESS BY TREATMENT GROUP

Percent	Frequency of face to face contact				
	Family GP	Chiropractor	Acupuncture	Naturopath	Reiki
Never	1	1	–	2	1
2x/year	7	10	10	12	11
Every few months	11	13	15	20	12
Monthly	10	12	10	15	15
Few times/month	22	12	16	15	21
Weekly	18	19	25	14	24
Few times/week	33	33	25	23	18
Percent	Frequency of phone contact				
	Family GP	Chiropractor	Acupuncture	Naturopath	Reiki
Never	2	2	1	3	3
2x/year	8	15	10	12	9
Every few months	7	10	7	16	8
Monthly	9	10	13	10	12
Few times/month	14	12	15	13	15
Weekly	19	19	22	22	25
Few times/week	40	32	32	24	28
Percent	Residential distance in minutes				
	Family GP	Chiropractor	Acupuncture	Naturopath	Reiki
Live together	16	20	14	14	10
About 10 minutes	32	36	26	28	27
About 30 minutes	29	26	31	28	39
About 60 minutes	14	8	16	12	13
60+ minutes	7	7	7	8	6
300+ minutes	2	2	6	11	5

therapies and practitioners. A typical patient had two confidants and one network member who provided general health information. Fewer people had networks that could provide them with information about alternative therapies and practitioners. (Reiki was the only exception: Almost every network had someone who could advise patients on alternative therapies and practitioners.) This low representation of providers of information about CAM may be a result of the fact that the data were collected in 1994–95; a time when the use of CAM had not yet spread so expansively to the larger population (see Valente, chapter seven).

More than half of the health ties of the patients of acupuncture, naturopathy and Reiki were with women. Indeed, women formed the great majority of Reiki ties. Given that many more women than men were patients of acupuncture/traditional Chinese medicine, naturopathy and Reiki, the predominance of women was not surprising. It may also be that women discuss and exchange information about health and health care more frequently than men, thus accounting for the predominately female composition of the health ties.

Patients revealed modest but real variations in their health networks depending on the type of health care provider patients were consulting. The networks of physician patients were made up almost entirely of family and friends, with some representation by physicians. Only one family physician patient mentioned an alternative practitioner in their health network. Similarly, the networks of CAM patients were also made up almost entirely of family and friends. Yet, all the CAM groups of patients had physicians in their networks, showing that the use of CAM did not imply that patients had turned their backs on physicians; a finding that has been demonstrated in a number of other studies (Crellin, Andersen and Connor, 1997; Eisenberg *et al.*, 1998; Vincent and Furnham, 1997). Only in the extreme situation of Reiki, did clients have many alternative practitioners in their networks.

But more importantly, regardless of the treatment group from which the patients in this study came, and the sectors represented in their networks, strong ties predominated in these health networks. Strong ties consisted not only of health confidants but they were also the ties that provided the patients in this study with general health information as well as specific information and advice about CAM practitioners and therapies. Granovetter's view on the function of weak ties providing new and diverse information was not supported here. Health seemed to be too important a matter to be dealt with by others who were not considered intimates. In short, health networks consisted of small networks of strong ties. This finding makes it clear that when it comes to health, people turn for support and information to their dearest and nearest.

Although Reiki clients had a higher percentage of acquaintances in their networks than other treatment groups, they too had a majority of strong ties in their networks. Why was it that acquaintances were not more influential, especially in the case of Reiki clients where, based on the strength of weak ties argument, we expected that they would play a stronger part? The explanation may lie in Friedson's concept of the lay referral group, and who people take seriously when they make inquiries about health and health care. Since health is an important and serious matter, people tend to rely on those they know and trust, (i.e., their strong ties). The patients in this study chose not only to confide in their close ties, but also to glean much of their information from these close relatives and friends (including some physicians and alternative practitioners). Acquaintances may have given them ideas about types of therapies and who to consult, but these suggestions required confirmation and legitimation from close ties in order to be taken seriously.

In support of Friedson (1960) and Chrisman and Kleinman (1983), the data show that different patients turned to different types of people in the various health care sectors for support and information. Patient ties of family physicians came mainly from the informal sector (family and friends) and to a lesser extent from the professional sector (physicians). Hardly any ties emanated from the folk sector (alternative practitioners). By comparison, the four alternative groups had health ties emanating from all three sectors: informal, professional and folk. But despite having ties emanating from the folk sector, these varied according to the type of CAM therapy they were using. For example, patients of chiropractors had health ties mainly with chiropractors, but hardly with anyone else. At the other end of the spectrum, Reiki clients had the most health ties with people from the folk sector. Their ties were not only with multiple Reiki practitioners but also with naturopaths, acupuncturists/traditional Chinese medicine doctors, chiropractors and several other types of alternative practitioners.

The health networks of all five treatment groups were embedded in family, especially immediate family. Strong ties with family members provided the most assistance and information for all types of patients, but especially for the patients of family physicians who had fewer weak ties in their networks. Next in importance came strong ties with friends. As expected for patients of family physicians, those physicians described as (very) close to them were also influential in their health care. Also as expected for Reiki clients, the CAM practitioners whom they regarded as (very) close influenced their health behaviour. Yet, contrary to expectations, CAM practitioners were not substantial components of the health networks of chiropractic, acupuncture, or naturopathic patients.

Being close also meant that patients of all groups usually lived near many of their health ties, saw them regularly, and spoke often by telephone. Access probably did have an indirect effect on support, for frequent contact and proximity helped keep strong ties strong and available to provide health support. Without access, strong ties could not exert an influence on health matters. Health confidants and providers of information and advice are needed on a regular basis and ready access is crucial.

CONCLUSION

The analysis presented here is one of the first attempts to use social network analysis to examine how people come to use alternative types of health care. We know that friends and family are important reference points in the search for health care; we also know that physicians have been a secondary although important source of support, information and advice. What we have not been able to ascertain until now is what kinds of people give specific kinds of support, and the extent to which the patients of physicians differ from the patients of alternative therapists. Are there overlaps in the sources of advice given? And does it make a difference if the people turned to are socially close or merely acquaintances?

We have found appreciable similarities in the health networks of physicians' patients and CAM patients. All their networks were small, and based on strong, informal ties with family and friends. With the exception of Reiki patients, all the patients in this study have about the same percentage of ties with physicians as they do with alternative practitioners. This suggests the intertwining of networks leading to physicians and to alternative therapies: the modalities of treatment are linked and often simultaneous, rather than separate and sequential.

The differences found suggest that those with somewhat larger, more diverse networks are more apt to be involved with alternatives. The larger the network and the greater the participation of friends, the more alternative therapies will be used. Although these networks are not built on weak ties, Granovetter was right in conjecturing that large, diverse networks provide a wider range of opportunities – in this case, leading patients to treatment options beyond the medical model. This was certainly the case for the Reiki patients whose high incomes and educational levels help to determine the breadth of their networks and the abundant information those networks provide. While these findings are derived from a sample of Canadian users of CAM, they are not bound by geographic location. Indeed, the same patterns are likely to be found in the United States, Britain and elsewhere.

This work represents an initial effort to identify who people turn to for specific kinds of health information and advice. It does not address the equally important considerations of who people in treatment turn to for emotional support, or for more concrete kinds of support such as financial help, assistance with tasks of daily life, and small health care services. Future research using network analysis has the potential to reveal the full range of health care supports that are available to protect health and manage health care.

REFERENCES

Alonzo, Angelo. 1979. 'Everyday Illness Behaviour: A Situational Approach to Health Status Deviations.' *Social Science and Medicine* 13:397–404.

Astin, John. 1998. 'Why People Use Alternative Medicine: Results of a National Study.' *Journal of the American Medical Association* 279:1548–53.

Badgley, Robin F., Fortin-Caron, Denyse and Marion G. Powell. 1987. 'Patient Pathways: Abortion.' pp. 159–171 in *Health and Canadian Society: Sociology Perspectives*, 2nd ed. Edited by David Coburn, Carl D'Arch, George Torrance and Peter New. Markham, Ont.: Fitzhenry and Whiteside.

Breton, Raymond. 1964. 'Institutional Completeness of Ethic Communities and the Personal Relations of Immigrants.' *American Journal of Sociology* 70:193–205.

Chrisman, Noel, and Arthur Kleinman. 1983. 'Popular Health Care, Social Networks, and Cultural Meanings: The Orientation of Medical Anthropology.' Pp. 569–590 in *Handbook of Health, Health Care and Health Professions*, edited by David Mechanic. New York: Free Press.

Coe, Rodney, Frederick Wolinsky, Douglas Miller, and John Prendergast. 1984. 'Social Network Relationships and Use of physician Services: A Reexamination.' *Research on Aging* 6:243–256.

Crellin, .J.K., R.R. Andersen, and J.T.H. Connor. 1997. *Alternative Health Care in Canada*. Toronto: Canadian Scholars' Press.

Eisenberg, David M., R.B. Davis, S.L. Ettner, S. Appel, S. Wilkey, M. Van Rompay, and R.C. Kessler. 1998. 'Trends in Alternative Medicine Use in the United States, 1990–1997: Results of a Follow-Up National Survey.' *Journal of the American Medical Association* 280:1569–75.

Eisenberg, David M., Ronald C. Kessler, Cindy Foster, Frances E. Norlock, David R. Calkins, and Thomas L. Delbanco. 1993. 'Unconventional Medicine in the United States: Prevalence, Costs and Patterns of Use.' *New England Journal of Medicine* 328:246–252.

Friedson, Eliot. 1960. 'Client Control and Medical Practice.' *American Journal of Sociology* 65:374–382.

Furnham, Adrian and Chris Smith. 1988. 'Choosing Alternative Medicine: A Comparison of the Beliefs of Patients Visiting a General Practitioner and A Homeopath.' *Social Science and Medicine* 26(7):685–89.

Granovetter, Mark. 1973. 'The Strength of Weak Ties.' *American Journal of Sociology* 78:1360–80.

Homans, George. 1961. *Social Behaviour: Its Elementary Forms*. New York: Harcourt Brace Jovanovich.

Kadushin, Charles. 1966. 'The Friends and Supporters of Psychotherapy: On Social Circles in Urban Life.' *American Sociological Review* 31:786–802.

Kelner, Merrijoy, Oswald Hall, and Ian Coulter. 1980. *Chiropractors, Do They Help?* Toronto: Fitzhenry and Whiteside.

Kelner, Merrijoy, and Beverly Wellman. 1997a. 'Health Care and Consumer Choice: Medical and Alternative Therapies.' *Social Science and Medicine* 45:203–212.

Kelner, Merrijoy, and Beverly Wellman. 1997b. 'Who Seeks Alternative Health Care? A Profile of the Users of Five Modes of Treatment.' *Journal of Alternative and Complementary Medicine* 3:1–14

Kleinman, Arthur. 1980. *Patients and Healers in the Context of Culture*. Berkeley: University of California Press.

Kleinman, M., L. Eisenberg, and B. Good. 1978. 'Culture, Illness and Care.' *Annals of Internal Medicine* 88:251–58.

Lee, Nancy Howell. 1969. *The Search for an Abortionist*. Chicago: University of Chicago Press.

Leventhal, Howard, and Robert S Hirschman. 1982. 'Social Psychology and Prevention.' Pp. 183–226 in *Social Psychology of Health and Illness*, edited by G.S. Sanders and J. Suls. Hillsdale, NJ: Erlbaum.

McKinlay, John. 1972. 'Some Approaches and Problems in the Study of the Uses of Services: An Overview.' *Journal of Health and Social Behavior* 13:115–152.

McKinlay, John. 1975. 'The Help-Seeking Behavior of the Poor.' in *Poverty and Health*, edited by J Kosa and I Zola. Cambridge: Harvard University Press.

Mechanic, David. 1968. *Medical Sociology*. New York: The Free Press.

Pescosolido, Bernice. 1986. 'Migration, Medical Care Preferences and the Lay Referral System: A Network Theory of Role Assimilation.' *American Sociological Review* 51:523–540.

Pescosolido, Bernice. 1991. 'Illness Careers and Network Ties: A Conceptual Model of Utilization and Compliance.' *Advances in Medical Sociology* 2:161–84.

Pescosolido, Bernice A. 1992. 'Beyond Rational Choice: The Social Dynamics of How People Seek Help.' *American Journal of Sociology* 97:1096–1138.

Pescosolido, Bernice A., Carol Brooks Gardner, and Keri M. Lubell. 1998. 'How People Get Into Mental Health Services: Stories of Choice, Coercion and 'Muddling Through' from 'First – Timers'.' *Social Science and Medicine* 46:275–286.

Pratt, Lois V. 1976. *Family Structure and Effective Health Behavior: The Energized Family*. Boston: Houghton Mifflin.

Ryan, Gery W. 1998. 'What do Sequential Behavioural Patterns Suggest about the Medical Decision-Making Process?: Modeling Home Case Management of Acute illnesses in a Rural Cameroonian Village.' *Social Science and Medicine* 46:209–225.

Salloway, Jeffrey, and Patrick Dillon. 1973. 'A Comparison of Family Networks and Friend Networks in Health Care Utilization.' *Journal of Comparative Family Studies* 4:131–42.

Sharma, Ursula. 1995. *Complementary Medicine Today: Practitioners and Patients* London: Routledge.

Suchman, Edward A. 1965. 'Stages of Illness and Medical Care.' *Journal of Health and Human Behaviour* 6:114–128.

Vincent, Charles and Adrian Furnham. 1997. *Complementary Medicine: A Research Perspective* Chichester: John Wiley & Sons.

Weimann, Gabriel. 1982. 'On the Importance of marginality: One More Step into the Two-Step Flow of Communication.' *American Sociology Review* 47 (December):764–73.

Wellman, Barry. 1990. 'The Place of Kinfolk in Personal Community Network.' *Marriage and Family Review* 15:195–228.

Wellman, Beverly. 1995. 'Lay Referral Networks: Using Conventional Medicine and Alternative Therapies for Low Back Pain.' pp. 213–238 in *Research in the Sociology of Health Care*, Volume 12 edited by Jennie J. Kronenfeld. Greenwich: JAI Press.

Wellman, Barry, and Milena Gulia. 1999. A Network is More than the Sum of Its Ties: The Network Basis of Social Support.' pp. 83–118 in *Network in the Global Village* edited by Barry Wellman. Boulder, CO: Westview Press.

Wellman, Barry, and David Tindall. 1993. 'How Telephone Networks Connect Social Networks.' *Progress in Communication Science* 12:339–42.

Wellman, Beverly, and Barry Wellman. 1992. 'Domestic Affairs and Network Relations.' *Journal of Social and Personal Relationships* 9:385–409.

Wellman, Barry, and Scot Wortley. 1989. 'Brother's Keepers: Situating Kinship Relations in Broader Networks of Social Support.' *Sociological Perspectives* 32:273–306.

Wellman, Barry, and Scot Wortley. 1990. 'Different Strokes From Different Folks: Community Ties and Social Support.' *American Journal of Sociology* 96:558–588.

ENDNOTE

1. Research for this paper has been supported by the Social Science and Humanities Research Council of Canada. I appreciate the advice and assistance supplied by Sivan Bomze and Barry Wellman. The 'we' used throughout this text reflects the close collaborative relationship I have with Merrijoy Kelner. This is a single-authored paper that is a product of our joint work.

2. 'Friends' includes network members identified as neighbours and coworkers. As almost all such ties were strong ties, we felt comfortable grouping them with friends *per se*.

3. Granovetter defines strong ties as having frequent contact, emotional intensity, feelings of intimacy, embeddedness and reciprocal social support.

4. In Canada, patients who use conventional medical services are reimbursed by the government, and patients neither see a bill nor have to fill out administrative forms..

5. Based on the information for each tie, a data set was created for the 300 patients and 1,344 health ties. Each patient tie had an identification number that was linked with the patient identification number. This enabled us to link information about ties and networks. The information collected for each tie such as relationship, gender, closeness, length of time known, frequency of contact and residential distance was coded and entered into SPSS/pc. The three questions which generated the names of the network ties were coded dichotomously: getting or not getting support. Each of the three questions became our dependent variables, and we were able to use logistic regression to examine the relationship between tie relation, tie strength and tie support.

Section Three: Researching CAM

This section proposes some of the diverse research approaches that need to be considered in the study of CAM. The chapters move from a single research focus on clinical efficacy to broader process-oriented and multi-layered research designs. The models used in this section represent the range of approaches currently being used in researching CAM. There are undoubtedly others which will prove fruitful in the future. Researchers need to think beyond the usual methods and employ innovative approaches which reflect the particular features of CAM therapies. It will also be important for research designs to employ a variety of methods from different disciplines and traditions. The social sciences can make a strategic contribution to the development of appropriate research in this area.

CHAPTER 9

Assessing the Evidence Base for CAM

E ERNST

INTRODUCTION

Complementary and alternative medicine (CAM) is often defined by what it is not rather than by what it is. Here it is delineated as '... diagnosis, treatment and/or prevention which complements mainstream medicine by contributing to a common whole, by satisfying a demand not met by orthodoxy or by diversifying the conceptual frameworks of medicine' (Ernst *et al.*, 1995) – a definition that has recently been adopted by the Cochrane field in this area (the Cochrane Collaboration is a worldwide organisation devoted to assessing, maintaining and disseminating the evidence-base in all fields of medicine).

CAM has become an important topic mostly because of its popularity in the general population. Estimates are that between 20% and 65% of all adults in industrialised countries have tried at least one type of CAM within the past year (Fisher and Ward, 1994; Eisenberg *et al.*, 1998; MacLennan *et al.*, 1996; Häusermann, 1997; Astin, 1998; Ernst and White, 2000). This high level of popularity renders it an ethical imperative to answer two key questions. Is CAM effective? Is CAM safe? The aim of this overview is to search for answers to these seemingly simple questions.

IS COMPLEMENTARY/ALTERNATIVE MEDICINE EFFECTIVE?

The current popularity of CAM therapies implies that many people have perceived it as effective. Moreover, it is reported to be associated with a high level of consumer satisfaction (Abbot and Ernst, 1997). A more difficult, yet ultimately more relevant, issue is whether CAM is superior to placebo, or to 'sham', or other treatment options such as conventional medical therapies. What is needed is good, systematic research that can shed some light on the ability of CAM therapies to help people with their health problems. Many obstacles to rigorous testing exist, yet there are no valid reasons why such research should not, in principle, be feasible.

To answer the question of the specific effectiveness of CAM (i.e. effectiveness over and above placebo or sham treatment), we ought to consult the evidence from controlled, preferably randomised clinical trials (RCTs) (Vickers *et al.*, 1997). This research strategy allows us to establish whether or not an observed effect can be linked causally to a specific intervention, with the highest degree of probability. Where possible, RCTs should be placebo (or sham)-controlled and (double) blind. For certain therapies, this is difficult or even impossible to achieve. Examples of this are massage therapy, hypnosis or autogenic training (note that sham-controlled trials of chiropractic do exist. In spite of these dilemmas, many scholars argue that RCTs are almost invariably feasible, usually desirable and often essential (Vickers *et al.*, 1997).

For several CAM therapies, some RCTs have been conducted which lend support to their effectiveness. Yet, at the same time, there are also other studies that cast serious doubt on this notion. Table 9.1 summarises the situation for the three most prevalent CAM therapies: acupuncture, homoeopathy and spinal manipulation. The picture that emerges is similar for all three treatments: when the totality of the available evidence is assessed in systematic reviews, the trial evidence is often contradictory and overall, the effectiveness is not proven beyond a reasonable doubt.

The importance of an objective assessment of all available trial data cannot be over-emphasised (Jefferson, 1999). The generally accepted way of achieving this is to conduct a 'systematic review'. Such an approach entails locating all pertinent studies and evaluating these according to pre-defined

TABLE 9.1: THE 'HIERARCHY OF EVIDENCE' APPLIED TO THREE POPULAR COMPLEMENTARY THERAPIES

Type of Evidence	Criteria fulfilled for		
	Acupuncture°	Homoeopathy	Spinal manipulation[X]
Systematic review or meta-analyses	Evidence positive but not compelling	Evidence positive but not compelling	Evidence not compelling
Randomised controlled trials	YES/NO*	YES/NO*	YES/NO*
Observational studies	YES	YES	YES
Case reports	YES	YES	YES

° as a treatment for chronic pain, (for which it is most commonly used)
* evidence in some trials positive in others negative
[X] as a treatment of low back pain
(Herbalism has been excluded from this table and Table 9.2 because each remedy needs to be assessed on its own merit and generalisations are therefore not possible).

Book extension form

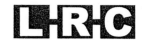

On the 28th May 2010 all books that have been taken out are due back in. If you need to take books out for longer than the 28th May and continue borrowing until the end of term you will need to take this form to your course tutor for signing.

End of term is Friday 9th July 2010.

You only need to fill out one form to continue loaning items until the end of term. Only your course tutor can sign this form.

When you are returning your books don't forget you can return them to the:

- Issue Desk
- Returns box (outside LRC entrance)
- Sheppey LRC
- HE Study Centre

··

Book extension form

Name of student   _____

Student number   _____

Name of course tutor   _____

Signature of course tutor   _____

Date   _____

Please return your completed form to the LRC issue desk or HE Study Centre. Thank you.

criteria of inclusion, exclusion and quality (Crombie and McQuay, 1998). Following this research design assures that systematic reviews minimise both selection bias and random error. Failure to insist on a systematic approach has been aptly criticised. As Vickers and Smith have phrased it: 'Narrative or unsystematic reviews, as they are called, are a proven danger to health' (Vickers and Smith, 1997).

Fortunately, authoritative systematic reviews or meta-analyses are available on subjects such as acupuncture as a treatment for chronic pain, its most prevalent indication (Patel et al., 1989), homoeopathy in general (homoeopaths treat individuals rather than diseases) (Linde et al., 1997), and spinal manipulation for low back pain (its main indication) (Assendelft et al., 1996). They usually conclude that the evidence is, on balance, insufficient to prove clinical effectiveness in defined clinical conditions, beyond a reasonable doubt. Table 9.2 quotes the verbatim conclusions from the above-cited publications (Patel et al., 1989; Linde et al., 1997; Assendelft et al., 1996). Of course, insufficient evidence can never mean that these therapies are ineffective, rather, in these cases, 'the jury is still out'. More and better quality RCTs are required to answer the important questions relating to effectiveness and efficacy of complementary and alternative treatments.

It should be stressed that the three therapies (acupuncture, homoeopathy and spinal manipulation) chosen to make this point here are only examples. They were selected because the number of RCTs available is substantially larger than for other forms of CAM. This is true with only one important exception: herbal medicine. In this area, we are in the fortunate position to have a substantial body of compelling evidence. The following list provides examples of recent systematic reviews of herbal treatments (Ernst, 1999).

- Hawthorne is helpful for early stages of congestive heart failure.
- Ginkgo biloba delays the clinical course of dementia.
- St John's Wort provides symptomatic relief of mild to moderate depression.
- Horse chestnut decreases signs and symptoms of chronic venous insufficiency.
- Yohimbine is effective for erectile dysfunction.
- Peppermint is useful as a symptomatic treatment of irritable bowel disease.
- Ginger alleviates nausea and vomiting of various causes.

In fact, the evidence for some plant-based medicines is so convincing that in several countries (e.g. Germany) phytotherapy is no longer seen as a form of CAM but rather as orthodox medicine which has to comply with all accepted standards and regulations of conventional synthetic drugs.

TABLE 9.2: CLINICAL TRIAL EVIDENCE IN COMPLEMENTARY MEDICINE – CONCLUSIONS FROM RECENT, AUTHORITATIVE SYSTEMATIC REVIEWS AND META-ANALYSES

	Acupuncture	Homoeopathy	Manipulation
Conditions	chronic pain	any	low back pain
Type of data summarised	14 RCTs of various forms of acupuncture	89 randomised and/or placebo-controlled trials	8 RCTs of chiropractic
Method of evaluation	systematic review	meta-analysis	systematic review
Conclusion (verbatim quotes)	various sources of bias, including problems with blindness, precluded a conclusive finding	clinical effects of homoeopathy (not) completely due to placebo chronic low back pain	(no) convincing evidence for the effectiveness of chiropractic for acute or
Reference (No)	Patel M et al. (13)	Linde K et al. (14)	Assendelft WJJ et al. (15)

RCT = randomised controlled trial

IS COMPLEMENTARY AND ALTERNATIVE MEDICINE SAFE?

Many users of CAM are convinced that CAM is entirely safe. It is perceived as natural, and 'natural' implies 'no side-effects'. Yet this misunderstanding, often encouraged by the mass media, can be dangerously wrong. There is nothing 'natural' in sticking needles into people or prescribing herbal remedies which may be natural but can be also highly toxic to the body. There is research that shows that most, if not all therapies are associated with *direct* risks and adverse effects (Ernst and De Smet, 1996). We therefore do know that serious complications can occur but, at present, we cannot reliably define their frequency (Table 9.3). One of the most urgent tasks for CAM research therefore is to conduct investigations that will adequately define the exact incidence figures of adverse effects. This research is by no means aimed at tarnishing the reputation of CAM, but rather it is meant to establish criteria for assessing whether or not the various CAM therapies are safe for patients.

In addition to direct hazards, it has been shown that there are *indirect* risks of CAM (e.g. Ernst and De Smet, 1996) which should be considered (Table 9.3). These include: misdiagnoses, disregard of contra-indications (Zimmer *et al.*, 1994), hindering access of patients to effective conventional medical interventions

TABLE 9.3: SAFETY OF COMPLEMENTARY THERAPIES

	Acupuncture	Homoeopathy	Manipulation	Herbalism
Examples of serious adverse effects	trauma, infections	allergies	fractures, stroke	toxic liver damage
Fatalities reported?	YES	NO	YES	YES
Frequency of adverse effects known?	NO	NO	NO§	for some herbs only
Complication avoidable?	NO*	NO	NO⊗	in some cases YES
Indirect dangers	potentially applicable to all complementary therapies • Missed diagnoses • Misdiagnoses • Disregarding contra-indications • Discontinuation, prevention/delay of effective therapy • Potentially hazardous diagnostic procedures			

* YES in case of infection
⊗ fracture rates might be minimised by excluding high risk patients (e.g. menopausal women) only for common, mild and transient adverse effects.
§ only estimates exists of serious adverse effects

(Abbot *et al.*, 1998; Ernst, 1997) or potentially harmful diagnostic practices associated with a given type of therapy (Ernst, 1998).

This issue is obviously most delicate, since it raises the following question: who is medically competent to take responsibility for patients and who is not (Ernst, 1995)? Competence can best be achieved by proper training and sufficient experience. Whenever training is insufficient, there are serious risks involved. Insufficient training or education may be a problem both with physicians (who may not be properly trained in a CAM procedure) or non-medically qualified CAM practitioners (who may not have sufficient knowledge in essential medical subjects like anatomy, physiology or pathology). If, for instance, a non-medically qualified acupuncturist causes a pneumothorax by puncturing a lung, one could argue that the lack of knowledge in anatomy was at the root of the problem and that a medically trained acupuncturist would have had sufficient formal teaching to prevent this complication. If, on the other hand, a physician with some superficial training in spinal manipulation causes a vascular accident through cervical manipulation, one could postulate that a chiropractor with adequate training in this method would have been less likely to have caused this damage.

An ineffective 'cure' for a treatable condition prevents or delays effective treatment and thus cannot be called truly safe. Thus, the issue of effectiveness is intimately associated with safety and it is clear that both are best researched in parallel.

BALANCING RISKS AND BENEFITS

Neither the potential risks nor benefits of a given therapy can be discussed meaningfully in isolation. Every time clinicians prescribe or administer a treatment they also carry out, either consciously or subconsciously, a 'mini risk/benefit evaluation'. If the benefit is potentially high (e.g. treating a life-threatening disease like cancer), substantial risks are acceptable. If the benefit is not decisive (e.g. treating a self-limiting condition like a common cold), hardly any risk at all is acceptable. In other words, if the potential risks outweigh the potential benefit, a therapy should be considered questionable and of no ultimate value.

If one agrees that the benefits of CAM are uncertain, it can be argued that substantial risks associated with it are unacceptable and that even small risks can be significant. This line of thought emphasises the fact that a rigorous investigation of the safety issue forms an essential part in defining the usefulness of CAM (Van Haselen and Fischer, 1998). Rigorous research into these areas therefore represents an ethical imperative (Ernst, 1996).

One could argue that the risks of conventional medicine are probably much higher than those of CAM. Yet, as outlined above, the absolute risk of a therapy is not ultimately relevant. It is the risk/benefit relation which must be considered. If, for example, the potential benefit of a treatment is to prolong a patient's life, as in cancer treatment, then considerable risks of a therapy are usually acceptable. If, on the other hand, the potential benefits are small, as in treating a common cold, hardly any risks will be acceptable. These considerations should apply to CAM as much as they do for conventional medicine. There is simply no room for double standards when dealing with the safety of patients.

WHO IS DEMANDING THIS EVIDENCE?

The current demands of the public seem largely untouched by concerns over the efficacy and safety of CAM. In spite of the considerable uncertainties related to efficacy and safety, CAM is more popular than ever before. Consumers are voting for it with their feet and their purses. Does this mean that trying to define efficacy and safety is meaningless? Most experts would insist that, on the contrary, efficacy and safety are the most important issues in any type of medicine. The supreme law of medicine is 'first do no harm'. In the context of the above discussion we would rephrase this: 'make sure that CAM does more good than harm'. Clearly this aim can only be reached by rigorously investigating both the efficacy and safety of CAM. Thus it seems that while the *wishes* of the public may be largely unaffected by the efficacy/safety debate, their *needs* are certainly not.

And who determines the needs of the public? This is a complex and provocative question which would generate different answers depending on who is being asked. In health care, however, the decision makers of mainstream medicine are likely to have the most influence over the decision. It is interesting, therefore, to note that two recent surveys (Van Haselen and Fisher, 1998; Ernst *et al.*, 1998) show that evidence relating to efficacy and safety ranks on top of the list of criteria that decision makers would apply when deciding whether or not to adopt CAM into routine care. Again, the plea here is for uniform standards. As mainstream medicine struggles to finally become evidence-based, it is inevitable that CAM will ultimately have to follow this same approach.

OBSTACLES TO RESEARCH

There are many reasons why, in spite of the often impressive tradition of CAM, our evidence is still so very fragmentary:

- lack of funds
- lack of scientific know how and infrastructure
- complexity of the subject area
- internal resistance

The most obvious obstacle to an adequate level of research activity lies in the lack of financial resources for carrying out research. Clinical trials are almost by definition expensive. In mainstream medicine the financial burden is often carried by the pharmaceutical industry. In the area of CAM there are no comparably interested parties. One exception could be the manufacturers of herbal and homoeopathic products. Yet, as plants are not patentable, the appetite to sponsor trials is usually not keen. It follows that government bodies ought to step into this void and start funding CAM research. To a certain extent this is already happening in some but by no means all countries. The driving force behind this is usually consumer demand.

CAM has no tradition of scientific investigation which is comparable to mainstream medicine. This means that both the know how and the infrastucture for research are largely missing. It is a challenge for the field to build this up. The limiting factor might again prove to be financial resources.

It has often been said that it is easy to carry out an RCT for a conventional drug but it is much more difficult to do the same for CAM. To a certain degree this is true. What, for instance, is a credible 'placebo' for acupuncture? How does one fit the need for individualization into the 'straight jacket' of an RCT? And how can one 'blind' a physical intervention like massage? These problems are usually solvable (Ernst and Fugh-Bernham, 1998), but they require innovation, an open mind and a solid training in research methodology. As stressed above the latter quality is a rarity in CAM.

Finally there still is a considerable resistance to CAM research. It comes from both the 'establishement' and CAM itself. The establishment might argue that, due to the low level of plausibility of the treatments involved, investigation into this area is a waste of resources (Vandenbrouk, 1997). Ardent proponents of CAM, on the other hand, might think that the application of science to CAM means 'throwing out the baby with the bath water' (Ernst, 1995). CAM, they believe is so special, subtle, holistic etc. that science would tend to destroy essential aspects of it. From the above discussion it is clear that this author disagrees with both of these views. I do, however, agree with Panatanowitz who wryly wrote that researching CAM seems like a 'veritable minefield where only fools rush in' (Panatanowitz, 1994).

CONCLUSION

At present, too little is known about the potential risks and benefits of CAM. Proponents of CAM have to demonstrate beyond a reasonable doubt that these therapies do more good than harm. The only way of achieving this is through rigorous research using the best methodology for the problem under investigation. To research these problems thoroughly is in the interests of patients, health policy planners and administrators, as well as health care providers of all kinds.

REFERENCES

Abbot NC, Ernst E. Patients' opinion about complementary medicine. *Forsch Komplementärmed* 1997; 4:164–8.

Abbot NC, Hill M, Barnes J, Hourigan PG, Ernst E. Uncovering suspected adverse effects of complementary and alternative medicine. *Int J of Risk & Safety* 1998; 11:99–106.

Assendelft WJJ, Koes BW, van der Heijden GJMG, Bouter LM. The effectiveness of chiropractic for treatment of low back pain: an update and attempt at statistical pooling. *J Manipul Physiol Ther* 1996; 19:499–507.

Astin JA. Why Patients Use Alternative Medicine. Results of a National Study. *JAMA* 1998; 279:1548–53.

Crombie IK, McQuay HJ. The systematic review, a good guide rather than a guarantee. *Pain* 1998;76:1–2.

Eisenberg D M, Trends in alternative medicine use in the United States, 1990–1997. *JAMA* 1998; 280(18):1569–1575.

Ernst E, Resch KL, Mills S, Hill R, Mitchell A, Willoughby M, White A. Complementary medicine – a definition. *Br J Gen Pract* 1995;45:506.

Ernst E, White A. The BBC survey of complementary medicine use in the UK. *Compl Ther Med.* 2000. 8:32–36.

Ernst E. The clinical efficacy of herbal treatments: an overview of recent systematic reviews. *The Pharmaceutical Journal* 1999; 262:85–87.

Ernst E, De Smet PAGM. Adverse effects of complementary therapies. In *Meyler's Side Effects*, Duke (Ed.) Elsevier, Amsterdam 1996.

Ernst E. The attitude against immunisation within some branches of complementary medicine. *Eur J Pediatr* 1997; 156:513–5.

Ernst E. Chiropractors' use of X-rays. A systematic review. *Br J Radiol* 1998; 71:249–51.

Ernst E. Competence in complementary medicine. *Comp Ther Med* 1995; 3:6–8.

Ernst E. The ethics of complementary medicine. *J Med Ethics* 1996; 22:197–8.

Ernst E, Armstrong NC, White AR, Pittler MH. Research is needed to determine how to integrate complementary medicine into the NHS. *BMJ* 1998; 317:1654.

Ernst E, Fugh-Berman A. Methodological considerations in testing the efficacy of complementary/alternative treatments (CATs). *Int J of Alt. & Complementary Med.*1998; 16(6).

Ernst E. Complementary therapies, the baby and the bath water. *Br J Rheumatol* 1995; 34:479–80.

Fisher P, Ward A. Complementary Medicine in Europe. *BMJ* 1994; 309:107–11.

Häusermann D. Wachsendes Vertrauen in Naturheilmittel. *Dtsch Ärzteblatt* 1997; 94:1857–1858.

Jefferson T. What are the benefits of editorials and non-systematic reviews? *BMJ* 1999; 318:135.

Linde K, Claudius N, Ramirez G, Melchart D, Eitel F, Hedges LV, Jonas W. Are the clinical effects of homoeopathy placebo effects? A meta-analysis of placebo controlled trials. *Lancet* 1997; 350:834–43.

MacLennan AH, Wilson DH, Taylor AW. Prevalence and cost of alternative medicine in Australia. *Lancet* 1996; 347:569–73.

Panatanowitz D. *Alternative medicine, a doctor's perspective.* South Cape Town 1994.

Patel MS, Gutzwiller F, Paccaud F, Marazzi A. A meta-analysis of acupuncture for chronic pain. *Int J Epidemiol* 1989; 18:900–906.

Vandenbrouk JP. Homeopathy trials, going nowhere. *Lancet* 1997; 350:824.

Van Haselen R, Fisher P. Evidence influencing British Health Authorities' decisions in purchasing complementary medicine. *JAMA* 1998; 280:1564–5.

Vickers A, Cassileth B, Ernst E, Fisher P, Goldman P, Jonas W *et al.* How should we research unconventional therapies? A panel report from the conference on Complementary and Alternative Medicine Research Methodology, National Institute of Health. *Int J Technology Assessment in Health Care* 1997; 13(1):111–121.

Vickers AJ, Smith C. Analysis of the evidence profile of the effectiveness of complementary therapies in asthma. Compl Ther Med 1997; 5:202–9.

Zimmer G, Miltner E, Maltern R. Lebensgefährliche Komplikationen unter Heilpraktikerbehandlung. *Versicherungsmed* 1994,46:171–74.

CHAPTER 10

Rethinking Models of Health and Illness Behaviour

BERNICE A. PESCOSOLIDO

INTRODUCTION

Models of health and illness behaviour are designed to answer a deceptively simple question: How do individuals come to recognize, understand and cope with health problems? Early research on this question was explicitly concerned with whether and why individuals turned to the new, 'scientific' forms of medical care instead of older, more indigenous methods and providers. By the 1950s, much of the research simply asked who used physicians, clinics and hospitals. In response to this question, models of 'health service use' evolved with few analyses of the use of any other sources of care outside the 'canopy' of formal, allopathic medicine (Pescosolido and Kronenfeld, 1995). Models of health service use have become the dominant approach to understanding illness behaviour and are used to understand not only the use of allopathic medicine but are often currently employed to describe the characteristics of individuals who turn to complementary and alternative medicine (CAM).

In this paper, I argue that utilization models have limitations for the study of illness behaviour, generally, and in particular, with regard to our ability to understand how individuals draw from different medical systems to provide advisors, advice and care. Specifically, these dominant approaches employ a set of assumptions that match the logic of a 'modern' society based more on the values of the Enlightenment that gave rise to allopathic medicine (e.g., rationality, progress based on science) than the realities of how individuals, even in these modern societies, respond to illness and disease. Using data from three studies that cross different kinds of societies and a range of illness problems, I illustrate the kinds of issues that should be included in models of health and illness behaviour. I offer a different model, the Network Episode Model (NEM) which attempts to respond to the limitations of other approaches. Rather than asking: 'How does an individual decide to use allopathic medicine instead of or in addition to CAM?', it asks: 'How does the 'community', both lay and professional influence 'illness careers'? That is, the NEM presents an approach which focuses on the entire set of responses a person has to the onset of illness, which includes access to diverse medical systems that cannot be studied apart from one another, and looks to their social network ties in day-to-day life as an underlying mechanism.

TRADITIONAL MODELS OF HEALTH AND ILLNESS BEHAVIOUR

Currently, four models of health service use dominate the literature: the Socio-Behavioural Model, the Health Belief Model, the Theory of Reasoned Action and the Theory of Planned Behaviour. One of the earliest, the **Socio-Behavioural Model** (SBM) detailed three basic categories: need, predisposing and enabling factors. Some *need* for care must be defined or individuals are not likely to consider whether or not to use services, what services to use and when to go. The nature of the illness and its severity (e.g., the 'hurt', 'worry', 'bother' or 'pain' that it causes) reflect not only important medical issues but also how people perceive this need and how symptoms are experienced. In the SBM, gender, race, age, education and beliefs, to name only a few, are defined as *predisposing* characteristics – those social and cultural factors that have been routinely documented in previous research to shape an individual's tendency to seek care. However, even in the presence of need and a profile of predisposing social characteristics, individuals must be able to act on a desire to receive care. *Enabling characteristics* are the means and knowledge to get into treatment. Geographical availability, having a regular source of care, travel time, financial ability (e.g., income, insurance) and geographical availability of doctors, clinics or hospitals can facilitate or limit the use of services. These latter factors, which target 'access', figure prominently among enabling characteristics. Andersen has revised the Socio-Behavioural Model by incorporating more variables that measure the allopathic system's organizational structure, goals and policies as well as those of the insurance industry and governments. The revised SBM considers the effects of service use, and in particular, how previous personal experience alters need, predisposing and enabling characteristics (Aday and Awe, 1997; Andersen, 1995).

The **Health Belief Model** (HBM) includes many of the same kinds of factors as the Socio-Behavioural Model, but its emphasis and intent are quite differ-ent. Where the SBM focuses on the influence of the system and issues of access on the use of curative services, the HBM examines the meaning of 'predispos-ing' characteristics for preventive services. Rather than looking generally at social and cultural factors, the HBM analyzes how an individual's general and specific health beliefs (e.g., beliefs about the severity of symptoms), their pref-erences (e.g., perceived benefits of treatment) as well as their experiences (with health problems and providers) and knowledge affect decisions to seek care, the adoption of health behaviours and outcomes (Strecher, Champion and Rosenstock, 1997).

The most recent model in this tradition is the **Theory of Reasoned Action** (TRA). 'Expectancy' becomes key as individuals rate how current and alternative actions can reduce health problems. Like the HBM, it focuses primarily on motivations, the individual's assessment of risk, and the desire to avoid negative outcomes. Individuals evaluate whether or not to engage in healthy (e.g., exercise) or risky (e.g. smoking) behaviours and whether to seek preventive (e.g. mammography) as well as curative (eg, medications) medical services. Like the SBM, it takes into account access to the system (Maddux and DuCharme, 1997; Weinstein, 1993).

Recently, however, the TRA has been revised sufficiently to evolve into a new model, the **Theory of Planned Behaviour** (TPB). The key differences with the TRA lie in two points. First, the TPB recognizes that individuals do not necessarily have total control over their behaviour. The amount of behavioural control that individuals perceive they have, or 'self-efficacy', becomes an important element in the model. Second, in the newest versions, for example, as pictured in Figure 10.1, 'cues' (in both an early phase of recognition and a later phase of action) or 'habits' become an important part of the decisions that individuals make to engage in health and illness behaviours (see Gochman, 1997).

THREE BASIC PROBLEMS

The general problems that these approaches share have been laid out in detail elsewhere (Pescosolido, 1992; Pescosolido and Kronenfeld, 1995). Here, I turn to an evaluation of their utility in understanding the use of alternative medicine. Clearly, each of these models can be tailored to look at beliefs about allopathic and alternative systems as the HBM suggests. They can focus on the relative access to allopathic versus alternative providers emphasized in the SBM. They can elaborate social norms and cues regarding various medical systems according to the TRA and the TPB. Despite this, I argue that the application of standard utilization models hinders our understanding of individuals' responses to illness in general, but especially for alternative medicine. Specifically, there are three fundamental problems that these models share.

The first, the which I refer to as the *'tyranny of use/no use'*, results from reliance on a strict, either-or conceptualization of 'choices' that people make when they confront illness. This reflects, in part, the analytic tools we have brought to the sophisticated, empirical study of health care choices. Originally, studies relied on simple cross tabulations, where the number of categories of care were laid out. Each table presented the effect of one, or sometimes two, factors on illness behaviours. As theories became more inclusive, recognizing

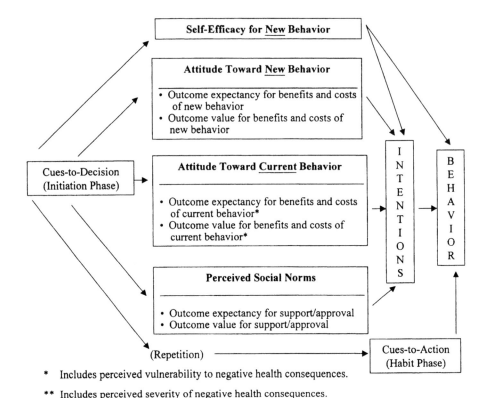

FIGURE 10.1: A REVISED THEORY OF PLANNED BEHAVIOR INCORPORATING CUES AND HABITS. REPRINTED WITH PERMISSION.

the influence of a whole range of factors, researchers took advantage of rapid developments in survey methodology and the importation of multivariate regression techniques into the social and socio-medical sciences. Ordinary least squares regression, and later logit regression, provided a way to consider the effects of any one factor, for example beliefs, while taking into account others, for example, an individual's access to care. This allows us to get a profile of users.

But the reliance on econometric models and traditional survey designs coupled with the low prevalence of use of particular kinds of alternative medicine translated into their virtual exclusion in empirical studies. Further, these analytic techniques forced a simplistic modeling of health and illness behaviour – either as the number of times an individual carried out a practice or visited a provider (i.e., the volume of use) or a simple 'zero/one' coding of whether individuals used these or they did not. There was no particular reason why these types of analyses could not target the use of allopathic versus alternative medicines; however, as described earlier, the general tendency was to be concerned almost exclusively with whether individuals accessed the allopathic system (Pescosolido and Kronenfeld, 1995).

Recently more complex models (e.g., multinomial regression) have allowed an expansion of categories (e.g., Frank and Kamlet, 1989). These approaches do allow for multiple categories in the dependent variable (e.g., individuals use allopathic, alternative, informal care). However, they face certain limitations. As the number of categories of the dependent variable increase, there are greater estimation and interpretation problems. More importantly, this approach cannot solve the major stumbling block that individuals *must* be forced into one and only one category. This stands in direct opposition to the clear documentation by anthropologists that individuals routinely draw simultaneously and sequentially from different medical systems (e.g., Press, 1969; Romannucci-Ross, 1997). So, for example, if individuals used an indigenous healer and then proceeded to an allopathic physician, the usual response is to 'code up'. In this case, they would be placed in the allopathic category. This approach continues the focus on a single choice, plucked out of an entire 'history' of responses to health problems places (Pescosolido, 1992).

The second problem arises from, but is not solved by, the rich tradition of ethnographic work on illness behaviour. Traditional models do not tend to draw from such studies which provide '*deep understandings of procedures and users*'. These studies provide great detail about the providers and patients of alternative medical systems. This information is central to our understanding of the meanings, processes and practices involved. While often rich, detailed and dynamic in nature, they are unable to provide a picture of why some individuals use alternative medicine and others do not. They tend to be limited in scope, the number of cases and generalizability. What we are faced with is a bifurcation of research by method (qualitative versus quantitative approaches), and often by discipline (e.g., economics versus anthropology) which impoverishes our ability to understand both the process of responding to health problems and the contingencies that shape illness careers (Pescosolido, 1991).

Third, the problem of the '*compartmentalization of illness*' leads to questions concerning how we ask individuals about who they consult, how they are referred to them and what they do about illness problems. Focusing solely on illness fails to recognize that many problems require an elimination of other possible definitions of the situation in the face of physical and mental health problems (e.g., moral failure, supernatural punishments, the 'ups and downs' of life). People often use a variety of responses which include, but are not limited to, medical care. Further, the unnatural separation of illness behaviour from social life is reflected in traditional models' reliance on *rational choice* as the underlying mechanism at work (Pescosolido, 1992). Even as more and more models have included routine and regular aspects of social life (e.g., the HBM now includes social networks as a 'box'), these are conceptualized as additional 'utilities' affecting the individual's weighing of the costs and benefits associated with this *conscious and voluntary decision.* These models, not surprising then, are referred to often as 'decision-making' models or 'help-seeking' models which duplicate the same set of values which gave rise to the professional dominance of allopathic medicine (i.e., rationality, individuality; Brown, 1979). This is the case despite extensive documentation that much medical care is routine, sometimes coerced, and presents a wide range of consequences and needs outside of the formal medical system (see Pescosolido, Gardner and Lubell, 1998 for a review). In fact, the public's embrace of CAM has been linked directly to this more inclusive perspective (see, for example, Kane *et al.,* 1974 on chiropractic).

The lack of congruence between the 'cognitive worlds' of allopathic medicine and individuals is reflected in the theoretical models that seek to understand why some individuals come to use the formal system, while others do not. However, addressing these problems does not require a model tailored only to the use of CAM. Rather, it suggests that we develop more integrated models of illness behaviour that would improve our understanding of the use of both allopathic and alternative medicine. Such a model would combine the correlational contributions of traditional models while incorporating the dynamic richness of ethnographic models. The model would view medical pluralism as an end in itself, even if the intent is to understand individuals' resort to allopathic medicine. It would allow for a more 'embedded' view of illness behaviour, allowing not only for a documentation of the effect of health beliefs on utilization but also for seeking out the meaning, origins, consequences and mechanisms of these beliefs. The model should allow for different 'engines of action' (Coleman, 1986) rather than debate the stale arguments over the nature and limits of rationality. Certainly, there are cases where this is the mechanism while, even as the TPB acknowledges, sometimes it is not. Dominant models, by assuming all use of providers and practices is rational and voluntary, detract from the interesting question of when and why individuals cannot rely on their tacit knowledge, cultural routines and pragmatic responses but must shift to a cost-benefit analysis (Pescosolido, 1992).

An important caveat is in order. There is little question that the dominant models can be seen as more process-oriented than I have depicted and, thus, able to accommodate many of these criticisms. In fact, they can also be seen as allowing for medical pluralism and some degree of communal rather than individual decision-making. The reality is, however, that in practice this is not the case. I would argue that, despite such potentially dynamic and inclusive depictions, the overriding *weltanschung* that pushed the development of these models has also set inherent limitations on how we have thought about and used them. For example, these models often attempt to document the degree to which individuals' beliefs are congruent with those underpinning allopathic medicine. To the degree that this is the case, they argue, individuals will use allopathic medicine. However, these approaches virtually assume that such beliefs are held to the exclusion of other possible belief systems. The underlying image is that with modern times or with more education, one set of beliefs are 'replaced' with another set. Yet, much research uncovers 'layers' to beliefs about illness causation across very different kinds of societies, across different health problem and even within one problem (e.g., Fosu, 1981; Hostetler, 1963).

SETTING THE PARAMETERS OF A THEORETICAL AND EMPIRICAL RESEARCH AGENDA: THREE ILLUSTRATIONS

In order to get a sense of the challenges we face, descriptive data from three studies are presented here to illustrate the complexity of how individuals experience and respond to illness. These three cases vary dramatically in their social and geographical context, the nature of the health problem and the types of study design. To the degree that they present us with similarities, despite these great differences, they provide an agenda for the next step in the development of models and methods.

The response to health problems in a Mexican village

Young's (1981) investigation of the 'decision process' in a small Mexican village followed the tradition of describing and modeling the illness process itself. Through detailed ethnographic and interview work, Young documented 323 'illness episodes' in a sample of 63 households in Pitchitáro, Mexico. Table 10.1 provides information, directly from his book, which shows the number of steps individuals used in coping with these health problems. Most individuals used only one source of care (61.6%) and very few (1.2%) opted for no treatment. While this latter figure is significantly lower than in most other utilization studies, it is important to recall that the scope of 'treatment' is much broader than in most studies. However, even with this considered, the use of two options captures almost 90% of how individuals respond to illness.

Table 10.2 indicates that while there were few choices, what individuals used first could be very different. Most individuals who used self-care did so as the first step in the sequence of care. However, the situation for curers, practicantes (local, non-physician practitioners of Western medicine) and physicians

TABLE 10.1:   NUMBER OF STEPS IN TREATMENT SEQUENCES, PICHATARO, 1975–1977

Number	Frequency (N)	Percentage %
No treatment	(4)	1.2
One alternative	(199)	61.6
Two alternatives	(80)	24.8
Three alternatives	(32)	9.9
Four alternatives	(6)	1.9
Five alternatives	(2)	0.6
Total	(323)	100.0

Young, James Clay, *Medical Choice in a Mexican Village*, copyright © 1981 by Rutgers, The State University. Reprinted with permission of Rutgers University Press.

and others is not so clear cut. There was a slight tendency for individuals to use curers as their second option and almost an even split in using practicantes first or second. Those who used physicians reported that they were slightly more likely to use them as the second option of resort but equally likely to use a physician as the first or third option.

In examining the factors that shaped the use, Young focused on fifteen cases, doing extensive observation and general interviewing. He asked a series of questions about the conditions under which individuals would use a practicante versus a physician, for example. He found four factors to be the most crucial in structuring the process of dealing with an illness – the seriousness of the illness; knowledge about an appropriate home remedy; faith in the effectiveness of folk treatment as opposed to medical treatment for that illness, and the balance of the expense of alternatives and available resources (p. 167).

TABLE 10.2:   DISTRIBUTION OF TREATMENT CHOICES, PICHATARO, 1975–1977.

Choice	Self-Treatment N	Curer N	Practicante N	Physician N	Other N
Initial	232	24	31	23	9
Second	7	34	35	38	6
Third	2	9	6	21	2
Fourth	0	2	0	5	1
Fifth	0	0	0	2	0
Total	241	69	72	89	18
Percentage (%)	(49.3)	(14.1)	(14.7)	(18.2)	(3.7)

Young, James Clay, *Medical Choice in a Mexican Village*, copyright © 1981 by Rutgers, The State University. Reprinted with permission of Rutgers University Press.

The response to mental health problems in Puerto Rico.

Table 10.3 reports on the extent of the use of a wide variety of practitioners and practices among those living in poor areas of Puerto Rico (which comprise 80% of the island) as reported in the Mental Health Care Utilization Among Puerto Ricans Study (Alegría *et al.,* 1991). In each of the two waves of data collection and after a series of psychiatric epidemiology questions, individuals were asked if they or others around them thought they had a mental health problem. If they responded 'yes', they were asked what they did and read a list of possible options. As indicated in Table 10.3, a wide variety of options are used by individuals reporting an 'episode'. Further, there is a fair amount of stability in the level of use across waves. A large percentage (40.1% in Wave 1 and 52.3% in Wave 2) talk to a relative. While this is relatively high among the options offered to respondents, it is, by no means, what all individuals 'decide' to do when they acknowledge that they have mental health problems (see below on sequencing). Fewer individuals report that they discuss their problem with friends (28.7 and 35.5% respectively). Over-the counter medications, religious practices and exercise or meditation are used by one-fifth to one-quarter of respondents. About one-fifth of respondents report consulting a general practitioner or mental health specialist. These levels are very much in line with studies on the U.S. mainland.

As one of the first, large-scale, population-based, representative sample survey studies that takes seriously a dynamic, community-based perspective in health care use, the Puerto Rico Study provides important information on the nature and extent of the use of a wide variety of advisors and practices encountered during the course of a mental health problem. It also allows a look at the order in which individuals draw from society's resources. Table 10.4 offers a quick glance at how individuals choose among advisors they contacted during their illness episode. What is surprising about the results in this table is the wide variety of advisors contacted first. While, almost two-thirds of those who talked to a relative did so first (65.4% in Wave 1 and 64.2% in Wave 2), over a third go first to physicians (36.3% in Wave 1 and 39.1% in Wave 2). Almost that many consult a mental health provider (e.g., psychiatrist, social worker, mental health clinician) as their preliminary medical care contact (30.6% in Wave 1 and 35.3% in Wave 2). In the only finding different between the two waves, 39% of those in Wave 1 and 26.7% of those in Wave 2 contacted a friend first. Finally, between one-fifth and one-quarter of those reporting mental health problems first went to a member of the clergy to discuss their problems (24.3% and 20%, respectively).

Finally, Figure 10.2 shows the actual pathways to different medical systems that these individuals reported in the first wave (1992–1993). What this shows is that of the statistically *possible* pathways to care, individuals in Puerto Rico

TABLE 10.3: PERCENTAGE OF INDIVIDUALS USING DIFFERENT ADVISORS AND PRACTICES FOR SELF-REPORTED MENTAL HEALTH PROBLEM (MENTAL HEALTH CARE UTILIZATION AMONG PUERTO RICANS STUDY, 2 WAVES)

	Wave of Data Collection	
	1992–1993 (N = 767) %	1993–1994 (N = 774) %
Advisors		
Relative	40.1	52.3
Friend	28.7	35.5
Clergy	14.8	14.1
General Practitioner	20.2	21.8
Mental Health Specialist	22.9	21.4
Espiritista, Curandero	*	3.1
Other	4.1	4.4
Practices		
Home Remedies	15.2	13.2
Over-the-Counter Medicines	28.7	34.6
Religious Practice	26.6	23.6
Alcohol	8.5	7.3
Exercise/Meditation	23.5	20.5
Other	6.7	3.3

* Not available as a category in Wave 1.

used 66% of them. That is, there appear to be 42 different pathways that individuals use in responding to mental health problems (43 once the 'Nothing' option is added). As Figure 10.2 indicates, these patterns can be simple, using only one advisor (e.g., 176 or 23.5% consult individuals in the lay sector only)

TABLE 10.4: PERCENTAGE OF INDIVIDUALS SELECTING EACH TYPE OF ADVISOR FIRST, BY INDIVIDUALS REPORTING MENTAL HEALTH PROBLEMS (MENTAL HEALTH CARE UTILIZATION AMONG PUERTO RICANS STUDY, 2 WAVES)

	Wave of Data Collection			
	1992–1993		1993–1994	
	%	N	%	N
Advisor				
Relative	65.4	(312)	64.2	(408)
Friend	39.0	(223)	26.7	(277)
Clergy	24.3	(115)	20.0	(110)
General Practitioner	36.3	(157)	39.1	(170)
Mental Health Specialist	30.9	(178)	35.3	(167)
Other	18.8	(32)	32.4	(34)

or complex, using three or more types of advisors (i.e., 87 or 11.6% consulting individuals in three or all four sectors; see Kleinman's 1980 typology of medical sectors).

Ending up in a mental health facility in Indianapolis.

This final table takes a different look, one that combines the coding of fairly open-ended accounts of how individuals report that they ended up making their first major contact with a mental health facility, with closed-ended checklists of social network ties, socio-demographic and diagnostic characteristics, etc. That is, a standard, structured interview schedule was altered to begin with personal 'stories' of the entry into the formal, speciality system. Again, we see that a large percentage (but not a majority, 45.1%) report a reliance on personal contacts in the lay system of care (Table 10.5, Panel A).

FIGURE 10.2:   PATHWAYS TO CARE, MENTAL HEALTH CARE UTILIZATION AMONG PUERTO RICANS STUDY, 1992–93, N = 747

Pathway	(N)	Pathway	(N)
Lay	(176)	GP → MH → Lay →Folk	(3)
MH	(43)	MH → GP → Lay → Folk	(1)
Folk	(11)	Lay → GP → MH	(14)
Folk → Lay	(11)	GP → Lay → MH	(2)
MH → Lay	(6)	Folk → GP → MH	(1)
Lay → MH	(35)	Lay → GP → MH → Folk	(3)
Folk → MH	(1)	Lay → MH → GP → Folk	(3)
GP → MH	(13)	Folk → Lay → GP → MH	(2)
MH → GP → Lay	(4)	Lay → MH → Folk → GP	(1)
GP → MH → Lay	(1)	MH → Lay → Folk → GP	(1)
Lay → GP	(23)	GP → Lay	(15)
MH → GP	(1)	Folk → GP → Lay	(2)
GP → Lay → Folk	(2)	Folk → GP	(3)
Lay → GP → Folk	(4)	Lay → MH → GP	(7)
Lay → Folk → MH → GP	(3)	Lay → GP → Folk → MH	(1)
Lay → Folk → GP → MH	(3)	GP → Lay → Folk → MH	(1)
Lay → Folk → GP	(8)	MH → Folk → Lay	(3)
Folk → Lay → GP	(3)	MH → Lay → Folk	(1)
Lay → Folk → MH	(7)	No Pathway (None)	(277)
Lay → MH → Folk	(5)		
Folk → Lay → MH	(1)		
Lay → Folk	(22)		
MH → Folk	(3)		

Almost a third of individuals (27.7%) engage in self-care and relatively few go 'through' medical providers (11.2%) or other professionals (11.0%). Even fewer use the social service system or other mental health providers (2.3% each). Too few individuals explicitly mentioned alternative medical systems to separate this out.

In this case, we see more steps in the illness career (Table 10.5, Panel B). Typically, and unlike Pitchátaro, individuals gave accounts that included an average of four options. No one indicated that they went directly to the formal mental health system and very few reported fewer than three steps in the sequence (8.2%). Whether this reflects protocol differences between the two studies or the differential nature of the health problem (general versus mental health) cannot be determined here.

TABLE 10.5:   SUMMARY OF SOURCES AND PATHWAYS TO CARE (INDIANAPOLIS NETWORK MENTAL HEALTH STUDY, WAVE 1, 1990–1994)

Panel A: Sources of care	%	(N)
Personal Network Contacts	45.1	(208)
Personal Coping (Independent Problem-Solving Action)	27.7	(128)
Medical Provider	11.2	(52)
Other Professional	11.0	(51)
Social Service Provider	2.3	(11)
Other Mental Health Provider	2.3	(11)
Total		

Panel B[1]: Number of steps in pathways to care	%	(N)
Two	8.2	(10)
Three	18.1	(22)
Four	18.1	(22)
Five	21.4	(26)
Six	15.7	(19)
Seven	8.2	(10)
Eight	2.4	(3)
Nine	3.3	(4)
Ten	0.0	(0)
Eleven	2.4	(3)
Twelve	.8	(1)
Mean	4.23	(2.41)
Unique Pathways	85	

[1] N = 121; 10 cases did not have useable data.

THE DYNAMIC, SOCIAL ORGANIZATION OF MENTAL HEALTH CONTACTS: THE NETWORK-EPISODE MODEL

What the above illustrations reveal is a complex set of responses and orderings that cannot be easily accounted for or even described in dominant approaches. Recently, we proposed the **Network-Episode Model** (NEM) that draws both from the strengths of traditional, contingency and more dynamic, ethnographic approaches (Pescosolido, 1991, 1992; Pescosolido and Boyer, 1999; see Figure 10.3). That is, this model combines a general search for systematic correlates with a focus on the meaning and process of individuals' use of different medical care systems. The essence of the model is that it moves away from 'boxes' of contingencies and stages to 'streams' of illness behaviour as people negotiate between changing community conditions and treatment system possibilities. It starts with a few basic ideas.

First, important research questions focus on understanding the illness career as the nature of contacts to and from the community and the treatment system, and the degree to which individuals use each. The NEM focuses on how these different combinations and sequences affect the continued use of services and outcomes. Finally, it explores when, how and under what conditions individuals shift from evoking standard cultural routines and move into a rational choice-based calculus.

Second, by their very nature, the focus on the series or set of contacts represents a dynamic view of the response to health and illness (see next section for detail). The NEM also suggests these responses are not random. Both the social support system(s) and the treatment system(s) are on-going streams which influence and are influenced by the illness career. Dealing with any health problem is a social process that is managed through the contacts (or social networks) that individuals have in the community and treatment systems. People are social – they face illness in the course of their day-to-day lives by interacting with other people who may recognize (or deny) a problem; send them to (or provide) treatment; and support, cajole or nag them about appointments, medications or lifestyle. What this social support system looks like and what it offers is critical to understanding whether individuals construct a problem as a medical one; what kinds of actions they see as appropriate; and how they react to contact with any lay or formal providers. Further, the treatment sector, itself, represents the provision of a *human* service that can be characterized by networks of people that provide care, concern, pressure and problems (Pescosolido, 1999). The NEM conceptualizes medical systems as a changing set of providers and organizations with which individuals may have contact when they are ill (bottom stream, right-hand side, Figure 10.3). Like the community and the episode of illness, they change over time in response to the health problems that people bring, technological and medical innovation, policy

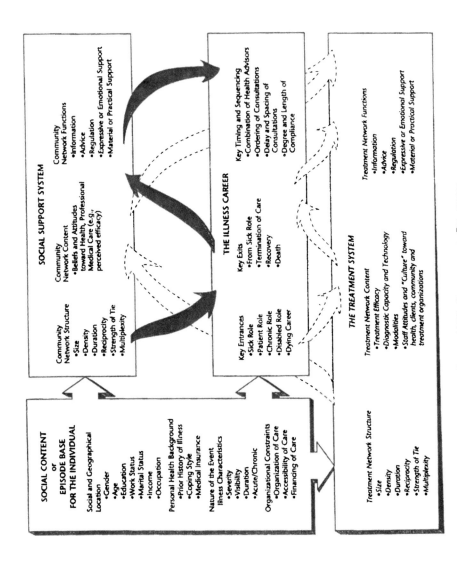

SOCIAL CONTENT
or
**EPISODE BASE
FOR THE INDIVIDUAL**

Social and Geographical
Location
• Gender
• Age
• Education
• Work Status
• Marital Status
• income
• Occupation

Personal Health Background
• Prior History of Illness
• Coping Style
• Medical Insurance

Nature of the Event
Illness Characteristics
• Severity
• Visibility
• Duration
• Acute/Chronic

Organizational Constraints
• Organization of Care
• Accessibility of Care
• Financing of Care

SOCIAL SUPPORT SYSTEM

Community
Network Structure
• Size
• Density
• Duration
• Reciprocity
• Strength of Tie
• Multiplexity

Community
Network Content
• Beliefs and Attitudes
  toward Health, Professional
  Medical Care (e.g.,
  perceived efficacy)

Community
Network Functions
• Information
• Advice
• Regulation
• Expressive or Emotional Support
• Material or Practical Support

THE ILLNESS CAREER

Key Entrances
• Sick Role
• Patient Role
• Chronic Role
• Disabled Role
• Dying Career

Key Exits
• From Sick Role
• Termination of Care
• Recovery
• Death

Key Timing and Sequencing
• Combination of Health Advisors
• Ordering of Consultations
• Delay and Spacing of
  Consultations
• Degree and Length of
  Compliance

THE TREATMENT SYSTEM

Treatment Network Structure
• Size
• Density
• Duration
• Reciprocity
• Strength of Tie
• Multiplexity

Treatment Network Content
• Treatment Efficacy
• Diagnostic Capacity and Technology
• Modalities
• Staff Attitudes and "Culture" toward
  health, clients, community and
  treatment organizations

Treatment Network Functions
• Information
• Advice
• Regulation
• Expressive or Emotional Support
• Material or Practical Support

FIGURE 10.3: REVISED NETWORK-EPISODE MODEL (PESCOSOLIDO AND BOYER, 1998). REPRINTED WITH PERMISSION

developments which set limits to resources and access and, in more recent times, to the preferences of consumers and insurance companies. Thinking about treatment in social network terms allows us to break down the treatment experience by charting the kinds and nature of experiences that people have in treatment which may affect whether they come back, take their medications or get better. Social support networks in treatment create a climate of care which affects both individuals and practitioners in different medical systems (Pescosolido, 1999).

Third, when health or illness problems arise, the person has certain characteristics (social, psychological, etc.); the illness problem itself has certain characteristics (severity, type); and the larger context in which they live has certain characteristics (good social welfare policies; poor treatment system, etc.). All of these characteristics have influence and can affect the trajectory of the social support system, the illness career and the treatment system. For example, we know that women tend to both have more social supports in the community and be more likely to become caretakers when illness strikes. Similarly, if the illness condition is serious and chronic it is more likely to impact the social support system. In sum, all three streams are anchored in the social locations, histories and problems that people and societies have (see Pescosolido, 1991, 1992 and Pescosolido and Boyer, 1999 for detail).

PATTERNS, PATHWAYS AND STEPS

At minimum, what the NEM suggests is that we consider a reconceptualization of the 'dependent variable' – that is, the nature and meaning of responses to illness. This is the case whether our interests lie in understanding how people get to mainstream medical care, CAM, or remain outside the reach of any formal practitioners. The basic idea here is that, if the response to illness is part of a whole set of actions (i.e., the illness career), the only way that we can truly understand why individuals use CAM, for example, is to demarcate where and when in the career a particular option is used.

Table 10.6 presents three possible ways of reconceptualizing the dependent variable along with some methods that have been or could be used to emprically describe them. *Patterns* of care target the combination of advisors, practitioners and systems of medical care that individuals bring together or are forced on individuals who appear to have health problems. For example, a 'singleton' pattern includes only one source of care. In Pichátaro, most individuals that Young interviewed reported using only one source of care (Table 10.1). In Puerto Rico, there are three singleton patterns – many individuals never consult 'advisors' outside of the lay system of care, some report the first and only contact with the speciality mental health sector, and few mention that the only source of care was in the folk system (Figure 10.2). 'Complex' patterns of care combine the use of medical care advisors and providers across other systems of care. In the Indianapolis study, for example, most individuals reported that they first had contact with *at least* one advisor outside the specialty mental health sector (Table 10.5, Panel B). In Puerto Rico, we found that individuals who use more complex patterns tend to have more serious mental health problems (Pescosolido *et al.*, 1998).

Pathways add the dimension of sequencing – that is, the order in which individuals access different medical care systems. For example, Romannucci-Ross' (1977) 'hierarchies of resort' study of health practices in Melanesia suggested that there were two main and distinctive sequences. An 'acculturative' sequence started with the allopathic system, in this case, Western physicians or nurses. If that failed to provide relief, individuals moved to the folk system, Western religious healers, practices and advisors. Finally, if the search continued, native religious practices and advisors were sought out. In the 'counter acculturative' sequence, home remedies (the lay system) were first tried, followed by visits to traditional, indigenous healers (the folk system) and finally going to a hospital (the allopathic system) in the event that all else failed. In the Puerto Rico study, Figure 10.2 shows that the most common sequences are those in which individuals move from the lay system of care to either the specialty mental health sector (Lay → MH) or to the general allopathic medical provider (Lay → GP).

Finally, *steps* follow most directly from Young's (1981) work in Mexico and Janzen's (1978) work in Zaire. Rather than focusing on the entire string of responses, this conceptualization takes apart sequences and tries to examine what factors are associated with each health care contact in order. For

TABLE 10.6:   RECONCEPTUALIZING THE DEPENDENT VARIABLE OF HEALTH CARE USE

Focus	Meaning	Examples
Patterns	The combination of advisors, providers, and/or practices used during the course of an illness episode.	Singleton: One contact Complex: Two or more contacts over the illness episode
Pathways	Sequence of advisors, providers, and/or practices used over the course of an illness episode.	Direct: Physician Only Multiple: Lay → Alternative → Allopathic
Steps	The conditional ordering of advisors and/or practices used over the course of an illness episode	Lay → Allopathic ↑ ↑ Severity Lay Advice

example, does the severity of the health problem influence which system of care individuals contact first? If individuals go on to consult a second advisor or provider from another medical system, is this affected by what happened in the last contact?

Each of these approaches has been used, at least to some extent, by adopting different analytic strategies and using statistical models outside of the usual multivariate models.

DISCUSSION AND IMPLICATIONS

In sum, this review suggests that individuals with health problems draw from a wide variety of sources of help. While we see some substantial differences in the number of options used across the studies, they all challenge the dominant utilization approaches and open the way to rethinking how to model the use of CAM as part of a total, embedded response to health problems. Are individuals who go to a physician the same as those who go to an alternative source of care and a physician in some combination? Are individuals who opt for the same sources of care but do so in different order the same? Both our theoretical work and research currently underway suggest not (Pescosolido *et al.,* 1998). Under which conditions do individuals use their contacts in the lay or informal system last? Issues of the voluntary versus involuntary use of services may help provide an answer (Bennett *et al.,* 1993; Gardner *et al.,* 1993; Hiday, 1992; Pescosolido, Gardner and Lubell, 1998). How might we depict the basic set of pathways? While we get a complete sense of the set of pathways in the Puerto Rico study, they resemble neither Romannucci-Ross' simple acculturative, non-acculturative typology nor any of the revised illness career models that have been offered. Clearly, no multivariate technique could deal with the long list of possibilities and the 'thin cells' that result in many of the pathways. This calls for more theoretical work to suggest ways to collapse them to match concerns of researchers, providers or policymakers. For example, from a clinical, treatment or health services research perspective, what matters about these pathways is whether individuals ever reach the formal health system, and if so, whether they turn to other types of advisors *after* they enter (see Pescosolido, Boyer and Lubell, 1999). From the standpoint of CAM, collapsing pathways to reflect the positioning of their use in a sequence might be useful. More sophisticated questions lie ahead about how to incorporate the content of care (the timing and duration of the use of each sequence) into theoretical propositions, protocols and analyses.

What the descriptive results presented in this paper do not reveal are the insights we have gained in our fieldwork in Indianapolis and Puerto Rico. Specifically, these studies, among the first of their kind, suggested to us that we may not be approaching the collection of data in the most effective way. Particularly in the Puerto Rico study, we suspect that individuals use 'espiritistas' to a much greater extent than our respondents reported in their attempts to deal with a recognized mental health problem. It may be the case that individuals consult these individuals in the course of their day-to-day lives and do not consider this in the same vein as other health care options, even when prompted with a structured list. This paper does not address these issues of measurement, particularly for alternative systems of care. They remain lingering questions in rethinking how individuals not only use options but respond to our inquiries and observations about how they face illness. The Network Episode Model offers a start at reconceptualizing individuals' responses to health and illness behaviour but it is only a beginning.

AKNOWLEDGEMENTS

Support for this project was provided by the ConCEPT 1 Program in Health and Medicine, funded by the President's Strategic Directions Charter Initiative at Indiana University; the Indiana Consortium for Mental Health Services Research (R24MH51669); and, Independent Scientist Award from the National Institute of Mental Health (K02MH01289)

REFERENCES

Aday, Lu Ann and William C. Awe. 1997. 'Health Service Utilization Models,' in David S. Gochman (ed.). *Handbook of Health Behavior Research III: Demography, Development and Diversity.* (New York: Plenum Press, 1997), pp. 153–172.

Alegría, Margarita, Rafaela Robles, Daniel H. Freeman, Mildred Vera, A.L. Jimenez, C. Rios, R. Rios. 1991. 'Patterns of Mental Health Utilization Among Island Puerto Rican Poor.' *American Journal of Public Health* 81:875.

Andersen, Ronald. 1995. 'Revisiting the Behavioral Model and Access to Care: Does It Matter?' *Journal of Health and Social Behavior* 36:1–10.

Bennett, N.S., C.W. Lidz, John Monahan, E. Mulvey, S.K. Hoge, L.H. Roth and W. Gardner. 1993. 'Inclusion, Motivation and Good Faith: The Morality of Coercion in Mental Hospital Admission.' *Behavioral Science and the Law* 11:295–306.

Brown, E. Richard. 1979. *Rockefeller Medicine Men: Medicine and Capitalism in America,* (Berkeley: University of California Press).

Coleman, James S. 1986. 'Social Theory, Social Research, and a Theory of Action', *American Journal of Sociology.* 91:1309–35.

Fosu, Gabriel. 1981. 'Disease Classification in rural Ghana: Framework and Implications for Health Behavior.' *Social Science and Medicine* 15B:471–480.

Frank, Richard G. and Mark S. Kamlet, 1989. 'Determining Provider Choice for the Treatment of Mental Disorder: The Role of Health and Mental Health Status.' *Health Services Research* 24:83–103.

Gardner, William, Steven K. Hoge, Nancy Bennett, Loren H. Roth, Charles W. Lidz, John Monahan and Edward P. Mulvery. 1993. 'Two Scales for Measuring Patients' Perceptions of Coercion During Mental Hospital Admission.' *Behavioral Sciences and the Law* 11:307–322.

Gochman, David S. 1997. 'Personal and Social Determinants of Health Behavior: An Integration,' in David S. Gochman (ed.). *Handbook of Health Behavior Research III: Demography, Development and Diversity,* (New York: Plenum Press), pp. 381–400.

Hiday, Virginia. 1992. 'Coercion in Civil Commitment: Process, Preferences and Outcome.' *International Journal of Law and Psychiatry* 15:359–77.

Hostetler, John. 1963. 'Folk and Scientific Medicine in Amish Society.' *Human Organization* 22:269–275.

Janzen, John M. 1978. *The Quest for Therapy in Lower Zaire*, (Berkeley: University of California Press).

Kane, Robert, Craig Leymaster, Donna Olsen, F. Ross Woolley and F. David Fisher. 1974. 'Manipulating the Patient.' *Lancet* 29:1333–1336.

Kleinman, Arthur. *Patients and Healers in the Context of Culture*, (Berkeley: University of California Press), 1980.

Maddux, James E. and Kimberley A. DuCharme. 1997. 'Behavioral Intentions in Theories of Health Behavior,' in David S. Gochman (ed.). *Handbook of Health Behavior Research I: Personal and Social Determinants*, (New York: Plenum Press), pp. 133–152.

Pescosolido, Bernice A. 1999 'Bringing People Back in: Why Social Networks Matter for Treatment Effectiveness Research.' Unpublished Manuscript. Indiana University.

—. 1992. 'Beyond Rational Choice: The Social Dynamics of How People Seek Help.' *American Journal of Sociology* 97:1096–1138.

—. 'Illness Careers and Network Ties: A Conceptual Model of Utilization and Compliance,' in Gary Albrecht and Judith Levy (eds.), *Advances in Medical Sociology, Vol. 2*, (Greenwich, CT: JAI Press, 1991), pp. 164–181.

Pescosolido, Bernice A. and Carol A. Boyer. 1999. 'How Do People Come to Use Mental Health Services? Current Knowledge and Changing Perspectives,' in Allan Horwitz and Teresa Scheid (eds.), *A Handbook for the Study of Mental Health: Social Contents, Theories and Systems*, (New York: Cambridge University Press, pp. 392–411).

Pescosolido, Bernice A., Carol A. Boyce and Keri M. Lubell. 1999. 'The Social Dynamic of Responding to Mental Health Problems: Past, Present and Future Challenges to Understanding Individuals' Use of Service', in Carol Aneshensel and Jo Phelan (eds.) *Handbook of the Sociology of Mental Health*, (Plenum Press)

Pescosolido, Bernice A., Carol Brooks Gardner and Keri M. Lubell. 1998. 'How People Get Into Mental Health Services: Stories of Choice, Coercion and 'Muddling Through' From 'First Timers'. *Social Science and Medicine* 46:275–286.

Pescosolido, Bernice A. and Jennie J. Kronenfeld. 1995. 'Health, Illness and Healing in an Uncertain Era: Challenges From and For Medical Sociology.' *Journal of Health and Social Behavior* 36 (Extra Issue):5–33.

Pescosolido, Bernice A., Eric R. Wright, Margarita Alegría, and Mildred Vera. 1998. 'Social Networks and Patterns of Use Among the Poor with Mental Health Problems in Puerto Rico. *Medical Care* 36:1057–1072.

Press, Irwin. 1969. 'Urban Illness: Physicians, Curers and Dual Use in Bogata.' *Journal of Health and Social Behavior* 10:209–218.

Romanucci-Ross, Lola. 1997. 'The Hierarchy of Resort in Curative Practices: The Admirality Islands, Melanesia,' in David Land (ed.), *Culture, Disease and Healing*, (New York: Macmillan), pp. 481–486.

Strecher, Victor J., Victoria L. Champion and Irwin M. Rosenstock. 1997. 'The Health Belief Model and Health Behavior,' in David S. Gochman (ed.), *Handbook of Health Behavior Research III: Demography, Development and Diversity*, (New York: Plenum Press), pp. 71–92.

Weinstein, Neil. 1993. 'Four Competing Theories of Health Protection Behavior.' *Health Psychology* 12:324–333.

Young, James C. 1981. *Medical Choices in a Mexican Village*, (New Brunswick, NJ: Rutgers University Press).

CHAPTER 11

Incorporating Symbolic, Experiential and Social Realities into Effectiveness Research on CAM

DEBORAH C. GLIK

INTRODUCTION

The current resurgence of alternative healing practices in the industrialized world has inspired research interest about why clinicians and patients have been drawn to these healing modalities, and what impact their utilization might have on health and health care (Eisenberg, Kessler, Foster *et al.*, 1993; Thomas, Carr, Westlake *et al.*, 1991; Vincent and Furnham, 1996). Given the sociopolitical realities and research funding opportunities in the health care field today, recent research has focused on efficacy studies, using strict research protocols to see if the treatments work. Efficacy studies by definition look at whether a specific measurable treatment or dose has a specific effect in a controlled environment. Thus to a large degree these studies of the efficacy of complementary and alternative medicine (CAM) have been framed as clinical trials with medical outcomes and have been conducted in clinical contexts.

While clinical approaches to the study of CAM are certainly appropriate and necessary to establish its efficacy, and utilization studies can assess who is using care, I will argue here that a holistic research agenda for CAM must also include broader effectiveness studies, that are defined as evaluative field studies in the naturalistic settings in which healing interactions occur. The use of evaluative field studies that assess effectiveness of CAM, not simply efficacy in clinical settings, can broaden our knowledge of how CAM works. Effectiveness studies can do this by including cultural, ideological, inter-personal, and contextual factors as part of the equation to determine how these systems work to facilitate individual healing.

To begin to frame the argument for a broader definition of outcome studies on CAM it is useful to categorize CAM practices. First there are the more developed forms of healing such as acupuncture, chiropractic, homeopathy or naturopathy which do use a clinical model of health care delivery, quite similar in context to medical care. Second there are more psychological forms of care such as massage, rolfing, reflexology, expressive therapies or guided imagery, which entail a relationship between client and provider with outcomes defined less in physical and more in psychological terms. Finally there are indigenous and religious practices such as folk and spiritual healing, Yoga, meditation, or prayer. These latter forms of CAM often take place in groups, communities, and other social networks, and they have goals and objectives that are much broader than improving the symptoms of clients. They include practices that may be more aptly conceptualized as social, psychological or even spiritual interventions, rather than medical transactions (Frank, 1973; Kleinman, 1980; Glik, 1988).

By defining CAM broadly, clinically based care is seen as only one practice model under which individuals can gain access to alternative therapies. Clinical trials have become the accepted way to evaluate clinical care. By definition clinical trials presume a medical understanding of CAM, with specific standardized treatments given for specific conditions. However as not all CAM modalities fit into a clinical definition of care, it becomes apparent that clinical trials may not be the only way to determine the efficacy of CAM. Such trials may provide misleading answers, especially for the psychological and indigenous or community-based forms of CAM.

In this paper I will review selected literature that exemplifies research on CAM in more naturalistic or 'field' settings. Second, I will explore some current issues concerning CAM efficacy studies, and review alternative research models from health services and social science research that can be used. Third, drawing on my own research in the areas of spiritual healing (Glik, 1988; 1990a; 1990b; 1993), homeopathic care (Goldstein and Glik, 1998), and applied social research in public health, I will frame the research I have conducted on healing. I will present a conceptual framework using health services research and program evaluation principles to show how healing processes and outcomes can be more fully studied by integrating specific social and contextual variables into efficacy and effectiveness research on CAM.

BACKGROUND STUDIES

The study of alternative healing is not new, and there has been a long and well developed research tradition in sociology, anthropology and cross-cultural psychiatry on the persons who use non-medical healing practices and beliefs. The literature cited here reflects my own bias towards the study of non-clinical forms of CAM, and much of it is descriptive and non-quantitative. However a number of good examples of field research approaches stand out, and within this body of work are some directives for more rigorous and appropriate studies of CAM.

For example in the 1970s and 1980s a number of psychiatric and sociological studies were carried out among Christian and Pentecostal healing groups (Pattison, Nikolajs and Doerr, 1974; Allen and Wallis, 1978; Ness, 1980; Poloma, 1982), and among persons who adhere to Eastern or New Age healing practices (Galanter and Buckley, 1975; Bird and Reimer, 1982; McGuire, 1988). Findings have suggested that healing serves both social (Pattison, Nikolajs and Doerr, 1974; Ness, 1980) and psychological functions for participants (Bird and Reimer, 1982; McGuire, 1988). There have been studies of a variety of healing practices of ethnic and cultural minorities (Harwood, 1977; Wardwell, 1973; Snow, 1974; Jilek, 1974; Griffith *et al.*, 1986). Practices that occur in indigenous groups and settings not only benefit participants, but are seen as a means of cultural identity and regeneration (Garrison, 1974; Kleinman and Sung, 1979; Galanter and Buckley, 1978; Ness, 1980; Finkler, 1980, 1981; Griffith *et al.*, 1986). While quantitative data are scarce and research designs weak, thick description and sociologically informed explanation abound in this literature (Frank, 1973; McGuire, 1988; Macklin, 1974).

These studies on faith or folk or spiritual healing suggest three important elements that have implications for designing a valid research approach. First, while many of the conditions presented in alternative care contexts are chronic and non-life threatening, many of the ailments are described in physical rather than mental or emotional terms, even though some of the underlying issues could be seen to be stress related (Kleinman, 1984). Second, the subjective impact of these healing systems for clients is multifaceted, with an array of changes reported, including symptom relief, changes in mental and emotional states, increased feelings of social connectedness and adjustment and instances of psychological and spiritual insight (Jilek, 1974, Galanter and Buckley, 1978; Griffith *et al.*, 1986). Third, it is important to consider the social location and cultural relevance of healing practices for seekers. Issues that must be considered include the specific social constructions and explanations for illness, the relationship of healer with clients, the role and status of the healer in the surrounding community and cultural belief systems that proscribe healing practices (Macklin, 1974; Ness, 1980; McGuire, 1988).

The factors described above are all essential elements in raising clients' expectations and beliefs about the efficacy of healing (Frank, 1973; Kleinman, 1984). Thus a strong case can be made that the social and contextual characteristics in which CAM is delivered are important elements in whether CAM is effective. As a result these factors must be incorporated into measurement models that attempt to determine the effectiveness of CAM, as well as understanding the client's attraction in the first place (Glik, 1988; 1993). These elements are critical for understanding CAM, but they are not unique to non-clinical forms of care as has often been assumed. As many have noted, contextual, cultural and interpersonal factors are also important in professional and medical care contexts (Frank, 1973, Benson and Friedman, 1996).

CONTEMPORARY DEBATES IN STUDYING CAM EFFICACY

Current attempts to validate or invalidate the utility of CAM therapies have created some debate about the most appropriate methods for its study. Despite the concerns raised above, there has also been a strong movement among CAM researchers to promote efficacy research using randomized clinical trials (RCTs). According to some, the RCT, preferably with a double blind design, represents the gold standard for assessing efficacy or effectiveness of healing (Bulpitt, 1983; Vickers, Cassileth, Ernst *et al.*, 1997). The intent of these experimental research designs within clinical contexts is to isolate some underlying mechanism of alternative healing modalities so that an effect can be measured in a way similar to evaluating the impact of drugs on symptoms or finding a 'dose – response' relationship between taking medications and health outcomes.

Adherence to this 'medicalized' view of testing treatments in a specific research paradigm has meant that experimental designs are imposed on healing interactions, and the interpersonal, contextual and cultural factors that seemed to be so important in earlier descriptive or ethnographic studies of folk or indigenous systems are relegated to 'confounder' status, specifically defined as factors which if 'uncontrolled' may impede understanding of a true or net effect of a specific 'dose' of healing on the client. Examples of confounders might be high expectations both on the part of healers and clients, or a mutually held belief system about the role of energy in healing. Rationalized clinical trials typically try to minimize the impact of 'confounders' by making treatment and control samples more comparable, controlling the frequency and intensity of interventions, using exclusion criteria to restrict samples to certain defined conditions and relegating 'treatments' to specific actions. This makes results more interpretable as well as more conservative (Bulpitt, 1983). Clinical trials are usually geared to measure impacts that are short term and symptom specific, rather than long term or general. Moreover within the clinical arena, the importance of placebo effects are subject to debate, with some discounting them as a legitimate effect (Bostrom, 1997) and others defending placebo effects as a positive aspect of the healing paradigm (Benson and Friedman, 1996)

Adopting RCTs to study healing implies that some specific transaction between any healer and any patient creates some effect. In clinical research it is assumed that the setting, context, or relationship between healer and patient is less important than the specific *modus operandi* of the transaction. RCTs, as indicated by their norm of random assignment of individuals into treatment and control groups, allow inferences to be made that eliminate the issue of selection bias or baseline differences between groups. In most alternative forms of healing, selection into care is an important variable influencing outcome.

Paradoxically, concurrent with arguments by some CAM researchers for a more conservative definition of 'legitimate' methods to do efficacy research (i.e. the RCT), the medical field itself has become much more liberal in its inclusion of certain outcome measures (Kaplan, Greenfield and Ware, 1989; Hays, Kravitz and Mazel *et al.*, 1994). Thus in the wider arena of clinical research on pharmaceuticals or medical procedures, there has been phenomenal growth in the incorporation of psychosocial and quality-of-life measures as important outcomes to measure in clinical trials over the past decade. In less technologically driven forms of care such as psychotherapy, counseling or patient education, the nature of the clinical encounter and variation in service delivery are compared with hypothesized outcomes. Given these developments, recent articles have recommended the need for an expanded definition of viable approaches to the study of CAM using both experimental and observational types of studies including epidemiological, evaluative and social survey types of designs (Levin, Glass, Kushi, Schuck, Steele and Jonas, 1997; Shuck, Chappell and Kindness, 1997).

To expand our thinking about efficacy research for CAM, it is important to look to some other fields that have made great progress in the development of viable evaluation research models. One area of relevance is health services research where over the past twenty years models to assess quality of care and medical care outcomes have grown greatly in sophistication and precision (Donabedian, 1980; Williamson, 1971; Fries, 1993). The other area of relevance is that of applied social research, where models and methods used to assess social programs more generally have also developed a great degree of refinement (Rossi and Freeman, 1993). Concepts derived from these research areas can be adopted to formulate a more contextual and 'sociological' approach to the evaluation of CAM.

USEFUL CONCEPTUAL MODELS FOR THE EVALUATION OF CAM

The area of health outcomes research has emerged from empirical studies of health care reimbursement, health care utilization, quality of care and health status outcomes. This type of research is based on the collection and analysis of large data sets and the creation of predictive causal models linking specific dimensions of care. This area of research has made extensive use of health status and quality-of-life measures designed for survey research within populations and for service delivery systems (Stewart *et al.*, 1989; Brown, 1984; Steinwachs, 1989), as well as explicit studies linking the amount and types of medical care that patients receive to both generic and disease specific outcomes (Reuben, *et al.*, 1995; Hays *et al.*, 1994; Yelin *et al.*, 1985; Greenfield *et al.*, 1995).

'Outcomes research' describes a set of concepts or models rather than a specific research design. That is, outcomes research designs can vary from controlled randomized trials to descriptive survey research. Typically these studies use survey research merged with patient record and reimbursement data as well as measures of quality of care. Moreover many are large scale studies, looking at data from multiple treatment sites or practice settings such as hospitals, clinics or doctors offices. What differentiates outcomes research from more traditional definitions of clinical trials (Bulpitt, 1983) is its orientation to real world conditions and its attempt to conceptualize and measure dimensions of health care that fall outside the clinical laboratory. Thus health outcomes research, also called effectiveness research, assesses how variations in treatments, types of practice, patient characteristics, types of patient care, quality of care, reimbursement and baseline conditions will impact treatment outcomes. In the broadest or most comprehensive designs, participation by patients and their interactions with clinicians are recorded since they are also seen as possible influences on outcomes (Kaplan *et al.*, 1989, Hohmann and Parron, 1996).

Within this tradition, one set of organizing concepts suggested by Donabedian (1980) has been adopted widely by outcomes researchers. They are dimensions of structure, process and outcomes of care, as well as characteristics of individuals themselves. Donabedian, interested in the quality of care and its impact on outcomes, defined 'structure' as the institutional arrangements in which care takes place, 'process' as what physicians do and how they interact with patients and how patients use the system and 'outcomes' as health status change indicators. Characteristics of patients such as chronicity of illness, age, or gender are also linked to process and outcome variables. These concepts can be integrated into the study of non-conventional as well as conventional care.

The second useful set of concepts comes from the field of applied social research. In this area, researchers have over the past few years shifted their focus away from strict experimental designs to encompass more explicitly fully elaborated, multivariate causal models. In other words, rather than using experimental manipulation primarily to test the impact of specific interventions on people, they have learned to rely on sophisticated statistical controls that can assess the relative contribution of a range of associated variables including predisposing, mediating, process and outcome variables. Thus the classic input – output, experimental 'black box' orientation to assessment first espoused by Campbell and Stanley (1966) is, to some extent, being superseded by theory-driven approaches. These approaches attempt to specify how a 'treatment input' will have impact on programmatic outcomes, using a range of experimental, quasi-experimental, comparative or full coverage designs (Chen, 1990; Chen and Rossi, 1980).

A key element in this type of evaluation is figuring out how a set of independent and treatment process variables link to outcome variables and to each other. Then, statistical methods are used to model the expected relationships between variables (Cordray, 1986 Chen, 1990; Chen and Rossi, 1980; Judd and Kenny, 1981; Wang and Walberg, 1983; Rossi and Freeman, 1993). Here too, methods have been developed to overcome inherent weaknesses in non-random or quasi-experimental designs, which interfere with uncovering causal effects. For example, if there is bias in who uses care (i.e. a selection bias) then techniques can be employed to control for such biases (Rossi and Freeman, 1993). Like health outcomes research, these methods often use longitudinal designs across multiple sites.

These approaches and techniques can also be adapted to the study of CAM efficacy. In the next section examples of my own CAM research where elements of evaluation and outcomes research were incorporated are presented, using dimensions of structure, process, outcomes and individual characteristics to define research elements (Donabedian, 1980).

ILLUSTRATRIVE EXAMPLES

Structure/outcome

One question that arises continuously in outcomes research is the relationships between the way care is delivered, the places where care care is delivered and the outcomes of interest. The structure of care delivery could include, types of institutions delivering care (e.g. private office, group setting), types of reimbursement (e.g. fee for services, third party payment) or cost recovery systems (e.g. third party billing). In a study on alternative healing carried out in Baltimore in the 1980s, persons' affiliations with specific types of healing groups were assessed in relation to their impact on beliefs and quality of life outcome indicators. Members of three groups, Christian charismatic groups, New Age groups and medical patients comprised the sample. Over 300 persons (approximately 100 per group) were followed over a six month period to assess their engagement in CAM or medical care and how that was related to an array of quality-of-life measures (Glik, 1986; 1988; 1990a).

It was hypothesized that these different healing contexts would be differentially related to outcome measures of quality-of-life controlling for illness severity, sociodemographic and religiosity variables. The analysis of these data showed that even when there were a large number of variables controlled, the type of healing groups persons were aligned with (CAM or medical) had a large impact on outcomes. Persons in some CAM groups had much more positive scores of quality-of-life outcome indicators than medical patients, even though CAM clients were generally at higher risk for poorer outcomes than the medical patients sampled. Specifically persons who attended services or were clients of either New Age or Christian Charismatic healers tended to be older, sicker, and more socially marginal than clients of a medical practice sampled; however they had higher scores of measures of adjustment and psychological well being than the medical patients.

Individual characteristics/outcome

Another issue that can be addressed through these models is to assess whether a person's pre-existing conditions or predispositions influence the outcomes of care. Whether individuals are randomly assigned or not or outcomes of different treatments compared or not, in both field trials or clinical studies, there are always variations in the outcomes individuals experience which can be linked back to something about the way things were at the beginning of the study. For example, some factors can be seen in research done on patients of homeopaths conducted at UCLA (Goldstein and Glik, 1998). Based on a sample of 81 patients and followed over a six month period, outcomes could be linked back statistically to some conditions of respondents at the beginning of the study.

Inspection of some relationships showed that between initial health and treatment effects, persons with worse physical health at Time 1 did not improve as dramatically as those with better health at Time 1. This is not a particularly revolutionary finding but one which is typical in most medical outcome studies, as all systems of care do better with less ill patients. A second finding was that patients who had higher expectations of successful outcomes at Time 1 had higher scores on all three outcome measures: physical health status change, perceived change in primary condition, and perceived change in outlook. Also sociodemographic measures were not consistently related to self-reported health change, perhaps more a reflection of lack of variability in these indicators in this sample, where a large number of patients had high socioeconomic status. The conclusion then to be drawn from this study is that how a person feels initially about a healing process, either positive or negative, can affect outcomes.

Process/outcomes

One important consideration in creating models to understand the dynamics of healing is the specification of processes, or the 'hows' of treatment, that may influence outcomes. Typically in more naturalistic studies where one cannot control 'dosage', processes described may have to do with how a practitioner interacts with a patient or the effects of such processes. For example in my own studies on healing one example of 'process' variables is called 'redefinition of the situation' (Glik, 1990b). This factor became apparent over the course of one study as persons were being healed of conditions they did not have at the outset of the study. For example, an individual might start the treatment process with a very specific condition such as chronic pain or indigestion. However when queried 3 or 6 months later about what was healed they might report that they had re-established a relationship with a family member or had learned to accept their medical condition. Assessing how the definition of primary condition changes over times implies some interaction of person with healer or system. Over the course of the study, symptoms and conditions reported were systematically redefined by respondents. Most notably conditions became more chronic and less medical, and those who had redefined their condition were more likely to report having experienced some form of healing. These findings suggest the subtle and pervasive influence of healing subcultures, where certain types of illness experiences are more culturally acceptable.

Multiple modes of assessment

A final set of issues is how effects are measured. That is, when assessing healing, change may be occurring on many levels. An interesting if unconventional measurement tool that has been used in clinical psychotherapy, though not in social science research, is the MARI Card test, which measures persons' cognitive propensities to experience certain states of consciousness that can be linked to arousal as well as altered states of consciousness. This test uses symbols and colors to assess cognitive states (Kellogg, 1978). For example there are specific selections that would indicate that a person has a propensity for 'peak' experiences or feelings of great excitement at the time measured, whereas other selections might indicate a certain degree of ambivalence towards their current situation. Typically these states, while felt, may not be consciously articulated.

Among study participants undergoing spiritual healing, I administered the MARI right before and right after a Christian charismatic healing service. It showed a great deal of psychic change, with persons going from a somewhat depressed outlook before the healing intervention to states of ecstasy after the intervention. When the same approach was attempted with a meditation group, the tendency was to go into meditative, low arousal states after the intervention. Thus different forms of healing may change states of consciousness of participants in very dramatic ways, and ultimately these underlying intra-personal dynamics may be correlated with both biological and social linkage processes. This test is one means to capture phenomenon that may be just outside of the conscious perception of the study participants and expand how we think about healing outcomes using unconventional measurements in research.

DISCUSSION

The findings presented here are only illustrative; they do not represent the whole spectrum of variables that can be used to show relationships between structure, process, outcomes and individual characteristics. They do represent some types of factors that might be used to develop a comprehensive approach to the study of CAM. To foster thinking about the approaches described above, I have devised a Conceptual Framework (see Table 11.1) that uses the structure, process and outcomes schema suggested by Donabedian (1980) and social programs evaluators (Rossi and Freeman, 1993, Chen, 1990).

Factors presented in Table 11.1 do not represent an exhaustive list. But this approach implies an inclusive research agenda using multiple sites and healers and data collected from individuals either through clinical records, survey research or both. The two starting points for research of this type are either 1) selecting members of a defined population, or 2) selecting patients with specific health conditions from participating providers. Study starting points do determine, to some extent, research objectives, study design and variables that are most important. Given the limitations of time and sample size, not all of these elements may be measured simultaneously in the same study.

Increasing the repertoire of research methods acceptable to evaluate CAM takes into account the variation in style and substance that characterizes the field of alternative healing today (Levin et al., 1997; Shuck, Chappell and Kindness, 1997). As has been discussed earlier, some CAM practices are more clinical and some are more akin to social interventions. Hence the evaluation of CAM needs to be expanded from over-reliance on 'medicalized' models based on clinical trials that may be appropriate for some types of healing only. Rather than expending time on creating experimental controls that may not be appropriate for other types of healing, the evaluation of healing can use quasi-experimental or multiple comparison or panel study designs. Design controls can be built in where possible if randomization is not possible. Weaker designs mean the research must rely on adequate theoretical and measurement models to account for variation, using multivariate techniques to control and adjust for baseline differences or differences in healing processes and conditions.

At present the health and human services research world is replete with studies on the social and health impact of programmatic interventions, some

TABLE 11.1: CONCEPTUAL MODEL FOR EVALUATION OF CAM

Characteristics of individuals	Structure of healing practice	Process of treatments	Outcomes of care
Sociodemographics (age, gender, status or QOL, ethnicity)	Clinic or group composition	Intensity, duration, frequency of treatment	Changes in health Psychological adjustment
Social structural factors (educ, occ, inc, religion)	Healer integration into mainstream medicine	Cognitive behavioural therapy	Changes in beliefs, values
Personality	Healer philosophical orientation	Indoctrination into worldview of healer	Health behaviours change, well role performance change
Spiritual orientation	Social support	Redefinition of illness, healing process	Stress reduction
Health status	Training, certification of healer	Group or interpersonal process	Psycho-neuro-immuno-logical markers
Expectations	Type of reimbursement	Incentives for adherence to regimen	Social/Psychological reintegration
		Quality, nature of interpersonal communications	
			Change in subjective perceptions of healing
			Change in states of consciousness

of which have no more strength or intensity than a series of CAM healing sessions. Examples include studies on the early detection and counseling of HIV/AIDS positives, diabetes self-care and follow up, cognitive behavioural interventions for drug addicts, creating healthy communities, outcomes of psychotherapy, the impact of day care on child health and well-being, community based programs in teen pregnancy prevention, welfare to work polices or new health insurance eligibility requirements for children of the working poor. These are all examples of social interventions hypothesized to have an impact on the health and well-being of participants.

More relevantly, how are these social interventions evaluated? None of these social and community interventions are conceptualized as clinical trials. Rather they are subject to a variety of evaluative designs adapted for field research that include surveys, quasi-experiments, and in some cases, true experimental designs. These designs can be small scale or large scale using population based or provider outcome data, based, for example, on Medicaid encounter forms, hospital discharge data or ongoing social survey research. Many of these studies are adequately funded so that large scale long term multi-site, multi-method data collection with adequate sample size and adequate comparisons are possible. If we conceptualize some forms of CAM as social interventions, we can begin to devise broader based more sociologically and culturally interesting evaluative research in this area. Research of this type will give insights into the importance of social, interpersonal and contextual variables linked to healing, and how healing fits in to broader social or cultural change, thus encouraging research that can influence theory, policy and practice.

REFERENCES

Allen, G. and R Wallis. 1978. 'Pentecostalists as a Medical Minority.' pp. 110–137 in *Marginal Medicine* edited by R Wallis and P Morley, Glencoe: The Free Press.

Benson, H.,and H. Friedman. 1996. 'Harnessing the power of the placebo effect and renaming it 'remembered wellness.' *Annual Review of Medicine* 47:193–199.

Bird, F and B. Reimer.1982. 'Participation rates in New religions and Para-religious Movements.' *Journal for the Scientific Study of Religion* 21:1–4.

Bostrom, Harry. 1997. 'Placebo-the Forgotten Drug.' *Scandinavian J Work Environ Health* 23 suppl 3:53–57.

Brown, J.H. 1984. 'The Dimensions of Health Outcomes: A Cross-validated Examination of Health Status Measurement.' *Am Journal Public Health.* 74:159.

Bulpitt, C.J. 1983. *Randomised Controlled Clinical Trials.* The Hague, Netherlands: Martinus Nijhoff Publishers.

Campbell, D.T. and J.T. Stanley. 1966. *Experimental and Quasi-experimental Designs for Research* Skokie, Ill, New York: Rand McNally.

Chen, H-t. 1990. *Theory Driven Evaluation* Newbury Park, CA: Sage.

Chen, H-t and Rossi PH. 1980. 'The Multi-goal Theory-driven Approach to Evaluation: A Model Linking Basic and Applied Social Science.' *Social Forces* 59 (3):106–122.

Cordray, D.S. 1986. 'Quasi-experimental Analysis: a Mixture of Methods and Judgment.' pp. 9–27 in *Advances in Quasi-experimental Design and Analysis* edited by WMK Trochim, San Francisco, CA: Jossey-Bass.

Diehl, D.L., G. Kaplan, I. Coulter, D.C. Glik and E.L. Hurwitz. 1997. 'Use of Acupuncture by American Physicians.' *The Journal of Alternative and Complementary Medicine* 3(2):119–126, 1997.

Donabedian A.1980. *The Definition of Quality and Approaches to its Assessment.* Ann Arbor, Michigan: Health Administration Press.

Eisenberg, D.M., R.C. Kessler, C. Foster *et al.* 1993. 'Unconventional Medicine in the United States: Prevalence, Cost and Patterns of Use.' *N Engl J Med* 328:246–252.

Finkler, K. 1980. 'Non-medical Treatments and Their Outcomes.' *Culture Medicine and Psychiatry* 4:271–310.

Finkler, K. 1981. 'Non-medical Treatments and their Outcomes: Focus on Adherents to Spiritualism.' *Culture Medicine and Psychiatry* 5:65–103.

Frank, Jerome. 1973. *Persuasion and Healing: A Comparative Study of Psychotherapy* Baltimore, MD: Johns Hopkins University Press.

Fordyce. E. 1976. *Behavioral Methods for Chronic Pain* W Mosby

Fries, J.F. 1993. 'The Dimensions of Health Outcomes: The Health Assessment Questionnaire, Disability, and Pain Scales.' *J. Rheumatology* 20:548–551.

Galanter, M. and P. Buckley. 1978. 'Evangelical Religion and Meditation: Psychotherapeutic Effects.' *The Jo of Nervous and Mental Disease* 166(10):685–691.

Garrison, V. 1974. 'Sectarianism and Psychosocial Adjustment: A Controlled Comparison of Puerto Rican Pentecostals and Catholics.' pp in *Religious Movements in Contemporary America.* edited by I.I. Zaretsky and M.P. Leone, Princeton, NJ: Princeton University Press.

Glik, D.C. 1986. 'Psychosocial Wellness Among Participants in Spiritual Healing Groups.' *Social Science and Medicine* 22(5):579–586.

Glik, D.C. 1988. 'Symbolic, Ritual, and Social Dynamics of Spiritual Healing.' *Social Science and Medicine.* 27(11):1197–1206.

Glik, D.C. 1990a. 'Participation in Spiritual Healing, Religiosity and Mental Health.' *Sociological Inquiry.* 60(2):158–175.

Glik, D.C. 1990b. 'he Redefinition of the Situation: The Social Construction of Spiritual Healing Experiences.' *The Sociology of Health and Illness* 12(2):151–168.

Glik, D.C.1993.'Beliefs, Practices, and Experiences of Spiritual Healing Adherents in an American Industrial City.' pp. 199–223 in *Yearbook of Cross-Cultural Medicine and Psychotherapy* edited W. Andritsky, Berlin: Wissenschafft and Bildung Press.

Goldstein, M.S. and D.C. Glik. 1998. 'Use and Satisfaction with Care among Clients of Homeopaths.' *Alternative Therapies in Health and Medicine.* 4(2):60–65.

Greenfield S., W. Rogers, E. Mangotich, M.F.Carney, A.R.Tarlov. 1995. 'Outcomes of patients with hypertension and non-insulin dependent diabetes mellitus treated by different systems and specialties: Results from the Medical Outcomes Study.' *JAMA:* 274(18):1436–44.

Griffith, E.H., G.E. Mahy and J.L. Young. 1986. 'Psychological Benefits of Spiritual Baptist Mourning.' *American Journal of Psychiatry.* 143:226–229,

Hays, R.D., R.L. Kravitz, R.M. Mazel, C.D. Sherbourne,M.R. DiMatteo, W.H.Rogers, S. Greenfield. 1994. 'The Impact of Patient Adherence on Health Outcomes for Patients with Chronic Disease on the Medical Outcomes Study.' *J Behav Med.* 17:347–360.

Harwood, A, 1977. 'Puerto Rican Spiritism.' *Culture Medicine and Psychiatry* 1:135–153.

Hohmann, A.A. and D.L.Parron. 1996. 'How the New NIH Guidelines on Inclusion of Women and Minorities apply: Efficacy Trials, Effectiveness Trials, and Validity.' *Journal of Consulting and Clinical Psychology.* 64(5):851–5.

Jilek, W.G. 1974. *Salish Indian Mental Health and Culture Change* Toronto: Holt, Rinehart and Winston.

Judd, C.M. and D.A. Kenny.1981. 'Process Analysis: Estimating Mediation in Treatment Evaluations.' *Evaluation Review.* 5(5):602–619.

Kaplan, S.H., S.Greenfield and J.E. Ware, Jr. 1989. 'Assessing the Effects of Physician-Patient Interactions on the Outcomes of Chronic Disease.' *Medical Care* Mar 27(3) Suppl.: s110–27.

Kellogg, J. 1978. *Mandala: Path of Beauty* Clearwater, FL: Atma Press.

Kleinman, A. 1980. *Patients and Healers in the Context of Culture:* Berkeley: University of California Press.

Kleinman, A. 1984. 'Indigenous Systems of Healing: Questions for Professional, Popular, and Folk Care.' pp. 138–164 in *Alternative Medicines: Popular and Policy Perspectives.* edited by JW Salmon, New York: Tavistock.

Kleinman, A. and L.H. Sung. 1979. 'Why do Indigenous Practitioners Succesfully Heal?' *Social Science and Medicine* 13 (B):7–26.

Levin, J.S., T.A. Glass, L. Kushi, J.R. Schuck, R. Steele and W.B. Jonas. 1997. 'Quantitative Methods in Research on Complementary and Alternative Medicine: A Methodological Manifesto. NIH Office of Complementary and Alternative Care.' *Medical Care* 35(11):1079–94.

Macklin, J. 1974. 'Belief, Ritual and Healing: New England Spiritualism and Mexican – American Spiritism Compared.' Pp. 383–417 in *Religious Movements in Contemporary America*. edited by I.I. Zaretsky and M.P. Leone, Princeton, NJ: Princeton University Press.

McGuire, M.B.1988. *Ritual Healing in Suburban America* New Brunswick, NJ: Rutgers University Press.

Ness, R.C.1980. 'The Impact of Indigenous Healing Activity – an Empirical Study of two Fundamentalist Churches.' *Social Science and Medicine* 14(b):167–180.

Pattison, E.M., A.L. Nikolajs, C. Lapins and CH Doerr.1974 'Faith Healing: A Study of Personality and Function.' *Journal of Nervous and Mental Diseases* 157:394–409.

Poloma, M. M 1982.*The Charismatic Movement: Is there a New Pentecost?*. Boston: Twain Publishers.

Reuben, D.B., L.A. Valle, R.D.Hays, A.L. Siu. 1995. 'Measuring Physical Function in Community Dwelling Older Persons: a Comparison of Self-administered, Interviewer Administered, and Performance Based Measures. *J Amer. Geriatr Society* 43:17–23.

Rossi PH and Freeman HE. 1993. *Evalution: A systematic approach* 5th Edition. New bury Park, CA: Sage.

Schuck J.R., L.T. Chappell and G. Kindness. 1997. Causal Modeling and Alternative Medicine. *Alternative Therapies in Health and Medicine.* 3(2):40–47.

Snow, L.F. 1974. Folk Medical Beliefs and their Implications for Care of Patients *Annals of Internal Medicine.* 81, 82–96.

Steinwachs, D.M. 1989. 'Application of Health Status Measurement in Policy Research.' *Medical Care* 27:12.

Stewart, A.L., S. Greenfield, R.B. Hays, K.Wells, W.H. Rogers, S.D. Berry, E.A. McGlynn, J.E. Ware, Jr.1989. 'Functional Status and Well-being of Patients with Chronic Conditions: Results from the Medical Outcomes Study.'*JAMA* Aug 18, 262 (7):907–13.

Thomas, K.J., J. Carr, J. Westlake, *et al.* 1991. 'Use of Non-orthodox and Conventional Health Care in Great Britain'. *Br. Med J.* 302:207,

Vickers, A., Cassileth, B., Ernst, E., Fisher, P., Goldman, P., Jones, W., 1997. 'How should we research unconventional therapies?' *International Journal of Technology Assessment in Health Care* 13:1, 111–121.

Vincent, C and A. Furnham. 1996. 'Why do Patients Turn to Complementary Medicine?: an Empirical Study.' *Br J Clin Psychology* 35:37.

Wang, M.C. and H.J. Walberg. 1983. 'Evaluating Educational Programs: an Integrative, Casual-Modeling Approach.' *Educational Evaluation and Policy Analysis* 5(3):347–366.

Wardwell, W. 1973. 'Christian Science and Spiritual Healing' pp. 72–88. in *Religious Systems and Psychotherapy* edited by R.H. Cox, Springfield, Mo: Charles C. Thomas.

Williamson, J.W.1971. 'Evaluating Quality of Patient Care: a Strategy Relating Outcome and Process Assessment.' *JAMA,* 218:564–569.

Yelin, E.H., C.J. Henke, J.S. Kramer, M/C. Nevitt, M. Shearn and W.V.Epstein. 1985. 'A Comparison of the Treatment of Rheumatoid Arthritis in Health Maintenance Organizations and Fee-for Service Practices.' *New England J Med.* 312:962–967.

Section 4 – The Future of CAM

Health care systems in industrialized countries are likely to change dramatically in the future, as they respond to shifts in demography, morbidity, rising costs and demands for consumer satisfaction. The future place of CAM in these evolving health care systems is intimately linked to the findings of current research in CAM. Governments are exploring ways of regulating CAM practitioners to ensure public safety. In this endeavour, they will be relying heavily on evaluation studies of individual patient outcomes. Therapies such as acupuncture which have been shown to work in selected conditions (National Institutes of Health, 1997) may then be able to find a secure place in the health care system of the future.

The future of CAM will be played out differently in different societies depending on their histories and the political, economic and social pressures that prevail (van der Grinten, 1997). For example, in Britain, the National Health Service (NHS) supports the use of osteopathy, acupuncture and homeopathy (Coates and Jobst 1998). Canada, on the other hand, although it has national health insurance, does not currently fund CAM practitioners with the exception of limited support for chiropractors. In the United States, where health maintenance organizations (HMO's) are providing most of the funding for health care, the picture is highly variable. Some HMO's support selected CAM therapies while others do not. Market demand seems to be the driving force in funding them.

Social science has the potential to supply knowledge about human behaviour in a constantly changing environment in which health care is only one element. Analyses of the structures and conditions under which health care providers are currently operating, the constraints placed on them by governments and budgets, and the effects of professional competition, all have implications for the future development of CAM.

Coates, J.R., and K.A. Jobst (Eds). 1998. 'Integrated Healthcare: A Way Forward for the Next Five Years? A Discussion Document from The Prince of Wale's Initiative on Integrated Medicine.' *Journal of Alternative and Complementary Medicine* 4:209–247.

National Institutes of Health. Consensus Development Conference Statement: Acupuncture. November 3–5. Revised Draft, 11/5/97. 1997:1–17.

van der Grinten, T.E.D. 1997. 'Governing Dutch Health Care: From Corporatism to New Ways of Cooperation.' Paper presented at the 92nd Annual Meeting of the American Sociological Association August 9–13, Toronto, Canada.

CHAPTER 12

Medical Pluralism and the Future of CAM

URSULA SHARMA

INTRODUCTION: THE FRAMEWORK

This chapter concerns the re-emergence of complementary and alternative medicine (CAM) and its likely significance in the overall pattern of health care in western societies. On the basis of empirical work which we have developed together over some years, Sarah Cant and I have tried to develop a comparative view that is more than just speculative, which is informed by other recent sociological work on changes in the role of medicine, patients, professions and the state, and which also takes into account work on society and culture in what sociologists have called high modernity (Cant and Sharma, 1999). This chapter draws on some of this work, treating the development of a new kind of medical pluralism mainly in relation to Britain – although the framework we have used can be applied to other western societies (with appropriate variations of emphasis).

Most sociological work on CAM has taken the concept of medical dominance as a starting point. Researchers have asked why and how biomedicine came to suppress or marginalise alternative medicines, focusing on the means which the medical profession has used to discredit the knowledge bases and therapeutic practices of particular forms of CAM (e.g. Saks, 1995; Nicholls, 1988), and to block the attempts of popular therapies to gain state recognition or tap into wider medical markets (e.g. Wardwell, 1988; Larkin, 1992). This approach has been very productive as a starting point. But there is a need to expand the framework within which research on CAM has taken place.

Firstly, whilst alternative and orthodox medicine still face each other in a sometimes antagonistic and occasionally co-operative engagement, the role of CAM in the health care system of Britain (and most other western societies) is not decided by the outcome of this engagement alone. The role of the consumers of alternative health care must be significant in an increasingly consumerist society, as must that of the state in a period where claims that the state has been 'rolled back' vie with claims that the state has taken on a stronger than ever regulatory and surveillant role. The recent re-emergence of CAM needs to be understood in the context of a wider web of relationships: the contest between orthodox medicine and CAM is not simply a self-contained 'zero sum game'.

The constituents of this 'wider web' are many and diverse; they might include, for example, health insurance companies (especially important in health care systems where – unlike Britain – most patients recover the costs of approved health care services from private or state sponsored insurance schemes). Health promoters and educators of various kinds, nurses and midwives, pharmaceutical companies and patient support/pressure groups could also be included. This chapter concentrates on four highly visible constituents – the users, the CAM professionals, the medical profession and the state. Their interactions are treated in terms of their embeddedness in wider social, political and cultural changes.

Expanding the geographical breadth and the historical depth of this problematic might encourage the conclusion that it is *medical monism* rather than *medical pluralism* that needs to be accounted for. Prior to the emergence of biomedicine as the dominant system of healing endowed with monopolistic powers by favour of the modern western state, many other forms of healing had flourished (Porter, 1989). In many postcolonial countries today biomedicine is far from being the only form of healing to obtain recognition by the state, even if it is the one which carries greatest prestige (Last, 1990). In others, biomedicine has never penetrated the rural areas, and has limited impact on the lives of the urban poor. In such situations the sick have never ceased to resort to forms of healing which pre-dated the arrival of biomedicine, as well as new forms which have developed since. If we use a wider lens than is usual in western medical sociology, we see that medical pluralism of one kind or the other has been the norm rather than the exception. The study of CAM today can benefit from being informed by the work of historians (such as Porter) and anthropologists (such as Last) whilst recognising the specific features of the form of pluralism emerging in western countries at the present time.

In what follows, the re-emergence of CAM is examined in terms of four major 'players' in the political field (users, the medical profession, the state, providers of CAM), using the illustrative case of Britain. I then attempt to appraise these developments.

USERS

Users of CAM have generally been studied through enquiry into the motivation for resort to CAM. In many such studies, users of CAM are contrasted, explicitly or implicitly, with people currently accessing biomedicine. Any differences discovered are held to throw light on why more people are using CAM (e.g. Harrison *et al.*, 1989; Astin, 1998). Most small scale studies have found what now seems rather unsurprising, namely that people using CAM generally do so in order to resolve chronic health problems for which they have already consulted their doctor. Users often describe specific dissatisfactions with biomedicine, but have seldom abandoned it. Some studies show differences in perceptions of health and health care between current users of CAM and biomedicine, but these differences are not such as to suggest that users of CAM represent a totally distinct subculture (Vincent and Furnham, 1997; 98–117). Nor are users themselves a single monolithic category; people who use osteopathy for a musculoskeletal problem need not have have much in common with people who access a spiritual healer for depression or emotional problems. As Furnham suggests, different therapies are by now likely to have distinct clienteles and trajectories. Now that CAM has been resurgent for a decade or two, we may also need to distinguish between motivation for first time use and motivation for habitual use. Long term exposure to CAM treatment or holistic ideologies of health care and patient role may actually be a factor in the developing situation (see Blais, chapter 6). In short, 'users' probably constitute too complex and diverse a category to be simply contrasted with 'non-users'.

It is likely that use of CAM is but one reflection of broad cultural and political changes. In as much as it reflects dissatisfaction with biomedicine, such dissatisfaction is not confined to users of CAM and there is a growing literature on 'challenges' to biomedicine (e.g. Gabe, Kelleher and Williams, 1994). Use of CAM may be just one of various manifestations of the growing confidence of the informed and increasingly consumerist patient (Cant and Sharma, 1999). In her critique of the myth of alternative health, Coward (1989) has shown that the notion of the individual's responsibility to strive for a perfectly balanced body/mind, which is embedded in much holistic health practice, is closely related to cultural trends which have diverse other manifestations (the health food movement, Crawford's 'healthism' [1980], what Coward calls the 'consciousness industries', stress on citizens' duty to limit their demands on the public health care system, etc). Perhaps use of holistic health care is just one way in which the individual can pursue what Shilling calls the modernist 'project' of the body:

> the body as an unfinished entity which is shaped and 'completed' partly as a result of lifestyle choices. (Shilling, 1993:200)

Finally there is another much more concrete factor which, as far as I know, no social scientist has considered, namely the increase in disposable income enjoyed by a large section of the middle class during the eighties. Although by the late eighties CAM was being accessed by most groups in Britain (MORI, 1989), the re-emergence of CAM started out as a middle-class movement (Fulder and Munro, 1985: 544) – the prerogative of those who could afford private consultations. The period in question certainly saw increased house-hold expenditure on health care services and products of all kinds. Increased income does not in itself explain the re-emergence of alternative medicines since consumers can spend their money on many other things besides health care. But when CAM is mainly accessed on the private market, it remains a relevant factor.

It may be that the time for asking the generic question 'why do people access CAM here and now?' has passed, and that it is much more appropriate to ask about specific therapies. In any case, usage of CAM appears to reflect complex cultural and social changes, of which it is not the only manifestation. Future empirical work on usage of CAM needs to explore and illuminate this embeddedness rather than cleave to what Pescosolido (chapter 10) calls the 'tyranny of use/non- use'.

CAM AND THE MEDICAL PROFESSION

Clearly those who have sought explanations for the fortunes of CAM in the self interested action of the medical profession are not wrong. The literature abounds in accounts of medical campaigns to discredit particular types of alternative medicine. The British Medical Association (BMA) report of 1986 was widely understood as an attempt to discredit alternative medicine in general. In this document the medical profession claimed the right, on the grounds of its scientificity, to act as arbiter of alternative therapies' claims. The report rehearses a triumphalist story of the rise of scientific biomedicine and requires alternative therapies to prove their efficacy through the means of the medical 'gold standard', the randomised double blind trial (BMA, 1986). In this respect the BMA was behaving similarly to national professional medical associations in many other western states (see Cant and Sharma, 1999:113ff).

Yet biomedicine has proved not to be the monolithic entity which it so often appears to be from the perspective of patients, and as it is often portrayed by social scientists. At the very time when the BMA was preparing the first report, researchers were amassing a body of evidence which suggested that GPs' attitudes to alternative medicine were far from uniform. A sizeable number claimed to be practising alternative medicines themselves, interested in training to practice one or more of them, or interested to know more about them so that they could refer patients. Perhaps this is not surprising, since biomedicine as found in the GP surgery has probably always been a rather pragmatic, even eclectic set of practices. Whatever the official standpoint, it has been clear that the medical profession in Britain and elsewhere included a wide range of attitudes to alternative therapies, with GPs (as opposed to hospital doctors – see Perkin, Pearcy and Fraser, 1994) being the group showing most interest.

One way of understanding these developments would be to see the presence of alternative medicine as drawing attention to contradictions in biomedicine as delivered in western countries like Britain, contradictions which are becoming more and more difficult to contain.

Firstly there is (as already noted) the contradiction between the idea of a highly personal professional and caring service in which patients' needs and feelings are taken into account, and the idea of a clinical practice which is scientific, highly rational and increasingly 'evidence-based' at all levels. There is also the contradiction between the need for patient 'compliance' as prerequisite for effective treatment (with all that this implies in terms of acceptance of the doctor's authority) and the consumerist tendencies already noted; patients were making demands for more care at just the moment when the medical profession was under pressure to give more value for money, more cost-effective services.

These tensions have been present all along and CAM is not the only factor which is bringing them to the surface. But they help us to understand why some doctors took a stance which was not entirely hostile to alternative medicine and many actually started to train and practice some forms of CAM during this period, even though they were unlikely to lose patients if they did not. Collectively the BMA turned to a more moderate position and was supportive of the legislation to register osteopaths and chiropractors in the early nineties. The second, much more sympathetic, BMA report (BMA, 1993) stresses the moral and professional authority of the doctor to help the public judge the competing claims of alternative medicine. Consumerist patients are liable to be critical of biomedicine's claims to absolute *clinical* authority, and so its *professional* authority as knowledgeable and disinterested arbiter of good practice needs to be reasserted. The role of the BMA is therefore to establish:

> the principles of good practice in non-conventional therapies which would safeguard the individual against possible harm to health and maximize the potential benefits of particular methods. (BMA, 1993:2)

In some parts of the western world (for example, the USA and Sweden) national medical associations have taken a more confrontational attitude (Cant and Sharma, 1999:117ff). However they have done this in spite of a growing practitioner interest in the integration of biomedical with certain forms of alternative health care, the growth of institutional channels for co-operation with certain types of alternative therapists, and doctors' acute awareness of the popularity of CAM with patients.

CAM AND THE STATE

In Britain the state has not taken a great deal of explicit interest in alternative medicine per se. In contrast to the situation in some other European countries, the practice of CAM by non-medically qualified practitioners was not illegal, so there was no demand for permissive legislation on the part of the public. The political questions for the British government were:

a) should alternative therapists be offered state registration or some other kind of recognition, and if so, how should these professions be positioned in relation to other health care professions?
b) should therapies be available under the National Health Service (NHS), thus receiving a much more direct imprimatur from the state?

A number of influential voices supported the idea of more registration, but this issue was slow to gain momentum since it took ministers a long time to understand that CAM professional groups were at very different stages of development and organisation. Whilst umbrella organisations formed in the eighties did continue to keep the issue in the public mind, generic approaches ceded to a 'therapy by therapy' approach on the part of government. Only two therapies were accorded state registration under the last Conservative government – osteopaths in 1993 and chiropractors in 1994. The Labour Party in opposition evinced some interest in CAM as a popular issue, but after a sweeping election victory in 1997 it became clear that its legislative priorities lay elsewhere.

This does not mean that government policy has not affected or will not in future affect the position of CAM in the overall health care system. Since 1991 the internal market system introduced by the Conservative Government has had profound effects on the delivery of health care. One major effect of this was to limit the professional autonomy of the medical profession by increasing the subjection of doctors at all levels to greater managerial and budgetary control. Yet at the level of primary health care it did permit GPs to opt to hold and manage their own practice budgets. This meant that they could now use the GP budget holding system to buy in the services of alternative therapists, set up integrated clinics, etc. These moves did not lead to anything like a full integration of CAM practitioners into the NHS; they did not have any kind of career ladder within the bureaucratic structures of the NHS, they were often paid by session only or hired rooms in GP surgery buildings. But it did address a public desire for free access to alternative health care evidenced in opinion polls (RSGB, 1984).

Thus some kinds of alternative medicine have become locally available on the NHS as a by-product of some government policies, without this having been explicitly intended by the policy makers. Future changes planned by the present Labour government are unlikely to lead to an immediate reverse in the gains made by CAM. This much change is probably enough to satisfy the articulate patients with purchasing power who were the main users of CAM in the seventies and early eighties and to reassure those users who had feared that European harmonisation would lead to the outlawing of CAM in Britain. Alternative medicine now has a modicum of legitimacy and some forms are available in the NHS, albeit on a very patchy and unsystematic basis. Poorer patients can only access it free of charge if they chance to have a GP who is interested or they are in the catchment area of a community-ased project which offers some form of alternative therapy.

In many postcolonial countries governments are now encouraging the professionalisation of traditional healers and herbalists of various kinds as one way of meeting the shortfall in health care provision – especially in Sub-Saharan Africa where the AIDS epidemic has created much strain on resources and a strong need for more health education. Some have suggested that in western countries also the re-emergence of CAM has provided a cheap health care option in the face of escalating public health care costs (e.g. Easthope's work on Australia. Easthope, 1993). In Britain, decisions about introducing CAM in the NHS have been made at the local or regional level by managers who have certainly had an eye to the potential savings which use of CAM might bring about in terms of reductions in drug prescription bills, GP appointments etc. On the other hand, it can also be argued that it is government ministers who have 'permitted' positive decisions about CAM to be taken. In any case it is certainly true that the strengthened position of CAM in Britain, as in many other countries, cannot be understood without taking into account the context of changing state health care policy.

CAM PROFESSIONS

The story of the resurgence of CAM has usually been told from the point of view of the demand side but it can also be told from the supply side (Why do more and more people set up shop as CAM practitioners?). As Saks has shown (chapter 13), many CAM groups have engaged upon a process of professionalisation, attempting to hasten the coalescence of (or at least co-operation among) professional associations for each therapy, with enforceable codes of ethics and agreed criteria for competence. However, whilst they need the support of the orthodox medical profession for this degree of legitimacy, a radically changed institutional environment means that they cannot follow a route comparable to that of orthodox medicine. Contemporary western governments tend to see themselves as regulating markets rather than constraining them, and to this end the accountability and governance of those who claim professional or occupational specialisation is important. From this point of view the CAM groups who attempt to get together and agree on competence and standards are, willy nilly, obliged to engage in a process which affects many other occupational groups – from travel agents to beauty therapists. In the realm of health care the relations between the dominant medical profession and professions supplementary to medicine are not as fixed as they might appear. Nurses are claiming greater and distinctive professional competences, are more likely to engage in research, and are qualified by university validated degrees and diplomas. Indeed hospital doctors are increasingly prepared to lighten their own load by permitting senior nurses to conduct procedures which were previously reserved for doctors. The medical profession is likely to give the CAM professions the support they need for registration or other kinds of state recognition if CAM practitioners are able to relieve GPs of patients with troublesome chronic problems unresponsive to orthodox treatments (as has happened with osteopaths and chiropractors in the UK and elsewhere).

Training in CAM is increasingly available in medical schools and universities in Britain, as in some other European countries and in the USA. This can be seen as the product of a conjunction between the demand for more academic and research oriented training in a number of paramedical professional groups (nurses, physiotherapists) and the demand that universities accommodate more students and undertake more different kinds of vocational education.

The opportunities for professionalisation therefore are more than just a product of the individual therapies' will to obtain more status and security (though this is undoubtedly important) but in part are a byproduct of a number of trends and policy developments both internal and external to the health care system.

Social closure would be a fine thing to protect the practitioners' position further. But in this respect some therapies are caught in something of a dilemma. For instance, in Britain many homoeopaths rely on income from teaching professional skills. It is not always easy to build up a full time practice, especially as practitioners tend to congregate in urban areas near colleges and are thus often in direct competition with each other for patients. Some training schools are established by practitioners after quite shallow professional experience and in some other therapy groups, schools have proliferated in advance of standardisation and professional self-regulation. So whilst closure and protection of boundaries are in the interest of the professional collectivities, they may be difficult to achieve at the present time.

DISCUSSION

To summarize what has been argued so far, the story of alternative medicine is incomplete if it is told only in terms of a heroic struggle between alternative practitioners and organised biomedicine. Its former rejection and the limited legitimacy it has now achieved have depended much on the changing attitudes of doctors, but also on the configuration of relationships between medicine and other groups and institutions. Not least of these is the state, even though (paradoxically) the British state has taken little explicit interest in alternative medicine. Alternative medicine has crept through a back door into the spaces opening up in other institutional structures. In Britain such 'spaces' include the opportunities for a greater consumer voice in the organisation of health care, or the changing relationships between health care managers and clinicians in the NHS. But CAM has also been limited by those spaces and, in Britain, is seeking ways to fit itself into the 'spaces' offered in the NHS without abandoning holistic ideals. Nobody explicitly decided that health care should become more pluralistic, but the outcome of these diverse currents is that the medical monism of the mid-20th century has been seriously eroded in Britain, as in many other countries.

In Britain there is greater diversity of therapies than was formerly the case and they are available to more people, if still patchy in distribution. Some patients do have increased choice in health care. But it is not like the pluralism Porter describes as characteristic of the period prior to the rise of biomedical hegemony where forms of healing competed in what was an entirely private market for the patronage of the wealthy (Porter, 1989).

For patients, the choices between CAM and biomedicine, or between different kinds of CAM, are still loaded. Alternative therapies still carry differing degrees of legitimacy and the costs will vary accordingly. Nor is there any reason to suppose that patients who use one form of CAM will be just as prepared to use any other. They will have their own ideas about what forms are more valid and trustworthy. However, some patients are behaving very like the South Indian patients described by Nichter (1989), having clear (if not always uniform) ideas about what kinds of healing are good for what kind of ailment (Sharma, 1995:55). Some may be like the subjects of Amarasingham's Sri Lankan study, moving from therapy to therapy in order to find treatment that addresses their need for both meaning and relief in chronic illness (Amarasingham, 1980). It is possible to see in this a kind of postmodern abjuration of absolute authority (Bakx, 1991). However, individual members of the public discriminate among the various alternative medicines according to which ones they are or are not prepared to use (RSGB, 1984; MORI, 1989). A hierarchy of therapies emerges, based on the degree of legitimacy they have attained through state and medical recognition, the degree of training their practitioners receive and the kind of fees they can command. The range of therapies regarded as legitimate or useful by any individual user may not be as wide as the total array of available CAM therapies may suggest. The appeal to postmodernism underestimates the mundane fact of prolonged discomfort and disruption of social life which chronic illness involves and which would appear to be the main immediate motivating factors for individuals accessing CAM.

Is all this a good thing or a bad thing? Curiously there has been little general public debate in Britain about what sorts of alternative therapy should be available, how they should be available and at what cost to the public. Most of the debate has been conducted around claims to efficacy of particular therapies and has not addressed wider political and ethical issues, or been integrated into debates about what kind of health care system we want in the twenty-first century.

An extreme libertarian view would allow people to have access to whatever kind of health care they desire, regardless of whether or not the treatments are regarded as efficacious by others. (If they want it then it must be good for them; they have the consumerist right to seek it out). If we take this view we do not have to worry about efficacy, only about who pays for the treatment. But if we accept that the state or insurance agencies will pay for some treatments, then issues of accountability must come in; efficacy (or cost effectiveness, or degree of professionalisation of practitioners or some other criterion for judgement) becomes relevant, given that no government expects to enjoy complete lack of accountability for public spending. Once we start to discriminate among therapies, issues of which criteria are relevant and who is to be the judge inevitably follow. Doctors, health service managers, practitioners and the public all have their views. The medical profession has the best developed and probably most influential 'machinery' already in place for judging treatments and evaluating knowledge. Some CAM practitioners have resisted medicine's insistence on the randomized controlled trial as the gold standard mode for judging efficacy. They fear that the price of legitimacy is submergence of their own distinctive knowledges and practices. But if public money is to be spent on CAM (through whatever institutional mechanism) then there needs to be some mode of discrimination. If the final result is to be more than a simple product of interaction between the current views of clinicians and their managers (which would probably restrict public provision to a very few therapies) then there needs to be a wider debate about who should discriminate and on what basis. The public could be drawn into decisions as to the grounds on which therapies should be available in a state-funded health care system, though there is no reason to suppose that the popularity of CAM in general will yield public unanimity on which sorts of therapy justify state expenditure.

Alternatively we could say that the provision of CAM should be left to the market; if people want alternative medicine, they can get it in the High Street even if they cannot get it at their GP surgery. A dual system of public/private provision will yield what people want one way or the other. The therapies that are totally useless or which nobody wants will atrophy and the ones which are useful will flourish and some will be supported by the state. Such market rhetoric is common in Britain as in other western states at the present time. But the trouble with both 'pure' market-based systems of health and welfare and with dual systems of provision is that, as we already know, they favour the rich over the poor. In Britain this is evident with education and social insurance already, not to mention biomedical healthcare provision. Alternative medicine could be made more accessible to the poor who wanted to use it through more community-based schemes (some of which seem to have been very successful in Britain. See e.g. Ritchie and Ritchie, 1991) or through more accessible forms of health insurance. But the latter option still involves the problem of discriminating among therapies since it is unlikely that insurance companies, any more than the state, will be prepared to pay for just any therapy which an individual feels like having.

My own view is that the issue of which therapies justify expenditure and which do not will trundle on regardless of such issues of equity. On the whole, the subjection of CAM treatments to scientific testing is to be welcomed provided that it is recognised that RCTs are more helpful in judging some forms of treatments than others, and that a creative approach to methodologies is sustained. Such debates should continue. What I would like is more debate about accessibility to the therapies which are becoming accepted. If osteopathy or chiropractic or acupuncture are any good at all, why are they only patchily available in Britain? Why does accessibility of these therapies for those who cannot pay for private treatment depend so much on the quirks of local decisions and the erratic geographical distribution of practitioners? We need a pluralism which will address the broadest patient needs and is respectful of the diversity of patient suffering and response, not one which has evolved as a compromise answer to problems of public health-care funding or in response to professional aspirations of different groups of healers – be they alternative or biomedical.

REFERENCES

Amarasingham, L. 1980. 'Movement among healers in Sri Lanka: a case study of a Sinhalese patient' *Culture, Medicine and Psychiatry* 4:71–94
Astin, J. 1998. 'Why patients use alternative medicine' *Journal of American Medical Association* 279 (19):1548–1553
Bakx, K. 1991. 'The "eclipse" of folk medicine in western society?' *Sociology of Health and Illness* 13 (1):20–38
British Medical Association 1986. *Alternative Therapy*. Report of the Board of Science and Education. London: BMA.

British Medical Association. 1993 *Complementary Medicine. New Approaches to Good Practice.* Oxford:Oxford University Press.

Cant, S. and U.Sharma. 1999. *A New Medical Pluralism?Alternative Medicine, Doctors, Patients and the State.* London: UCL Press.

Coward, R. 1989. *The Whole Truth: the Myth of Alternative Health.* London: Faber and Faber.

Crawford, R. 1980. 'Healthism and the medicalization of everyday life' *International Journal of Health Services* 10 (3):365–88.

Easthope, G. 1993 'The response of orthodox medicine to the challenge of alternative medicine in Australia' *The Australia and New Zealand Journal of Sociology* 29(3):289–301

Fulder, S. and R.Munro 1985. 'Complementary medicine in the United Kingdom: patients, practitioners and consultations', *Lancet* 8454:542–5.

Gabe, J., G. Kelleher and G.Williams (eds) 1994. *Challenging Medicine.* London:Routledge

Harrison, C.,J. Dewison, P. Davies and P. Pietroni. 1998. 'The expectations, health beliefs and behaviour of patients seeking homoeopathic and conventional medicine' *British Homoeopathic Journal* 78 (Oct):210–218

Larkin, G. 1992. 'Orthodox and osteopathic medicine in the inter-war years' pp. 112–123 in M. Saks (ed) *Alternative Medicine in Britain.* Oxford:Clarendon Press.

Last, M. 1990. 'Professionalization of Indigenous Healers' pp. 349–366 in (eds) T. Johnson and C. Sargent *Medical Anthropology.* New York: Praeger

MORI (Market and Opinion Research International) 1989. *Research on Alternative Medicine* (conducted for *The Times* newspaper).

Nicholls, P. 1988. *Homoeopathy and the Medical Profession.* London: Croom Helm.

Nichter, M. 1989. *Anthropology and International Health.* Dordrecht: Kluwer Press.

Perkin, M., R. Pearcy and J.Fraser 1994. 'A comparison of the attitudes shown by general practitioners, hospital doctors and medical students towards alternative medicine'. *Journal of the Royal Society of Medicine*, 41:5–19.

Porter, R. 1989. *Health for Sale. Quackery in England 1650–1850.* Manchester: Manchester University Press.

Ritchie, R. and D.Ritchie 1991. 'The Craigmillar health project: helping people to define their own health needs', *Complementary Medical Research* 5 (3):460–164.

RSGB (Research Surveys of Great Britain) 1984. *Omnibus Survey on Alternative Medicine.* (Prepared for Swan House Special Events). London.

Saks, M. 1995. *Professions and the Public Interest. Medical Power, Altruism and Alternative Medicine.* Routledge:London.

Sharma, U.M. 1995. *Complementary Medicine Today. Practitioners and Patients.* Routledge: London. (Revised Edition).

Shilling, C. 1993. *The Body and Social Theory.* London: Sage Publications.

Vincent, C. and A. Furnham. 1997. *Complementary Medicine. A Research Perspective.* Chichester:Wiley.

Wardwell, W. 1988. 'Chiropractors: Evolution to Acceptance' pp. 157–191 in N. Gevitz (ed) *Other Healers. Unorthodox Medicine in America.* Baltimore: John Hopkins Press.

CHAPTER 13

Professionalization, Politics and CAM

MIKE SAKS

PROFESSIONALIZATION IN CONTEXT

This chapter looks at the politics of professionalization of complementary and alternative medicine (CAM) in the Anglo-American context – focusing primarily on Britain and the United States, in relation to North America. As will be seen, one of the most striking developments in CAM on both sides of the Atlantic has been the growth in the numbers of CAM groups – from acupuncturists and homoeopaths to chiropractors and osteopaths – that are striving, to varying degrees, to become professionalized. The political implications of this trend for the future development of CAM are explored in this chapter. As a starting point, though, it is necessary to discuss briefly how the notion of a 'profession' is best conceived, to provide a framework for understanding the current move towards the professionalization of CAM. This is a much contested area, for there are a range of differing models in the Anglo-American social scientific literature. Some of the more developed of these are now considered here.

Trait and functionalist commentators have historically viewed professions as different from other occupations, playing a positive and important role in the wider society (Saks, 1998b). The trait model is based on the listing of characteristics of a profession, as drawn up by contributors like Greenwood (1957) and Wilensky (1964). The most commonly cited attributes in this approach include a qualifying association, long training, ethical codes of conduct and skill based on esoteric knowledge (Millerson, 1964). However, this model is weakened by the fact that the elements are theoretically unrelated, with little agreement between individual authors on their exact configuration. Functionalist contributors like Goode (1960) and Barber (1963), though, have put forward a tighter and more conceptually integrated view of professions. They stress that a complex body of expertise, of great importance to society, is central to the definition of professions. This expertise, they argue, is accompanied by a collectivity orientation which ensures that it is applied in a non-exploitative manner that meets the functional needs of the social system and/or the relationship between professionals and their clients. It is claimed that in exchange for protecting the public in this way, occupations that succeed in the professionalization process gain a privileged social and economic position, as well as occupational autonomy.

The trait and functionalist approach to the definition of professions, however, downplays the conflictual political aspects of professionalization in terms of occupational self-interests (Saks, 1998b). This approach has been challenged in recent years for too readily leading its largely deferential proponents to link the ideology and reality of such groups. Interactionists such as Becker (1962) and Hughes (1963) were amongst the first social scientists to open up the knowledge base and altruism of professions to empirical scrutiny. In so doing, they saw professionalism not as so much as an intrinsic distinguishing feature of such occupations, but as a socially negotiated label carrying high prestige. Treating the term 'profession' in this way enabled them to look beyond conventional meaning and to emphasize the politics of work. However, in basing their notion of professionalization on the symbol which some occupational groups strive to attain, they did not focus sufficiently on the structural location of professions in society. This difficulty, however, is overcome by the now in vogue definitional framework of neo-Weberian writers on the professions, the work of whom underpins this chapter.

The neo-Weberian perspective on professions is represented by authors like Parkin (1979) and Collins (1990) and is based on the notion of social closure. This refers to the process by which occupations seek to regulate market conditions in their favour, in face of competition by outsiders, by restricting access to a limited group of eligibles. In this framework, professions are defined as occupations with a legal monopoly of social and economic opportunities in the marketplace, based on credentialism (Macdonald, 1995). While avoiding the self-fulfilling assumptions of trait and functionalist writers, this definition also highlights the privileged position of professions, underwritten by the state. This is crucial in examining trends in the professionalization of health care from the viewpoint of public policy. At the same time, neo-Weberians recognize the role of such factors as the development of ethical codes and the establishment of educational programmes in the political process involved in professionalization. This is seen to take place in a market-based context in which occupational groups seek to gain and maintain social closure through interest-based turf battles between professionalized and professionalizing groups (Saks, 1998b).

Central to the neo-Weberian notion of professions and professionalization is the emphasis given to the fluidly changing boundaries between professions and other occupational groups. As with the other approaches so far considered, the medical profession is viewed as a classic profession, alongside that of law. This is significant because it was the professionalization of conventional medicine that originally created the realm of CAM in the Anglo-American context. In this sense, CAM is defined not so much in terms of the content and philosophies of the therapies involved – which vary considerably – as by its political marginalisation. This is exemplified by the fact that CAM has not usually been substantially funded from official research sources, centrally included as part of the medical curriculum, widely practised by conventional health personnel or generally referred to extensively or positively in mainstream medical journals (Saks, 1992a). The professionalization of conventional medicine will now be considered in order to contextualise further the recent move of alternative therapists to professionalize.

THE PROFESSIONALIZATION OF CONVENTIONAL MEDICINE

The form of the exclusionary market regulation that defines professions varies across national boundaries and within nation states. Different emphasis is given to such areas as policing market entry, controlling competing practices, and the restrictiveness of its coverage (Moran and Wood, 1993). These variations are particularly significant internationally, given the political differences between Britain and the United States, which – like Canada – has a less federal structure (Naylor, 1993). Although some professional groups are licensed directly by the American federal government, this principle is not as extensively applied as in Britain. Differential state and other territorial jurisdiction of licensing and certification is the norm. There has, however, been much greater unity in the United States over the state regulation of medicine than other occupational areas (Freidson, 1986), even if it is still not as coherent as in Britain (Levitt, Wall, and Appleby, 1995). The different patterns of professionalization of medicine nonetheless gave rise in both countries to CAM, which could not be so clearly identified as a distinct field in the more pluralistic health system that prevailed earlier (see, for example, Gevitz, 1988b; Saks, 1992a).

In Britain, the medical monopoly was founded on the 1858 Medical Registration Act which placed the profession for the first time on a national self-governing basis by creating one register, with unified control over the standards of medical education (Waddington, 1984). The practice of the profession, moreover, increasingly came to be centred on biomedicine, based on the division of mind and body in which drugs and surgery were pivotal (Stacey, 1988). The developing medical profession, which won exclusive rights to the title of doctor, employed a range of sanctions – from ideological attacks to disciplinary action – against insiders and outsiders who departed from the orthodox fold (Saks, 1996). The medical-Ministry alliance at this time also meant that its leaders could block the attempts of groups like the osteopaths to gain state recognition, as they did in the 1920s and 1930s (Larkin, 1992). This enhanced the marginalisation of such occupational rivals as the hydropaths and the herbalists. They had operated on a more equal footing in the open, competitive environment up to the mid-nineteenth century, when the differentiation between orthodoxy and unorthodoxy had been far less clear.

Although CAM practitioners could still practise privately under the Common Law in Britain, their legitimacy declined as a result of the professionalization of conventional medicine. The medical monopoly also precluded them from operating on a paid basis within the state system (Saks, 1992a). This loss was reinforced in Britain through the developing health care division of labour, in which a procession of other occupations in the health sector gained professional standing in the first half of the twentieth century – from midwives and nurses to physiotherapists and radiographers (Donnison, 1977; Dingwall, Rafferty, and Webster, 1988; Larkin, 1983). The success of such occupations underlined the strength of conventional medicine as they were only granted a semi-professional legal status, subordinate to the medical profession (Turner, 1995). As the number of CAM practitioners outside the orthodox health care professions diminished (see *Report as to the Practice of Medicine and Surgery by Unqualified Persons in the United Kingdom* 1910), they were marginalised further by the extension of the monopoly of state medical practice through the 1911 National Health Insurance Act and the 1946 National Health Service Act and legislation restricting the claims of unorthodox practitioners to treat conditions like cancer, diabetes and epilepsy (Larkin, 1995).

In the United States, similar trends occurred in the professionalization of orthodox biomedicine following its rivalry with competing practitioners of CAM, including adherents of Thomsonism and homoeopathy in the nineeenth century. This took place, however, on a later timescale in a political context more strongly characterised by competitive individualism and physician self-employment (Starr, 1982). There is some similarity with Canada here, where the medical licensing system was also not standardised until shortly after the turn of the century, under significant challenge from the healing sects (Torrance, 1987). In the United States, the medical profession established licensing boards in most states by the start of the twentieth century, which were generally dominated by doctors (Moran and Wood, 1993). The American Medical Association had the power to approve and restrict entry to medical schools, in a system where physicians regulated other health professionals as well as themselves (Berlant, 1975). The medical monopoly was therefore derived from the developing state licensing system that supported the exclusive practice of doctors. This complemented the market shelters provided by specialty boards which offered certification for medical practitioners and institutional credentialing (Freidson, 1986).

In contrast to Britain, it is technically illegal for unlicensed competitors of CAM to practise in the United States, unless there is a separate licensing board (Freidson, 1986). This type of monopoly – paralleled by the growth of other subordinated health professions – took its toll of CAM therapists as they became more marginalised. Their marginality was accentuated by the vigorous public education campaign waged against them by the American Medical Association (Burrow, 1963). The transitional period of unification with the homoeopaths at the turn of the century (Rothstein, 1988) was rapidly transcended with the Flexner reforms, which set minimum standards for medical training schools (Kaufman, 1988). Similar legislation to Britain was introduced soon thereafter to limit the claims made by the 'quacks' associated with the wide range of drugs and devices available outside establishment medicine (Gevitz, 1988b). This led to a reliance by the medical profession on the courts and police to exclude outsiders such as chiropractors (Wardwell, 1994a).

This highlights that in both countries – as in Canada (Clarke, 1990) – the medical profession gained a substantial legally underwritten monopoly in the marketplace. Educational standards and ethical codes were also established in the political processes involved, following the classic neo-Weberian model. As has been seen, the form of the professionalization of medicine and the political implications for CAM were not the same in Britain and the United States in the first half of the twentieth century. The American medical profession, for example, historically tended to adopt a less stringent line on incorporation compared to its British counterpart, as illustrated by its early, more open, stance towards homoeopathy. This contrasts with the more consistently tough exclusionary position taken by leaders of the profession in Britain at a comparable point in time (Nicholls, 1988). The currently fast rising interest in CAM in the Anglo-American context, though, will now be documented as this has been an important precursor to the growing commitment of its practitioners to professionalize.

THE RECENT GROWTH OF CAM AND THE AGENDA OF PROFESSIONALIZATION

The 1960s was a watershed in the growth of public interest in most of the CAM therapies in Britain and North America – from acupuncture, aromatherapy and crystal therapy to healing, massage and naturopathy (Saks, 1997). Evidence on both sides of the Atlantic suggests that interest in CAM has since escalated sharply. In Britain even the most conservative estimate indicates that one quarter of the population now use CAM, with around one in seven visiting a CAM therapist every year (Sharma, 1995). In the United States about a third of the population currently employ CAM each year, with approximately a third of those consulting directly with practitioners (Eisenberg *et al.*, 1993) – the numbers of whom are still increasing (Eisenberg *et al.*, 1998). Further growth appears inevitable, as in the rest of Europe (Fisher and Ward, 1994) and Canada (Kelner and Wellman, 1997). A substantial majority of the British public now wish to have the main types of CAM available on the National Health Service (Saks, 1992a) and many insurers in the more privatised United States health system are prepared to cover these (Fulder, 1996).

This expansion has been parallelled by an increase in the number of CAM therapists. In the United Kingdom this has risen to around 45,000 (Mills and Peacock, 1997). These numbers are put in perspective by the scale of practice in the more populated United States where there are some 50,000 chiropractors alone, even if not all groups of North American CAM practitioners are as large or have expanded so fast (Wardwell, 1994a). In addition, doctors and allied health professions are increasingly employing CAM actively themselves on both sides of the Atlantic, although their professional bodies have not always been positively disposed towards them. This form of employment of such therapies can lead to the dilution of their underpinning philosophies and raise questions as to whether they are still 'alternative' to orthodox theory and practice (see, for example, Saks, 1992b). Whatever the interpretation, their mainstream usage is likely to expand further as educational instruction in them is gradually introduced into the curriculum for students of medicine and the allied health professions in Britain and North America (Fulder, 1996).

The reasons given for such growth, despite the longstanding professionally marginalised position of CAM up to the 1960s, are many. Rapidly increasing client demand at a time when the consumer has become more highly valued in the politics of health care seems to be part of the explanation in the Anglo-American context (see Light, 1993; Allsop, 1995). CAM certainly too holds the promise of being safer and more effective than conventional medicine in some areas, particularly for chronic conditions (Saks, 1994). The recent expansion of demand may also be linked to the public desire for a more holistic approach to health based, amongst other things, on the more subjective involvement of the client and the greater engagement of the whole person (Bakx, 1991). How far current public interest in such therapies reflects a wholesale countercultural shift or simply a practical desire to sidestep the limitations of biomedicine when it fails to bring about improvement is a question not yet fully resolved (Coward, 1989).

Recent political support for CAM has also been influential in its growth. Such support has been symbolised at the federal level in the United States by the establishment of the Office of Alternative Medicine, founded in 1992 through the National Institutes of Health. This has now become the National Center for Complementary and Alternative Medicine with a much enhanced annual budget of more than $50 million (Marwick, 1998). Prince Charles has provided parallel support for CAM in Britain by not only prompting a major medical enquiry into alternative therapy (British Medical Association, 1986), but also facilitating the production of a national discussion document to promote integrated health care (*Integrated Healthcare*, 1997). These initiatives have complemented a wide range of political lobbying on both sides of the Atlantic – from the Boston Women's Health Collective efforts to demedicalize women's lives in the United States (Phillips and Rakusen, 1996) to the more generic work of the all-party Parliamentary Group for Alternative and Complementary Medicine in Britain (Saks, 1992a).

Such lobbying has been crucial in view of the opposition to CAM from the medical establishment and the pharmaceutical companies in terms of the challenge that it poses (Walker, 1994). In this context, many of the CAM groups have sought to strengthen their position by endeavouring to professionalize. This move follows in the footsteps of conventional medicine which, as has been seen, took this route several decades before in Britain and North America, with devastating effects on the standing of CAM practitioners. The irony of the current situation is accentuated by the potential conflict of some aspects of the professionalization of conventional medicine based on state underwritten social closure, with the model that has traditionally underpinned CAM. This is exemplified by the tension between the formally educated expert at the heart of medical professionalization and the concept of the individual apprenticeship in CAM, which is usually ideologically rooted in a holistic notion of equal partnership with the client (Sharma, 1995).

Some CAM groups like the osteopaths sought to professionalize earlier in the century, with varying outcomes. In the case of the osteopaths, this resulted in acceptance and professional incorporation into medicine by the late 1960s and early 1970s in the United States and longstanding state rejection of their claims until very recently in Britain (Baer, 1987). What is distinctive about the present period, though, is the extent of interest in professionalizing amongst CAM bodies. This has been associated with a level of development of organizational unity, codes of conduct and educational standards usually reserved for the more established professions. Admittedly, not all CAM practitioners at grassroots level believe this to be a desirable and unambiguous path for future growth (see, for example, Cant and Sharma, 1995). Potential reasons for the rising interest in professionalization, though, are not difficult to find.

One major explanation has been a desire to gain greater legitimacy for CAM, at a time of expanding public interest. This is very important in the

British context at present where the European Union is perceived to be a threat to the rights of the medically unqualified to practise under the Common Law. This situation has led to fears that policies of harmonisation may lead to restrictive legislation, as in most of the rest of Europe (Huggon and Trench, 1992). The search for legitimacy has also been significant for groups like chiropractors in the United States, particularly since until recently they have endured the threat of jail sentences and the stigma of being labelled an 'unscientific cult' by the American Medical Association (Wardwell, 1992). Professionalization, however, cannot be seen simply as a defensive reaction to the medical challenge in a more favourable climate of public opinion in Britain and North America. It can also bring positive benefits to those involved in terms of the enhanced income, status and power associated with exclusionary closure, as well as the satisfaction of working in a well-regulated profession. That said, groups of CAM therapists have followed a number of different avenues to professionalization.

TRENDS IN THE PROFESSIONALIZATION OF CAM

CAM therapies are frequently incorrectly presented as a unified whole. The sometimes profound variations between them, however, are clearly apparent in the pattern of professionalization to date of this field. This is one of the main criticisms of using the term 'the holistic health movement' in blanket fashion in relation to CAM in the United States (see, amongst others, Alster, 1989). An appreciation of the weaknesses of applying such a concept has been fundamental to moving forward the standing of CAM in Britain. Here the initial efforts of some groups of unorthodox practitioners to professionalize were politically frustrated up to the late 1980s because the government wanted a common approach (Sharma, 1995). However, the potential umbrella bodies involved – the Institute for Complementary Medicine, the Council for Complementary and Alternative Medicine and the British Complementary Medical Association – were not able to heal the rifts both within and across specific therapies to enable this to happen (Fulder, 1996). This situation, though, was resolved when the government decided in the early 1990s that each area should determine its own place in the health sector (Sharma, 1995).

One of the main CAM groups on the road to professionalization in Britain today are the non-medical acupuncturists who have sought voluntarily to establish a common code of discipline, education and ethics. This was achieved in the early 1980s following the formation of the Council for Acupuncture, overcoming splits between the British Acupuncture Association and Register, the Chung San Acupuncture Society, the International Register of Oriental Medicine, the Register of Traditional Chinese Medicine and the

Traditional Acupuncture Society. This arrangement was further developed with the founding of the British Acupuncture Accreditation Board laying down minimum educational standards, together with the British Acupuncture Council which serves as the registering body (Saks, 1995a). There are parallels in the equally popular area of homoeopathy, in which the Society of Homoeopaths has taken the lead as a focus for medically unqualified practitioners. It established a register and code of ethics following its formation in 1981. Although this field is not yet as unified as that of acupuncture, many homoeopathic colleges have been formally accredited by the Society. This has helped to provide a recognised, systematic body of expertise centred on a three year full-time (or equivalent) educational basis (Cant and Sharma, 1996). In neither case, however, has the state yet underwritten a position of exclusionary closure.

Osteopathy and chiropractic are now at an even more advanced stage of professionalization in Britain in terms of obtaining state sanction. In the former, internal divisions were sufficiently overcome in 1993 for the Osteopaths Act to be passed, facilitated by the strengths of existing osteopathic training. Legislation has now established a General Osteopathic Council which polices a register set up to enable professional self-regulation, upholds ethical and educational standards, and provides statutory protection of title (Standen, 1993). In the smaller field of chiropractic, the majority of practitioners have buried their differences and agreed to accept the standards of the British Chiropractic Association in relation to the length and content of their education and the form of their practice. This is enshrined in the 1994 Chiropractic Act which established a parallel basis for state registration to that of the osteopaths, pivoted on a General Chiropractic Council (Cant and Sharma, 1995). While at the leading edge of professional development in CAM in Britain, though, there are nevertheless limits to the position of osteopathy and chiropractic. Although they have gained a legal monopoly, they have not yet won privileged access to National Health Service practice like doctors and other conventional allied health professionals.

The timescale involved also highlights that Britain lags behind the United States in the professionalization of CAM. This is well illustrated by the case of osteopathy in the United States. It was initially subjected to attack from the American Medical Association, including opposition to licensure and the prohibition of professional interactions with physicians. Its practitioners, however, are now licensed in every state and are eligible for a range of positions, from medical residencies to certification as medical specialists (Wardwell, 1994b). This is the culmination of a long and gradual process of incorporation, in which the curriculum of osteopathic colleges started closely to follow that of medical schools from the 1930s onwards (Gevitz, 1988a). A seminal event was the merger of the Californian Medical Association and the Californian Osteopathic Association in the early 1960s. This was followed by a growth in the number of state-sponsored osteopathic colleges and a flurry of state licensing arrangements of osteopaths as professional equals to physicians (Baer, 1987).

While this established osteopathy as a profession in neo-Weberian terms, chiropractic has followed suit in the United States, after a more turbulent history. It has now won wide-ranging state licensure and the right to reimbursement under Medicare and Medicaid. Its position was confirmed by a court ruling in the late 1980s in which chiropractors were given consultation rights with doctors and access to hospital diagnostic assistance. The American Medical Association was also required to end its boycott of their services (Wardwell, 1994a). This outcome is partly related to the professionalization strategy increasingly adopted by chiropractors in the United States from the late nineteenth century onwards. This has included the claim to scientific expertise and the progressive establishment of a long education, with stringent entry requirements and a growing research base (Martin, 1994). While ultimately successful, this also illustrates the variable nature of the licensing arrangements which underpin the professionalization of CAM in specific fields in the more fragmentary American political system. Despite gaining licensure, there are substantial differences between states over how far chiropractors are allowed to practise obstetrics and naturopathy, to sign death certificates and to undertake school examinations (Wardwell, 1994b).

The development of bodies such as the Canadian Chiropractic Association and the Canadian Naturopathic Association underline the trend in North America towards professionalization (Clarke, 1990). Some forms of CAM in the Anglo-American context, such as aromatherapy and crystal therapy, however, have not yet moved strongly in this direction. Reflexology in Britain, for instance, has many thousands of practitioners, but is centred on a limited knowledge base and a variable length of training, rarely exceeding a few weeks. With over one hundred separate training schools and eleven associations, it has been difficult to reach agreement on standards despite attempts to bring them together in a common framework. That most reflexologists do not wish to claim the autonomy or authority of the medical profession has also reduced the degree to which professionalization can be seen to be in process (Cant and Sharma, 1995). This illustration shows that professionalization is still only part of the picture as far as CAM is concerned, especially since studies in the United States and elsewhere indicate that its largest use is focused on self-care rather than practitioner-based delivery (see, for instance, Eisenberg *et al.*, 1993; 1998). What, though, are the implications of the growing trend towards professionalization in this area for health policy in the future?

THE IMPLICATIONS OF PROFESSIONALIZATION FOR HEALTH POLICY

While it should not be assumed – as trait and functionalist writers have some-times done – that further professionalization is inevitable (Wilensky, 1964), the implications of the current trend to professionalize CAM are potentially very great. This development poses a major political challenge to conventional medicine in terms of group self-interests. This is in part because it sharpens competition for the increasing number of orthodox practitioners of CAM, in view of the escalating market popularity of CAM on both sides of the Atlantic. The challenge is well exemplified in Britain by the tensions between exclusively medical bodies of practitioners such as the Faculty of Homoeo-pathy and the British Medical Acupuncture Society and their increasingly professionalized lay counterparts operating under the Common Law (see Cant and Sharma, 1995; Saks, 1995b). This raises questions about who should be able to practise CAM in future – the answer to which ranges from only those with a medical qualification to any practitioner with prescribed certification in the therapy concerned. The latter scenario points to an even greater challenge, as the professionalization of some forms of CAM may impinge on the current dominance of the medical establishment in the health care division of labour itself.

This challenge to medical hegemony is underlined by the broad ranging claims about the efficacy of CAM made by many of its proponents in the Anglo-American context. Such claims conflict with those of conventional med-icine. So too do their typically holistic philosophies, which can be seen to subvert the principles on which the system of orthodox biomedicine is primarily based (McKee, 1988). In view of the growing legitimation and increasing legally underwritten privileges now being gained by CAM therapists through professionalization, it is not surprising that the American Medical Association should have waged war against such rival practitioners for much of the twentieth century (Gevitz, 1988b). Nor is it too surprising that CAM should initially have been condemned as witchcraft in a report on this subject by the British Medical Association (1986). Nonetheless, the extent to which medical dominance has been eroded by the increasing professionaliza-tion of CAM should not be overstated, in view of the success the medical establishment has had in incorporating such threats.

This is illustrated by the response of the American Medical Association to the osteopaths. Recognition of this group was traded for control over their supply, once the strategy of complete exclusion was no longer viable. Incorporation also had the benefit of helping to resolve the problem faced by the medical profession of filling its surfeit of intern vacancies (Blackstone, 1977). A similar strategy is apparent in the latest report of the British Medical Association (1993) in which the professionalization of CAM therapists is welcomed as long as their research base is centred on the narrow orthodox touchstone of randomized controlled trials, a significant biomedical component is included in their education programmes and they are locked into medically-controlled referral relationships. These strategies of incorporation minimize the threat to the income, status and power of the established profession. As such, they mirror the earlier stance taken by conventional medicine in Britain and the United States to absorb the potentially damaging challenge of the occupations allied to medicine, with the support of the state (see Turner, 1995).

The continuing success of conventional medicine on both sides of the Atlantic despite such challenges means that the integrated health care of the immediate future is likely to continue to be primarily underpinned by orthodox biomedical science, with physicians still calling most of the shots – for all the current political attacks on their position (see Moran and Wood, 1993). This may not ultimately make the best use of the potential of CAM within the health care division of labour, especially if it develops on a strictly hierarchical semi-professional basis exclusively under the medical authority so respected by most functionalist writers on the professions (see, for example, Etzioni, 1969). The professionalization of CAM, however, has many potential advantages for the public in this and other foreseeable scenarios for the future. One of these is that the associated raft of education, research and ethical codes could help to protect the community, particularly when efficacy, cost and safety are central considerations (Saks, 1994). At the same time, the greater rigour and restrictiveness promoted by the professionalization of CAM may fruitfully encourage more collaboration and referrals between orthodox and unorthodox health care practitioners (Vincent and Furnham, 1997).

However, caution is also needed about the professionalization of CAM from the standpoint of health policy. The exclusive nature of professionalism may generate unacceptable barriers in the relationship of its practitioners with clients that conflict with their holistic, egalitarian philosophies. This may be accentuated by the incorporationist pressures greatly to increase the biomedical basis of their practice (Cant and Sharma, 1996). From a neo-Weberian viewpoint, there are also dangers that parochial, self-interested tribalism will come to the fore as monopolisation strategies are pursued, to the detriment of the public. This is highlighted by the professionalization strategy pursued by medicine itself in Britain and North America in the latter half of the nineteenth century. In this case, exclusive rights to practice were sought before medicine had much to offer by way of a scientific underpinning, prior to the introduction of antibiotics and the development of surgery (see Porter, 1987; Starr, 1982; Torrance, 1987). Stepping outside the neo-Weberian framework, there is also a possibility that the professionalization of CAM may draw the therapists involved into an undesirable institutional role in surveillance and control through state sponsorship, as suggested for different reasons by contemporary Marxists and Foucauldians in their analyses of Western societies (see, for instance, Navarro, 1986; Nettleton, 1992).

This latter eventuality needs to be weighed against the positive role that professions, based on exclusionary closure, can play in a neo-Durkheimian sense as intermediary groups acting as a buffer between the individual and the state (Saks, 1998a). A lot ultimately depends, though, on the form that professionalization takes in the CAM field. As was seen earlier in this chapter, there is much scope for variation on this count. It is important too to note that the future outcome in terms of health policy will not just depend on such bodies as the state, consumers, the private investment sector and the medical and allied professions, but also the position taken by CAM organizations themselves about the most appropriate way forward. In charting this future in the contemporary Anglo-American context, however, it would seem that – as more and more CAM associations move from the marginal to the mainstream in terms of professionalization – a more integrated health care system is likely to emerge which will bring more benefits than costs for users. This is at the heart of the challenge posed by CAM in the currently rapidly changing framework of health care in Britain and North America.

REFERENCES

Allsop, Judith. 1995. *Health Policy and the NHS: Towards 2000*. London: Longman.
Alster, Kristine. 1989. *The Holistic Health Movement*. Tuscaloosa: University of Alabama Press.
Baer, Hans A. 1987. 'The Divergent Evolution of Osteopathy in America and Britain.' pp. 63–99 in *Research in the Sociology of Health Care*, vol. 5, edited by J. Roth. Greenwich: Jai Press.
Bakx, Keith. 1991. 'The "Eclipse" of Folk Medicine in Western Society.' *Sociology of Health and Illness* 13(1):20–38.
Barber, Bernard. 1963. 'Some Problems in the Sociology of Professions.' *Daedalus* 92(4):669–88.
Becker, Howard. 1962. 'The Nature of a Profession.' pp. 27–46 in *Education for the Professions*, edited by National Society for the Study of Education. Chicago: University of Chicago Press.
Berlant, Jeffrey L. 1975. *Profession and Monopoly: A Study of Medicine in the United States and Great Britain*. Berkeley: University of California Press.
Blackstone, Erwin A. 1977. 'The AMA and the Osteopaths: A Study of the Power of Organized Medicine.' *The Antitrust Bulletin* 22:405–40.
British Medical Association 1986. *Report of the Board of Science and Education on Alternative Therapy*. London: BMA.
British Medical Association 1993. *Complementary Medicine: New Approaches to Good Practice*. London: BMA.
Burrow, James G. 1963. *AMA: Voice of American Medicine*. Baltimore: Johns Hopkins Press.
Cant, Sarah and Ursula Sharma. 1995. *Professionalisation in Complementary Medicine*. Report on a research project funded by the Economic and Social Research Council.
Cant, Sarah and Ursula Sharma. 1996. 'Demarcation and Transformation within Homoeopathic Knowledge: A Strategy of Professionalization.' *Social Science and Medicine* 42:579–88.

Clarke, Juanne N. 1990. *Health, Illness and Medicine in Canada*. Toronto: McClelland and Stewart.

Collins, Randall. 1990. 'Market Closure and the Conflict Theory of the Professions.' pp. 24–43 in *Professions in Theory and History: Rethinking the Study of the Professions*, edited by M. Burrage and R. Torstendahl. London: Sage.

Coward, Rosalind. 1989. *The Whole Truth: The Myth of Alternative Medicine*. London: Faber and Faber.

Dingwall, Robert, Anne Marie Rafferty, and Charles Webster. 1988. *An Introduction to the Social History of Nursing*. London: Routledge.

Donnison, Jean. 1977. *Midwives and Medical Men*. London: Heinemann.

Eisenberg, David M., Ronald C. Kessler, Cindy Foster, Frances E. Norlock, David R. Calkins, and Thomas L. Delbanco. 1993. 'Unconventional Medicine in the United States: Prevalence, Costs, and Patterns of Use.' *New England Journal of Medicine* 328:246–52.

Eisenberg, David M., Roger B. Davis, Susan L. Ettner, Scott Appel, Sonja Wilkey, Maria Van Rompay, and Ronald C. Kessler. 1998. 'Trends in Alternative Medicine Use in the United States, 1990–1997.' *Journal of the American Medical Association* 280:1569–75.

Etzioni, Amatai. 1969. *The Semi-Professions and their Organization*. New York: Free Press.

Fisher, Peter and Adam Ward. 1994. 'Complementary Medicine in Europe.' *British Medical Journal* 309:107–110.

Freidson, Eliot. 1986. *Professional Powers: A Study of the Institutionalization of Formal Knowledge*. Chicago: University of Chicago Press.

Fulder, Stephen. 1996. *The Handbook of Alternative and Complementary Medicine*. Oxford: Oxford University Press, 3rd edition.

Gevitz, Norman. 1988a. 'Osteopathic Medicine: From Deviance to Difference.' pp. 124–56 in *Other Healers: Unorthodox Medicine in America*, edited by N. Gevitz. Baltimore: Johns Hopkins University Press.

Gevitz, Norman. 1988b. 'Three Perspectives on Unorthodox Medicine.' pp. 1–28 in *Other Healers: Unorthodox Medicine in America*, edited by N. Gevitz. Baltimore: Johns Hopkins University Press.

Goode, William J. 1960. 'Encroachment, Charlatanism and the Emerging Profession: Psychology, Sociology and Medicine.' *American Sociological Review* 25:902–14.

Greenwood, Ernest. 1957. 'Attributes of a Profession.' *Social Work* 2:45–55.

Huggon, Tom and Alan Trench. 1992. 'Brussels Post-1992: Protector or Persecutor.' pp. 241–49 in *Alternative Medicine in Britain*, edited by M. Saks. Oxford: Clarendon Press.

Hughes, Everett. 1963. 'Professions.' *Daedalus* 92:655–68.

Integrated Healthcare. 1997. London: Foundation for Integrated Medicine.

Kaufman, Martin. 1988. 'Homeopathy in America: The Rise and Fall and Persistence of a Medical Heresy.' pp. 99–123 in *Other Healers: Unorthodox Medicine in America*, edited by N. Gevitz. Baltimore: Johns Hopkins University Press.

Kelner, Merrijoy and Beverley Wellman. 1997. 'Health Care and Consumer Choice: Medical and Alternative Therapies.' *Social Science and Medicine* 45:203–212.

Larkin, Gerald. 1983. *Occupational Monopoly and Modern Medicine*. London: Tavistock.

Larkin, Gerald. 1992. 'Orthodox and Osteopathic Medicine in the Inter-War Years.' pp. 112–23 in *Alternative Medicine in Britain*, edited by M. Saks. Oxford: Clarendon Press.

Larkin, Gerald. 1995. 'State Control and the Health Professions in the United Kingdom: Historical Perspectives.' pp. 45–54 in *Health Professions and the State in Europe*, edited by T. Johnson, G. Larkin, and M. Saks. London: Routledge.

Levitt, Ruth, Andrew Wall and John Appleby. 1995. *The Reorganized National Health Service*. London: Chapman and Hall, 5th edition.

Light, Donald. 1993. 'Countervailing Power: The Changing Character of the Medical Profession in the United States.' pp. 69–80 in *The Changing Medical Profession: An International Perspective*, edited by F.W. Hafferty and J.B. McKinlay. Oxford: Oxford University Press.

Macdonald, Keith. 1995. *The Sociology of the Professions*. London: Sage.

McKee, Janet. 1988. 'Holistic Health and the Critique of Western Medicine.' *Social Science and Medicine* 26:775–84.

Martin, Steven C. 1994. '"The Only True Scientific Method of Healing": Chiropractic and American Science 1895–1990.' *Isis* 85:206–27.

Marwick, Charles. 1998. 'Alterations are Ahead at the OAM.' *Journal of the American Medical Association* 280:1553–54.

Millerson, Geoffrey. 1964. *The Qualifying Associations*. London: Routledge and Kegan Paul.

Mills, S. and Peacock, W. 1997. *Professional Organization of Complementary and Alternative Medicine in the United Kingdom*. Report to the Department of Health, University of Exeter.

Moran, Michael and Bruce Wood. 1993. *States, Regulation and the Medical Profession*. Buckingham: Open University Press.

Navarro, Vincente. 1986. *Crisis, Health and Medicine: A Social Critique*. London: Tavistock.

Naylor, C. David. 1993. 'The Canadian Health Care System: A Model for America to Emulate?' pp. 25–66 in *North American Health Care Policy in the 1990s*, edited by A. King, T. Hyclak, S. McMahon, and R. Thornton. Rexdale: John Wiley and Sons.

Nettleton, Sarah. 1992. *Power, Pain and Dentistry*. Buckingham: Open University Press.

Nicholls, Phillip A. 1988. *Homoeopathy and the Medical Profession*. London: Croom Helm.

Parkin, Frank. 1979. *Marxism and Class Theory: A Bourgeois Critique*. London: Tavistock.

Phillips, Angela and Jill Rakusen. 1996. *Our Bodies Ourselves: A Health Book by and for Women*. Harmondsworth: Penguin, 3rd edition.

Porter, Roy. 1987. *Disease, Medicine and Society in England 1550–1860*. London: Macmillan.

Report as to the Practice of Medicine and Surgery by Unqualified Persons in the United Kingdom. 1910. London: HMSO.

Rothstein, William G. 1988. 'The Botanical Movements and Orthodox Medicine.' pp. 29–51 in *Other Healers: Unorthodox Medicine in America*, edited by N. Gevitz. Baltimore: Johns Hopkins University Press.

Saks, Mike. 1992a. 'Introduction.' pp. 1–21 in *Alternative Medicine in Britain*, edited by M. Saks. Oxford: Clarendon Press.

Saks, Mike. 1992b. 'The Paradox of Incorporation: Acupuncture and the Medical Profession in Modern Britain'. pp. 183–98 in *Alternative Medicine in Britain*, edited by M. Saks. Oxford: Clarendon Press.

Saks, Mike. 1994. 'The Alternatives to Medicine.' pp. 84–103 in *Challenging Medicine*, edited by J. Gabe, D. Kelleher, and G. Williams. London: Routledge.

Saks, Mike. 1995a. 'Educational and Professional Developments in Acupuncture in Britain: An Historical and Contemporary Overview.' *European Journal of Oriental Medicine* Winter:32–34.

Saks, Mike. 1995b. *Professions and the Public Interest: Medical Power, Altruism and Alternative Medicine*. London: Routledge.

Saks, Mike. 1996. 'From Quackery to Complementary Medicine: The Shifting Boundaries between Orthodox and Unorthodox Medical Knowledge.' pp. 27–43 in *Complementary Medicines: Knowledge in Practice*, edited by U. Sharma and S. Cant. London: Free Association Books.

Saks, Mike. 1997. 'East Meets West: The Emergence of a Holistic Tradition.' pp. 196–219 in *Medicine: A History of Healing*, edited by R. Porter. London: The Ivy Press.

Saks, Mike. 1998a. 'Deconstructing or Reconstructing Professions? Interpreting the Role of Professional Groups in Society.' pp. 351–64 in *Professions, Identity and Order in Comparative Perspective*, edited by V. Olgiati, L. Orzack, and M. Saks. Onati: Onati Institute.

Saks, Mike. 1998b. 'Professionalism and Health Care.' pp. 174–91 in *Sociological Perspectives on Health, Illness and Health Care*, edited by D. Field and S. Taylor. Oxford: Blackwell Science.

Sharma, Ursula. 1995. *Complementary Medicine Today: Patients and Practitioners*. London: Routledge, revised edition.

Stacey, Margaret. 1988. *The Sociology of Health and Healing*. London: Unwin Hyman.

Standen, Clive S. 1993. 'The Implications of the Osteopaths Act.' *Complementary Therapies in Medicine* 1:208–10.

Starr, P. 1982. *The Social Transformation of American Medicine*. New York: Basic Books.

The Prince of Wales Initiative on Integrated Medicine, 1997. Integrated Healthcare: *A Way Forward for the Next Five Years?* London: The Foundation for Integrated Medicine.

Torrance, George M. 1987. 'Socio-Historical Overview: The Development of the Canadian Health System.' pp. 6–32 in *Health and Canadian Society: Sociological Perspectives*, edited by D. Coburn, C. D'Arcy, G.M. Torrance, and P. New. Richmond Hill: Fitzhenry and Whiteside.

Turner, Bryan S. 1995. *Medical Power and Social Knowledge*. London: Sage, 2nd edition.

Vincent, Charles and Adrian Furnham. 1997. *Complementary Medicine: A Research Perspective*. Chichester: Wiley and Sons.

Waddington, Ivan. 1984. *The Medical Profession in the Industrial Revolution*. London: Gill and Macmillan.

Walker, Martin J. 1994. *Dirty Medicine: Science, Big Business and the Assault on Natural Health Care*. London: Slingshot Publications.

Wardwell, Walter I. 1992. *Chiropractic: History and Evolution of a New Profession*. St Louis: Mosby.

Wardwell, Walter I. 1994a. 'Alternative Medicine in the United States.' *Social Science and Medicine* 38:1061–68.

Wardwell, Walter I. 1994b. 'Differential Evolution of the Osteopathic and Chiropractic Professions in the United States.' *Perspectives in Biology and Medicine* 37:595–607.

Wilensky, Harold. 1964. 'The Professionalization of Everyone?' *American Journal of Sociology* 70:137–58.

CHAPTER 14

Research as a Tool for Integrative Health Services Reform

ALLAN BEST AND DEBORAH GLIK

INTRODUCTION

Why do we need to understand the paths people follow to complementary and alternative medicine (CAM), and the outcomes they experience there? How do health care policy makers, CAM practitioners and conventional physicians, respond to the dual use depicted in the chapters of this book? A compelling and pressing reason for pursuing these questions is that we can apply our knowledge to influencing current health care reforms, as well as to designing health services tailored to the needs of people.

Britain, the United States, and Canada are all in the midst of profound changes in health care, driven by at least two forces. The first is the broader drive to restructure health care that is more efficient and cost-effective. Canada's National Forum on Health (1997) was created to provide a far-reaching and visionary review of state funded health care as we head into the twenty-first century, looking at experience since it was born in the 1960s. The Forum concluded that the core values and foundations of the national insurance plan remained largely unchanged, but it called for more evidence-based decision-making, greater continuity of care, truly patient-centered care, more emphasis on prevention, and a genuinely integrative form of healthcare. Similar sentiments are expressed in the most recent British National Health Service White Paper, 'The New NHS: Modern, Dependable' (Department of Health, 1997). In the United States, managed care and the demand for greater efficiency are driving reform, although there too, there is increasing acceptance of evidence-based practice and prevention approaches (Light, 1996; Pelletier *et al.*, 1997).

The second, more specific force is the escalating public demand for CAM. In Britain, the Prince of Wales's Initiative on Integrated Medicine (1997) provides a thoughtful analysis of how these two forces converge. In the United States, President Clinton is appointing a Commission that will undertake a similar study of CAM, following the recent establishment by Congress of a National Center for Complementary and Alternative Medicine. Health Canada recently established an Office of Natural Health Products and is forming advisory committees to provide in-depth study of other aspects of CAM.

This chapter argues that there can be a high degree of consistency between the two objectives of reforming health care and meeting the growing public interest in CAM. A conceptual framework that positions CAM research as health services research can help us to meet both objectives. This agenda must address such questions as the utilization of CAM, the circumstances under which CAM is cost-effective, when it is (and when it is not) evidence-based, and the degree to which it is preventive. Looking at issues of evidence-base, cost-effectiveness, utilization, and preventive aspects sets the stage to promote true integration of CAM into the health care system, whatever form that might take.

Of course, research is only one factor in health care reform, and it is important to distinguish between integrative health services research and integrative health care reform. At the same time, we propose here that integrative CAM research might foster better and more rapid integrative health services reform. To this end, this chapter:

- Presents a preliminary model for research on integrative health services.
- Discusses the need for measurement development.
- Summarizes selected research priorities identified throughout this book.
- Recommends action for a CAM health services research agenda.

A WORKING MODEL FOR INTEGRATIVE HEALTH SERVICES

The goal of integration is for every person to have access to the full range and combination of health care services that contribute to reduced sickness and increased health-related quality of life and longevity. From a health services perspective, this goal requires not only equal access for everyone, but also a health care system that enables and supports this quest for optimal health. O'Donnell (1989) defines 'optimal health' as a balance of physical, emotional, social, spiritual, and intellectual health. It is clear from the research reported in this book that CAM users have a remarkably similar view. However, there are important theoretical debates about the definition of health and the best way to measure it (Frankish et al., 1999). Therefore, we highlight the need for clarifying concepts and devising ways of measuring them as an integral part of the proposed health services research agenda.

Figure 14.1 presents a working model for integrative health care services. It illustrates the complexity between levels of analysis and strategies for delivering integrated care, and incorporating different health care philosophies. The aim is to clarify the meaning and delineate measures of integration for health care delivery. The word 'integration' is used differently at each of three *levels*: health systems, care delivery, and personal health.

The goal of delivering integrated health care services requires at least four distinct *strategies*:

- development of safe, effective, and efficient clinical/healing strategies,
- development of reliable, accessible, and effective information and learning strategies,
- orchestration of a co-ordinated, programmatic, research-development-diffusion agenda to test specific methods and provide the necessary data for health reform decisions.
- realignment of health care structures to ensure equitable access.

This list of strategies is not exhaustive. For example, regulation might well be added as a fifth strategy ~ the pros and cons of regulation are presented by Sharma in chapter 12 and Saks in chapter 13.

Finally, integration draws from distinct health care traditions, from preventive to palliative care, each with their own theoretical frameworks, histories, language, methods, and knowledge base.

INTERACTIONS BETWEEN LEVEL AND STRATEGY DIMENSIONS

Health systems

The *healing* strategies within health systems include both formal health care systems, and the informal systems that provide access to CAM products and services. The term 'healing' is used rather than 'clinical' because it is recognizes that some important elements of care may occur outside clinical contexts (see Glik, chapter 11 for a fuller discussion). For example, the psychosocial dimensions of palliative care are increasingly being recognized, highlighting the critical role of family and community in contributing to increased quality of life, reduced cost, and perhaps greater longevity. As another example, the health promotion tradition places the role of the individual, and personal health management or self-care, at the heart of optimal health strategy. These examples underscore the importance of viewing integration as extending beyond the normal bounds of health care. A more effective and efficient system might aim to integrate these different aspects of health systems. Thus, the focus of the healing strategy at a health systems level is depicted as health reform. Integration might be measured by the efficiency with which a defined population's needs are met. Note that infrastructure issues such as training, reimbursement, and accessibility all must be considered within such outcomes research design, for they interact to determine outcomes and efficiency. In this manner, they define the generalizability of efficiency research within the delivery system in which the research is conducted.

The *learning* strategy at the health systems level focuses on policy issues around integration. There are key issues concerning how the public, health professionals, and policy makers each learn to play their respective roles in working towards the goal of optimal health. There is already a very strong demand from the public, professionals and policy makers for better information about CAM. Clearly the interest and motivation are there. However, effective public education and health promotion require enabling policies, and investment in resources and infrastructure. Policy is identified here as a major focus because Canada and Britain's public policies on universal health care have done so much to shape understandings of health and health care. In the United States, managed care is having an equally profound influence. Greater integration at a systems level will require major rethinking of the healing versus learning perspectives and their reciprocal roles in determining health outcomes. In Canada and Britain, the primary measures of integration at this level might assess the degree to which public policy documents adequately address the healing-learning-research balance. In contrast, in the United States, the relevant health systems measure might be the degree to which insurers provide coverage for integrated services which balance healing and learning components (Weeks, & Layton, 1998).

The focus of *research* at the health systems level is on health services research. Already it is clear from the preceding discussion that the meaning and measures of healing and learning at the health service level are somewhat imprecise and arbitrary. Measures of integration are complicated because both healing and learning affect outcomes. For example, public/professional education and provincial funding for health care must be co-ordinated at a policy level to maximize efficiency and outcomes. Conventional measures of outcomes such as total morbidity or total health utilization must be weighed against the combined costs of healing and learning services in order to determine efficiency. As is typical of health services research, as we move into a new area of investigation, there must be a significant investment in definition of key terms, as well as in methodology and measurement development.

The issue of *structure* at the systems level has to do with the distribution of services to persons, organizations, and populations. In an integrated system, service delivery will not be more concentrated in affluent enclaves, but equally distributed across socioeconomic strata.

To summarize, when we look at the four strategies across the health systems level, the challenge of understanding the concept of integration becomes apparent. There is a need to clarify meaning and measurement, specific to the context in which the term is being used. If the mission of better integration is to be achieved, we must make it a priority to collaborate across different traditions to develop a common language.

This debate and conceptual evolution are urgently important in the current health policy and reform environment. For example, in Canada, there is a growing policy priority being placed on a people-oriented system, a recognition of the need to integrate CAM, a push for greatly enhanced health information services, improved funding for health research and evidence-based decision making, as well as an emphasis on self-care and prevention. These trends create a policy environment which supports the shared decision making model outlined in Kelner's chapter 4, but the transition will not happen without careful thinking through of the implications of this model, good will, and a concerted multi-sectoral effort. The thinking must be bottom-up, beginning at the care team level (Best and Herbert, 1998), but also top-down, guided by an evolving understanding of health planning issues such as population health, the relationship between clinical and other care, and continuity of care and integration of services (Department of Health, 1997; National Forum on Health, 1997).

CARE DELIVERY

The care delivery level focuses on the team of those working together. The word team obviously is used loosely, since often this is exactly what they are not, and that is the challenge for integration (Becker, 1999). For the *healing* strategy, the team minimally will include the client and all her or his professional care providers. However, the term team also might be used to include family, product providers such as pharmacists and herbalists, etc. Measures might include efficiency, minimization of risks and side effects, strains on family and client satisfaction.

The focus of *learning* at the team level might be on the professional knowledge and skills required for them to perform their role, including the co-ordination or integration of the team members' efforts so as to maximize the team's effectiveness in managing the healing outcomes (Owens, 1995). Clearly, this requires an understanding of the skills and scope of practice for other team members (The Prince of Wales's Initiative on Integrated Medicine, 1997; see Leathard, 1994 for a review).

The *research* focus for the care team will be on outcomes research designed to assess and continuously improve the safety, effectiveness, and efficiency of integrated care models for specific health problems.

Finally, the *structural* dimension refers to the challenge that inter-professional collaboration poses to the autonomous standing of the various health care professions (Carrier and Kendall, 1995). Specifically, in an integrated system (and this may be idealistic), conventional physicians will not necessarily have higher status than CAM practitioners.

PERSONAL HEALTH

Individuals seeking integrative services typically combine healing and learning strategies to achieve better management of their health and illness. As elaborated throughout this book, they recognize the limitations of conventional medicine, and they add other philosophies to their personal health plan. Their *healing* objective is better health and can be measured by objective indicators and subjective assessments of health status and health-related quality of life. They typically want to take greater control over their own health, and seek *learning* strategies that will increase their knowledge, decision-making, and their personal health management skills (Wellman, chapter 8). This includes learning about environmental risks and solutions to those risks. The *research* focus might be specified as the study of the process by which individuals make health-enhancing changes in their lifestyle and health management practices, or the degree to which there are pragmatic shifts in how we conceptualize health and illness. The *structural* issue at this level is access to care; quality care needs to be available both to individuals and specific population subgroups who may have special needs or difficulty obtaining appropriate services.

HEALTH CARE PHILOSOPHIES

Next we turn to a third dimension of Figure 14.1 which illustrates the impact of different health care philosophies in both health care and health promotion. Four philosophies are shown ~ conventional (e.g. Western, biomedical), alternative (e.g. naturopathy, traditional Chinese or Ayruvedic medicines, chiropractic, massage), behavioural medicine, and health promotion. These four are not meant to be mutually exclusive or well defined themselves, but simply to illustrate the diversity of health care philosophies and the importance of thinking through the meaning of integration across disciplines.

Successful integration of philosophies requires that there be a full and concerted effort to provide clients and providers with a pragmatic and full menu of options for safe and effective healing and learning strategies, whatever their philosophical origin. Managed care in the United States is explicitly market driven in this regard (e.g. Pelletier, *et al.*, 1997). In Canada, it is more consumer driven as clients search for both better integration of healing strategies and greater personal control over health. Either way, the measure is greater efficiency and satisfaction, whether assessed at a systems, care team, or personal health level. In principle, the questions are empirical and can be

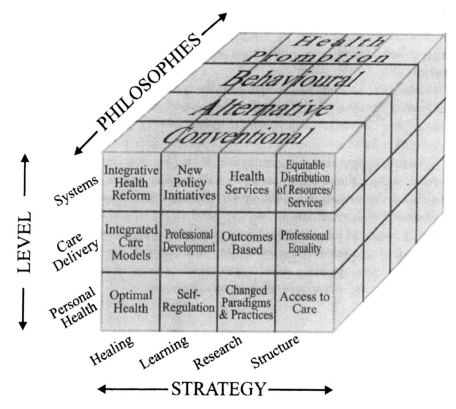

FIGURE 14.1: A WORKING MODEL FOR INTEGRATIVE HEALTH SERVICES

measured in a variety of ways and by a variety of disciplines. The difficulty is that these judgements always have a normative component, hence the debate in this book over philosophies that may conceptualize their measurement yardsticks differently.

A more profound, and more challenging way to view integration of philosophies is with respect to their theoretical underpinnings. Differences between traditions often appear overwhelming initially. With time, we may be able to overcome differences in assumptions, language, and values, but this kind of integration certainly will take much longer than pragmatic integration of strategies as measured by efficiency and satisfaction. Finally, there is a need to take into account structural variations within and between levels and traditions, and how a truly integrated system will begin to ameliorate some of the inequities in access and status that have plagued modern medicine for the past fifty years. For now, it is important to recognize that this conceptual integration of traditions is not amenable to empirical methods (and perhaps not possible by any means), but that we can work towards pragmatic integration without requiring conceptual integration as well. This does not mean that even pragmatic integration will come easily – for example, some degree of conceptual integration is required even to reach agreement on the balance between rigor and relevance in measuring key outcomes such as quality of life.

In sum, this working model highlights the fact that both the language and methods of integration vary across level, strategy, and philosophical dimensions. There currently is an important debate over language as researchers, practitioners, and policy makers work to improve our health delivery systems. It is proposed here that integrative health services is a concept that might nurture co-operation rather than conflict among key stakeholders. It opens a window of opportunity for CAM researchers and practitioners.

However, if the term integration is to prove useful in fostering this co-operation, it must be better defined and more finely measured. The different philosophies and stakeholders must agree on a common language and indicators in a common quest for more person-centered, more evidence-based, more cost-effective, and more equitably distributed services.

MEASURING INTEGRATION

Throughout the book, a myriad of measures is shown, based on theoretical or empirical grounds, to be important in the study of CAM utilization. There are two prerequisites for good use of these suggestions in fostering thinking about integration:

- Researchers, practitioners, and policy makers need a conceptual map that organizes these various constructs. In time, this complexity may be incorporated in a more parsimonious and elegant theory, but for now a road map will at least start to make sense of an otherwise bewildering array of elements.
- There needs to be shared understanding of at least the key constructs across diverse disciplines and perspectives.

Figure 14.2 sketches a provisional road map that (looking from left to right) begins with distal, general factors known to influence health choices and outcomes such as need, predisposing and enabling factors, demographics, personality, and developmental stage (Andersen, 1995). It then moves through more immediate, proximal aspects of the person such as knowledge and beliefs, motives, readiness for change (Gochman, 1997) and environment such as practitioner/client relationship, social support, structural arrangements (Wellman, 1995), to suggest short and long-term effects (e.g. self-care practices, utilization, health status). In principle, causal modeling research methods might pinpoint which of these factors are most important to study

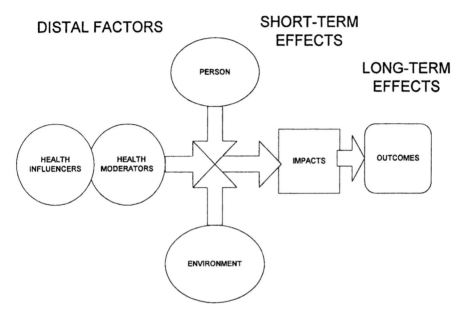

FIGURE 14.2: DETERMINANTS OF CARE CHOICES AND OUTCOMES

for CAM within an integrative health services agenda, and how these factors relate to one another, but for now this map allows us to organize some of the factors discussed in this volume.

The difficulty with Figure 14.2 is that it makes integration sound easy. There are at least two fundamental problems. The first is the positivistic suggestion that we can, in principle, sort out the temporal and interactive relationships among the host of variables that influence utilization and outcomes. The truth is that there is too much complexity and too little time to think this will happen soon. Second, there is a tension between utilization and effectiveness research. Some researchers are more interested in process issues around why people use CAM and the features of the care they receive. Such research tends to favor descriptive methodologies. Other researchers are more focused on the outcomes of safety and effectiveness, and tend to give greater weight to experimental designs. Figure 14.2 can suggest ways in which this duality might be redressed if a blend of descriptive and experimental methods is chosen, depending on the research question.

Table 14.1 is an initial attempt to organize the relevant elements alluded to in Figure 14.2 and throughout this book. Several observations are warranted:

	Influencers	Moderators	Proximal	Impacts	Outcomes
Individual	• Demographics • Health concerns • Personality • Care history • Care model	• Worldview • Life stage • Model of body and health • Morality	• Knowledge/beliefs • Health motives • Readiness for change • Risk factors • Risk aversion • Attitudes towards conventional medicine • Mind-body-spirit concepts • Self-efficacy • Outcome expectations	• Health promoting behaviour • Self-care practices • Self-regulation/restraint • Belief/behaviour coherence	• Health status • Quality of life • Transcendence

Interpersonal	• Information sources
	• Nature of therapy
		• Innovation champions	• Relationship with practitioners
			• Degree of choice
			• Social support/ties
			• Social cohesion
			• Diffusion promoters
			• Practitioner acceptance
				• Subculture norms	• Utilization
					  – patterns
					  – pathways
					  – steps

Community/ society	• Socio-political context • Market forces • Health care reform • Government attitudes and policy • Professional associations • Accessibility	• Population ageing/ chronic disease rates • Media	• Cultural attitudes • Compensation/ incentives • Role of practitioner	• Practitioner utilization patterns	• Care outcomes • Population health status • Efficiency

- Factors do not fit cleanly and neatly into the map. A closer examination of the meanings and theoretical underpinnings for each construct is necessary.
- Our disciplinary language creates a major challenge. There is no shared terminology for these constructs. Clearly, there is overlap between many of the terms, but until we again have looked at the underlying theories, we cannot reach consensus on how to bring together the different perspectives in a more co-ordinated health services research agenda.
- Without shared language, common measures are impossible. Yet, if we are to move the integrative health services mandate forward quickly (and we must, given the current pace of health reform), our credibility will hinge, at least in part, on the use of common, well-standardized measures.

RESEARCH PRIORITIES

What are the research priorities for integrative health services? Three areas are delineated here: conceptualization, design, and analysis and application.

Conceptualization

Research is needed on how change happens and how it can be fostered at each level in Figure 14.1: health systems, care, and personal. The different chapters in this book tend to focus at one of these levels to the exclusion of others, and this focus is important, to gain a thorough understanding of the complexity involved. A future step is to articulate the links between theory, research, and application across these three levels.

CAM research unfolds in a socio-politico-economic environment, whether or not we tie it to integrative health services and a reform agenda. The context shapes our research questions and methods, but there is support in the CAM research community for the notion that the standards of science must be common for conventional and complementary medicine. The recent (November 11, 1998) special issue of the *Journal of the American Medical Association* will become a landmark in the progression towards an evidence-based medicine that turns the blind eye of justice to the tradition from which the therapy comes, and looks instead to the safety, efficacy, and efficiency of the practices assessed.

Finally, on a conceptual level, research into why people use CAM needs to separate the content of the therapy from the delivery. As we reflect on the various influences on the use of CAM discussed in this book, we note that sometimes it is factors inherent in the treatment itself (e.g. adverse effects) that are important, sometimes it is not specific to a particular treatment at all but rather the (biomedical, reductionistic) nature of the health care philosophy or the way health care is structured (e.g. publicly-funded or managed care), and sometimes it's the relationship or the setting in which the care is provided. It is this complexity we need to untangle and understand if we want to move towards better, more integrated care. In other words, research on why people use CAM needs to separate out aspects of (1) help seeking behaviours, (2) the characteristics of the delivery system, and (3) the nature of the therapy (content, frequency, intensity).

Design

There has not been much research on the operation and outcomes of integrated health care services. There are many ways of designing research in the health field (Aday, 1998). One of the most important forms of design for this area is longitudinal research. While there is agreement among CAM researchers that this is a major priority, the issue of research paradigm is more divisive. It is common in biomedical circles to hear talk of 'the scientific method' and the importance of establishing safety and effectiveness before CAM can be acceptable to conventional medicine. What is less commonly highlighted is the reality that the questions we choose shape the answers we discover. There is very little serious discussion about the fundamental fact that the questions we ask and the methods we choose draw from the well of our preferred paradigm. Other chapters in this book explore these issues in greater detail.

The two most commonly contrasted paradigms are the reductionistic/positivist paradigm and the holistic/social-constructive paradigm. Patients often use a holistic paradigm when they talk about wanting to be seen as a whole person rather than as symptom or an organ. They have made their choice of paradigm. They are challenging researchers and practitioners to take a fresh and open-minded look at our own paradigm choices.

The reductionistic logic and tools of the randomized, double-blind, placebo-controlled clinical trial are not *the* scientific method, but only one of many. Scientific traditions as different as astronomy and anthropology do not use this method. Increasingly, such foundational disciplines to the study of medicine as physics and biology are using a new partnership perspective that brings together the best of both reductionistic and holistic paradigms. Even strong advocates of the reductionist paradigm recognize that there are occasions when other designs are superior (Gatchel and Maddrey, 1998; Levin *et al.*, 1997).

ANALYSIS AND APPLICATION

International comparisons between utilization patterns and reasons for choosing CAM are both necessary and feasible. It will be more challenging, but also important, to make a priority of international comparisons among health reform initiatives ~ there is much to be learned from each other's successes and failures.

A key challenge for outcomes research is to agree on what is important, and how health and system performance should be assessed. There is growing agreement that quality of life is as important as biologic measures of health status (Brooks, 1995; Lancet, 1997). Efficiency also clearly is key to health reform. But how about greater accessibility and choice? Better co-ordination and distribution of services? Are they truly being valued in the health reform process? How can we study them in ways that are most likely to influence practice and policy decisions?

RECOMMENDATIONS FOR INTEGRATIVE RESEARCH

The call for integrative research is a call to action. Scientists and practitioners frequently shun the messy world of health reform. Too often the critical importance of collaboration between research producers and research consumers is not appreciated (cCameron, Brown, and Best, 1996). More particularly, researchers often see their job as complete when they publish their findings in scientific journals. Based on what we know about the role of policy in creating a practice and research environment, clearly more must be expected if the evidence base we want is to be available and accessible to decision-makers in health reform.

Here are some recommendations to facilitate integrative research:

1. **Common Factors and Measures.** Core factors should be defined for priority research areas. Research funders must support the research on methods that is necessary to ensure measures with reliability, which balance considerations of rigor and relevance for both conventional and complementary researchers. To be fully integrative, both healer and client ideas about expectations for health and care, and what works and does not, need to be included in the process of developing measures. Multi-centre teams are one key to success; indeed, transnational efforts would do much to accelerate progress.

   This exercise of developing measures provides a good arena for different disciplines and perspectives to learn to work together, and try to move beyond their ideological differences. Both qualitative and quantitative methods are required for a well-rounded research agenda and a balanced set of measures. We need to incorporate the best from fields as disparate as psychoneuroimmunology and social evaluation.

2. **Shared Data Sets.** Research in this area is wonderfully rich and complex. There is more information than any one researcher or team can fully explore. Particularly as we begin to have common measures, there will be great value in posting and sharing data sets. Targeted funding for full analysis of data sets would stimulate fuller utilization of data and greater impact on health services reform.

3. **Virtual Research Community**. The confluence of a small but critical mass of dedicated researchers in this arena, the high policy relevance of the work, and the urgent need for timely research to inform the health reform taking place in our respective countries, builds a strong case for more international co-operation. Ideally, funding would be available specifically to support collaboration. However, there is much that researchers can do now to work together through Email and the Internet.

4. **Integrative Care Models**. The importance of multidisciplinary, integrative care teams that include the client as full partner already has been described. We have noted how essential it is that the artificial distinction between healing and learning be broken down, and that health services focus not only on clinical settings but also on the larger community in which health and healing occur. The social sciences provide strong evidence that quality information is a necessary but not sufficient condition for health behaviour change and self-care. Information needs processing before it provides true knowledge and understanding, upon which people can build personal health decisions and practices. High tech capabilities must be complemented by high touch caring in an integrated health system (Naisbett, 1982). People need to develop values, learning and self-regulation skills, and support systems, before they have the necessary capacity to take charge of their own health. If the information age is to realize its potential for empowering the individual, we need tools and systems for people to use in developing their capacities.

We need ways of supporting conventional professionals to learn about CAM and how they can encourage co-ordination, just as we need ways to help CAM practitioners work more effectively with their conventional counterparts. The research literature on continuing medical education underscores the difficulties of creating behaviour change in practice (Saks, 1996). The current push for evidence-based practice guidelines is encountering significant challenges; efforts to disseminate guidelines and ensure their adoption have progressed slowly. It is clear that the challenge is inherently difficult (Best, 1999).

5. **Partnerships Between Research Producers and Consumers**. Practitioners and researchers both have important roles to play. We need outcomes research to evaluate new and creative ways for multidisciplinary teams to work together. The data from these kinds of studies will provide important hypothesis-generating case studies that researchers then can evaluate more systematically once promising models have been identified. Researchers need to ensure that the complexity of the data (as suggested by Figure 14.2 and Table 14.1) are woven into their research.

CONCLUSION

This is an exciting time for researchers, practitioners, and policy-makers committed to the importance of more integrative health systems. A shared vision, a mutual agenda, and collaborative projects can accelerate the rate and quality with which health care reform embraces CAM. Effective and enduring partnerships between research producers and research consumers are essential if the trend toward better, more integrated health services is to achieve its promise. A carefully constructed collaborative research agenda will add value to these efforts.

REFERENCES

Aday, Lu Ann. 1998. *Evaluating the Healthcare System: Effectivemess, Efficiency and Equity.* 2nd ed. Chicago: Health Administrative Press.

Andersen, R.M. 1995. 'Revisitiing the Behavioral Model and Access to Medical Care: Does It Matter?' *Journal of Health and Social Behavior* 36(1):1–10.

Becker, B. 1999. 'Integrated Health Care in an International Context: An overview of Complementary and Alternative Health Practices in Four Health Delivery Systems.' Technical report prepared for Health Canada by the Tzu Chi Institute for Complementary and Alternative Medicine, Vancouver, B.C.

Best, A. 1999. Tracking and Co-ordinating Innovations in Medical Education. Focus on Alternative and Complementary Therapies, 4:62–63..

Best, A., and Herbert, C. 1998. 'Two Solitudes of Complementary and Conventional Medicine:. Roles for the Family Physician.' *Canadian Family Physician,* 44:2611–14.

Brooks, R.G. 1995. *Health status measurement: A perspective on change.* Toronto: MacMillan Press.

Cameron, R., Brown, K.S., and Best, J.A. 1996. 'The Dissemination of Chronic Disease Prevention Programs: Linking Science and Practice.' *Canadian Medical Association Journal* 8 (Supplement 2): S50-S53.

Carrier, T. and Kendall, J. 1995. 'Professionalism and Interprofessionalism in Health and Community Care: Some Theoretical issues.' Pp 36 in 'Interprofessional Issues in Community and Primary Health Care' edited by P. Owens, J. Carrier and J. Horder. London: Macmillan.

Department of Health. 1997. The New NHS: Modern, Dependable. London: Department of Health.

Frankish, J., Veenstra, G., and Moulton, G. 1999. 'Population Health in Canada. Issues and Challenges for Policy, Practice abd Research.' *Canadian Journal of Public Health.* 90 Supplement 1:S72–S74.

Gatchel, R.J. and Maddrey, A.M. 1998. 'Clinical Outcomes Research in Complementary and Alternative Medicine: An Overview of Experimental Design and Analysis.' *Alternative Therapies and Health* 4:36–42.

Gochman, David S. 1997. 'Personal and Social Determinants of Health Behavior: An Integration.' in David S. Gochman (ed.) *Handbook of Health Behavior Research III: Demography, Development, and Diversity.* New York: Plenum Press.

Lancet Editorial 1997. 'And Now All This.' *Lancet* 349:1.

Leathard, A. (Ed.) 1994. *Going Inter-Professional: Working Together for Health and Welfare.* London: Routledge.

Levin, J.S., Glass, T.A., Kushi, L.H., Schuck, J.R., Steele, L., and Jonas, W.B. 1997. 'Quantitative Methods in Research on Complementary and Alternative Medicine: A Methodological Manifesto.' *Medical Care* 35:1079–1094.

Light, D.W. 1996. 'Managed Competition: Theory vs. Reality.' Presented to the meetings of the American Sociological Association, New York City.

Naisbett, J. 1982. *Megatrends: Ten New Directions Transforming Our Lives.* New York: Warner.

National Forum on Health. 1997. 'Canada Health Action: Building on the Legacy.' Final Report B Volume 1. Ottawa: Health Canada.

O'Donnell, M.P. 1989. 'Definition of Health Promotion: Part III: Stressing the Impact of Culture.' *American Journal of Health Promotion* 3:5.

Owens, P., J.and H. Petch. 1995. 'Professionals and Management.' Pp. 37–55 in *Interprofessional Issues in Community and Primary Health Care,* edited by P. Owens, J. Carrier and J. Horder. London: Macmillan.

Pelletier, K.R., Marie, A., Melissa, M., and Haskell, W.L. 1997. 'Current Trends in the Integration and Reimbursement of Complementary and Alternative Medicine by Managed Care, Insurance Carriers, and Hospital Providers.' *American Journal of Health Promotion* 12:112–23.

Saks, M. 1996. 'The Interprofessional Agenda in Health and Welfare'. *Journal of Interprofessional Care* 10(2):189–94.

The Prince of Wales Initiative on Integrated Medicine, 1997. *Integrated Healthcare: A Way Forward for the Next Five Years?* London: The Foundation for Integrated Medicine.

Weeks, J. and Layton, R. 1998. 'Integration as Community Organizing: Towards a Model for Optimizing Relationships Between Networks of Conventional and Alternative Providers.' *Integrative Medicine* 1:15–25.

Wellman, B. 1995. 'Lay Referral Networks: Using Conventional Medicine and Alternative Therapies for Low Back Pain'. Pp. 224–238 in *Research in the Sociology of Health Care* edited by Jennie J. Kronenfeld. Greenwich: JAI Press.

Index

Acupuncture, 2–3, 6–11, 18–21,
69–71, 83–8, 102–5, 109,
116–18, 132, 146–58, 166–8,
172, 195, 230–3. *See also*
Traditional Chinese medicine
Aescalapius, 29–30
Age. *See* Characteristics of CAM
users
Alternative medicine. See Definition
of CAM
American Medical Association, 227,
230–3, 249. *See also* Government
Anthroposophical medicine, 48–50
Arthritis, 68
Australia, 2

Back pain, 68, 109, 118–19, 149
Beliefs. See Health beliefs
Biomedical model, 13, 19, 43, 45,
48, 52–53, 91
Body, 5–6, 11, 13, 19, 22, 28–33,
36, 39–57, 63, 65, 104–6,
110–12, 169, 213–14, 225
Britain. See United Kingdom
British Medical Association, 10,
214–15, 229, 233–4. *See also*
Government; National Health
Service

California Medical Association,
232
California Osteopathic Association,
232
Canada, 71–2, 79, 83–94, 102,
115–27, 143–59, 239–40, 242–4.
See also Canadian Chiropractic
Association; Canadian
Naturopathic Association;
National Forum on Health; Office
of Natural Health Products;
Quebec; Toronto
Canadian Chiropractic Association,
232
Canadian Naturopathic Association,
232
Cancer, 102
Cardiovascular disorders, 149
Characteristics of CAM users, 70–2,
83–5, 99, 105–10, 115–27, 148,
211–14
Chinese medicine. See Traditional
Chinese medicine
Chiropractic, spinal manipulation,
1, 4, 6, 9–10, 18, 29, 35, 55,
69–71, 83, 86, 96, 102–4, 106,
116–18, 132, 146–58, 166–8,
180, 195, 221, 231–2, 244

Lightning Source UK Ltd.
Milton Keynes UK
06 September 2009

143385UK00012BA/17/P